# Qualitative Gerontology

## Second Edition

### A Contemporary Perspective

Graham D. Rowles, PhD, is Professor of Geography, Behavioral Science and Nursing, Director of the Ph.D. Program in Gerontology, and Associate Director of the Sanders-Brown Center on Aging at the University of Kentucky. Dr. Rowles' research focuses on the experience of aging in different environmental contexts. A central theme of this work is exploration, using qualitative methodologies, of the changing relationship between elders and their environment with advancing age and the implications of this relationship for health and wellbeing. He has conducted in-depth ethnographic research with elderly populations in urban (inner city), rural (Appalachian), and nursing home environments. His publications include *Prisoners of Space? Exploring the Geographical Experience of Older People*, and three co-edited volumes, *Aging and Milieu: Environmental Perspectives on Growing Old, Qualitative Gerontology*, and *Long-term Care for the Rural Elderly*, in addition to more than 50 book chapters and articles. He is a Fellow of the Gerontological Society of America and the Association for Gerontology in Higher Education and received the 1997 Distinguished Academic Gerontologist Award of the Southern Gerontological Society. He was Editor of the *Journal of Applied Gerontology* from 1995–1999.

Nancy E. Schoenberg, PhD, is Associate Professor of Behavioral Science, Anthropology, and Internal Medicine (Cardiology) and a faculty member in the Sanders-Brown Center on Aging and Associate of the Center for Health Services Management and Research at the University of Kentucky. Dr. Schoenberg, a medical anthropologist and gerontologist, examines the illness experience in the context of local cultures and the wider array of structural arrangements. Incorporating anthropological principles, including holistic, critical, and grounded perspectives, she attempts to understand how older adults respond and adjust to chronic illness. Dr. Schoenberg particularly is interested in examining health disparities in the United States, specifically focusing on the experiences of African-American, rural and female elders and health threats of hypertension, diabetes, food insecurity, and coronary heart disease. Her research interests include self-care decisions of older adults toward heart disease, hypertension, and diabetes, qualitative and combination methods, and culturally appropriate long-term care options for elders. She currently is involved in research on self-care decision-making for coronary heart disease, experiential dimension of health care utilization for congestive heart failure, and a multi-ethnic comparison of diabetes self-care beliefs and behaviors.

# Qualitative Gerontology

## Second Edition

## A Contemporary Perspective

**Graham D. Rowles, PhD**
**Nancy E. Schoenberg, PhD**
**Editors**

 *Springer Publishing Company*

Springer Publishing Company, Inc.
536 Broadway
New York, NY 10012-3955

*Acquisitions Editor: Helvi Gold*
*Production Editor: Janice Stangel*
*Cover design by Susan Hauley*

01 02 03 04 05 / 5 4 3 2 1

**Library of Congress Cataloging-in-Publication Data**

Qualitative gerontology : a contemporary perspective / Graham D. Rowles, Nancy E. Schoenberg, editors.
    p. cm.
  Includes bibliographical references and index.
  ISBN 0-8261-1335-4
  1. Gerontology—Research.  2. Old age—Research.  3. Aging—Research.  I. Rowles, Graham D.  II. Schoenberg, Nancy E.
RA564.8 .Q355 2001
362.6'07'2—dc21
                                      2001 020646
                                             CIP

Printed in the United States of America

# Contents

# Contributors

**James E. Birren,** Center on Aging, University of California Los Angeles, Los Angeles, California

**Juliet M. Corbin,** Department of Nursing, San Jose State University, and Research Associate, Department of Social and Behavioral Sciences, University of California San Francisco, San Francisco, California

**J. Kevin Eckert,** Departments of Sociology and Anthropology, University of Maryland Baltimore County, Baltimore, Maryland

**Lisa Groger,** Department of Sociology, Gerontology and Anthropology, Miami University of Ohio, Oxford, Ohio

**Jaber F. Gubrium,** Department of Sociology, University of Florida, Gainesville, Florida

**James A. Holstein,** Department of Sociology, Marquette University, Milwaukee, Wisconsin

**Sharon R. Kaufman,** Department of Anthropology, University of California, San Francisco, San Francisco, California

**Gary M. Kenyon,** Gerontology Program, St. Thomas University, Fredricton, New Brunswick, Canada

**David L. Morgan,** Institute on Aging, Portland State University, Portland, Oregon

**Margaret A. Perkinson,** Program in Occupational Therapy, Washington University in St. Louis, St. Louis, Missouri

**Hege Ravdal,** PhD Program in Gerontology, University of Kentucky, Lexington, Kentucky

**Robert L. Rubinstein,** Department of Sociology, University of Maryland Baltimore County, Baltimore, Maryland

**Ronald M. Schmid,** Professional Photographer, Downingtown, Pennsylvania

**Johannes J. F. Schroots,** European Research Institute on Health and Aging, University of Amsterdam, Amsterdam, The Netherlands

**Dena Shenk,** Gerontology Program, University of North Carolina Charlotte, Charlotte, North Carolina

**Jane K. Straker,** Scripps Foundation, Miami University of Ohio, Oxford, Ohio

**Maria D. Vesperi,** Division of Social Sciences, New College of the University of South Florida, Sarasota, Florida

**Sheryl I. Zimmerman,** Department of Epidemiology and Preventive Medicine, Sheps Center for Health Services Research and School of Social Work, University of North Carolina at Chapel Hill, Chapel Hill, North Carolina

# Preface

It is now more than a decade since the publication of the first edition of *Qualitative Gerontology*. At the time of publication of the original volume in 1988, qualitative approaches to the study of older people and the experience of aging had begun to gain wide acceptance. Yet most practitioners of qualitative research still felt obliged to engage in elaborate and extensive justification of their epistemology and methodology. Little more than a decade later, much has changed. Few question the legitimacy of qualitative methods to revealing the richness of lives. Major journals in gerontology now routinely publish qualitative contributions. New styles of qualitative research have risen to prominence, including the extensive use of focus groups, studies of biographies and personal histories, and the use of photography and the visual arts to convey more subtle dimensions of the aging experience.

Along with new methods, new issues have arisen that require deliberation and thoughtful debate. What is the contribution of qualitative research to the progress of science? Do qualitative approaches require acceptance of a way of viewing the world that is incompatible with logical empiricism and more traditional scholarship? Is it possible to reconcile qualitative research with quantitative studies in a manner that allows findings to be complementary? How do we address the plethora of ethical concerns that arise when conducting such research? To what extent does the growing quantification of qualitative methods represent the co-option and sanitizing of the approach and a threat to continuing innovation? What is and should be the relationship among qualitative research, social action, and public policy? And, perhaps most important, what is the unique contribution of a qualitative approach to the study of growing old? As these compelling issues have come into focus, the time has come to revisit *Qualitative Gerontology* and update our perspective on the role and contribution of qualitative work in gerontology.

In the spring of 1998, the first author, Graham D. Rowles, was contacted by Helvi Gold (Acquisitions Editor at Springer Publishing Company) with a request to consider developing a second edition of *Qualitative Gerontology*. Subsequent contact with sociologist Shulamit

Reinharz, co-editor of the original project, revealed that in her own highly successful career, Shula had moved on to other issues and was loathe to revisit the volume. By chance, anthropologist Nancy E. Schoenberg had recently assumed a position at the University of Kentucky. Representing a new cadre of qualitative scholars and trained in a discipline with a long heritage of such inquiry, Nancy belonged to a second generation of qualitative gerontologists that had not been marginalized by their involvement in qualitative work. The issue for her was not one of defending the viability of qualitative gerontology but rather concern with more substantive epistemological issues in its employment to address key questions regarding aging and health. An extended series of conversations revealed that we both were dealing with key intellectual dilemmas in the use of qualitative methods in our own work. For Graham, a degree of angst emanated from ambivalence regarding a perceived trend toward the ritual quantification of qualitative studies and loss of their existential value. He feared the devaluing of intuition and the potential for the emergence of a limiting orthodoxy that was inherent in a flood of "how to" publications on qualitative methods. Nancy, recognizing that the once steady trickle of interest in qualitative approaches was now giving way to a flood, felt the need to enhance rigor and to demystify qualitative methods. Our discussions generated lively exchanges. In the end, despite our fear that a sequel rarely lives up to the success of the original, we decided to proceed with a second edition of *Qualitative Gerontology*.

As we pondered the content of what came to be known as "QG II," we realized that it was important for the new edition to clearly represent contemporary trends in qualitative gerontology. At the same time, we wanted the work to be more than merely an anthology of recent studies. Rather, as in the original volume, we sought to provide an integrative perspective on contemporary qualitative gerontology—to stand up and be counted with respect to our views. Hence, this book, as did its predecessor, commences with a review chapter laying out our shared perspective on the status of qualitative gerontology as we enter a new millennium. We hope our perspective will provoke lively ongoing debate regarding the evolution and potential of qualitative gerontology.

As was noted in the original volume, it is easy to talk a good game. The proof of any pudding lies in the eating. In this context, it lies in documenting how the use of qualitative gerontology has resulted in genuine insight that enriches and deepens understanding both of the aging experience and the way in which we derive insight into this experience. To accomplish this, and move to the next level in expanding the horizons of qualitative gerontology, we invited a group of the most eminent scholars in the field to contribute original essays. Three of our contributors—J. Kevin Eckert, Sharon R. Kaufman, and Robert L. Rubinstein—contributed to the original volume. Each scholar provides a fascinating glimpse into the progression and maturation of his or her thinking as he or she explores new themes in their work. Other contributors are leaders in gerontology whose names and visionary perspectives over the past decade have helped to forge the identity of distinctive schools of thought within qualitative gerontology: Gary M. Kenyon and pioneers Johannes J. F. Schroots and Jim Birren contribute essays on guided autobiography; David L. Morgan, an acknowledged expert on focus groups in gerontology, shares a recent perspective; Maria D. Vesperi contributes an essay that confirms her status as a leading scholar in the domain of aging and the written arts; Dena Shenk and Ronald M. Schmid reflect on more than a decade of employing photography as a qualitative research medium; Jay Gubrium and Jim Holstein continue their critical explorations of the passive and active subject and the nature of qualitative discourse; and Julie Corbin provides a reflective interpretive essay on participant observation.

Established luminaries are joined by representatives of a new generation of qualitative gerontologists whose contributions take us in exciting new directions. Lisa Groger and Jane K. Straker develop and discuss a fascinating typology of the relationship among alternative forms of qualitative and quantitative research. Margaret A. Perkinson takes us into the realm of cyberspace as she reveals the potential of "on-line ethnography" and points to the promise of the digital age to transform human communication and group dynamics.

The essays in this volume are organized in several sections representing distinctive domains of qualitative scholarship. While this book is definitely not a cookbook on qualitative research (there are now a plethora of such texts), and we do not claim the volume to be comprehensive, we do hope that it will be of value to persons entering this field for the first time as well as those at more advanced stages of inquiry. Each section is prefaced by a brief commentary that provides the reader with a synthesis of major issues in the domain and refers them to key works that they may wish to pursue in more depth. Commentaries are provided on biographical, life-history, and life-course perspectives; on participant observation; on in-depth interviewing; on the employment of mixed methods; and on approaches that utilize art, photography, and literature in the quest for gerontological insight.

Overall, our purpose is to reaffirm the richness of qualitative gerontology as an approach to exploring the aging experience. As will be elaborated in our concluding chapter, we are at the dawn of a new era in the study of aging. The emergence of the elderly population as a major component of society in the developed world, and increasingly in the developing world, is a fait accompli. We are learning more every day about the physiological, psychological, and social processes of aging. There is a growing volume of literature in critical theory that probes the social structures and institutions that condition the experience of growing old. Indeed, the outlines of a self-supporting, free-standing discipline of gerontology are beginning to take shape. But as substantive insights become more detailed and sophisticated, much larger existential questions come into ever-clearer focus. We contend that expanding knowledge is not paralleled by increased wisdom: we continue to lack insight into the meaning and significance of the aging experience. It is our belief that a liberated, risk-taking, quizzical, adventurous, even playful, qualitative gerontology provides a means to delve deeper into the aging experience in a manner that will enable us to transcend the limits of traditional science. It will offer the possibility of revealing dimensions of "being in the world" that will take gerontology to a new level of understanding of the later phases of life.

This volume would never have appeared without the input of many people. We thank Helvi Gold for her patience in waiting for the delivery of a manuscript that seemed to be "almost finished" for an eternity. Thanks are also due to our contributors for their willingness to consider multiple revisions requested by two finicky editors. A special debt of gratitude is owed to Hege Ravdal, a member of the new and ascending generation of qualitative gerontologists for whom this volume is written. Over the 2-year period of the project, Hege, a doctoral student in gerontology, served as our research assistant. She handled correspondence, made cajoling phone calls to authors, critically reviewed submitted materials, wrote one of the introductory sections, and handled the day-to-day administration of the project with grace and aplomb. Finally, we thank our spouses, Ruth Anderson Rowles and Mark Swanson, for their ongoing understanding of frequent dinner-time disruptions and late-night visits as we delivered the latest version of a chapter and sometimes lingered longer than we should have. While both are long familiar with our academic vocations and have, perhaps, become immune to our quirks, we nonetheless are pleased to acknowledge all they so selflessly contribute to enriching our lives.

We dedicate this book to the memory of Anselm Strauss.

Graham D. Rowles
Lexington, Kentucky

Nancy E. Schoenberg
Lexington, Kentucky

November 2000

# PART I

# Introduction

# CHAPTER ONE

# Back to the Future

## Nancy E. Schoenberg and Graham D. Rowles

> "We are not saying that there is only one way to do research, or that our way is best, or that the so-called old ways are bad. We are just saying that this is one way to conceptualize this field, and it is a way that we find useful."
>
> Denzin & Lincoln (2000, p. xiii)

In 1907, when the first ball began its descent into Times Square, approximately 3.7 million persons 65 years of age or older in the United States potentially could have enjoyed the event (Schick, 1986). Ninety-three years later, about 35 million older Americans might have tuned into their television sets and vicariously participated in the revelry as, completing its descent, the ball flashed its greeting to the new millennium. More than 52,000 of these elders could have been centenarians whose lives now spanned three centuries (Treas, 1995). Some elders would have participated in the daylong celebration in the excited Times Square throng. Many would have watched the event from the comfort of their homes with spouses and family. A significant number probably would have decided that a good night's sleep was more important than disruption of an ingrained "early to bed and early to rise" routine. Some, suffering from dementia, would have been unable to comprehend the significance of the moment. And for others, languishing in the quiet and darkened recesses of rooms in a skilled-care facility, the event might have passed unnoticed. Worldwide, a population of 595 million elders (60 years and older) in an increasingly global and communications-linked society would be alive to potentially celebrate the turn of the century (Tout, 1989).

Whatever their circumstances, the population of elders at the dawn of 2000 differed both quantitatively and qualitatively from that which celebrated the 1907 New Year. In the United States and elsewhere, this population had grown in size and proportion of the total population— 9.7% of the global population (Tout, 1989). Indeed, in the United States, the 20th century could be characterized as an "age of age," as life expectancy increased by close to 30 years over the 100-year period. The emergence of elders as a major component of society has resulted in demographic, economic, social, and political changes that have transformed the nature of the world in which we live. This growth has created a new and increasingly diverse constituency within humankind (Achenbaum, 1983; Cole, 1992; Haber, 1983; Markides & Black, 1996).

Over the past century, we have come to know much about the process of aging and about the lifestyles and life circumstances of elders. Indeed, the rapidly growing field of gerontology, reflected in the emergence of geriatric medicine, the creation of gerontology research institutes, and the proliferation of certificate, bachelors', masters', and even doctoral programs at universities and colleges throughout the world, parallels and contributes to an explosion of scholarship on aging and the aged (Achenbaum, 1995; Katz, 1996). Once widely, albeit implicitly accepted perspectives on growing old that were premised on the tension between polar opposite theories of disengagement and activity have been critically reexamined (Cumming & Henry, 1961; Rosow, 1967; Longino & Cart, 1982). A wider and more informed repertoire of beliefs and constructs about aging now embraces notions of continuity (Atchley, 1999), the staging of adult development (Erikson, Erikson, & Kivnick, 1986; Levinson, Darrow, Klein, Levinson, & McKee, 1978), life course and biographical perspectives (Birren, Kenyon, Ruth, Schroots, & Svensson, 1996; Hagestad, 1990; Hockey & James, 1993; Kenyon, Ruth, & Mader, 1999), meaning and identity as a motif of old age (Kaufman, 1986), socioemotional selectivity (Carstensen, 1991), and gerotranscendence (Tornstam, 1994, 1997). This more diverse armamentarium of constructs and orientations underscores the maturation of gerontology. Expanding the array of gerontological constructs, developing a wider range of viable theories (Bengtson & Schaie, 1999), and deepening levels of understanding (Birren & Deutchman, 1991; Birren et al., 1996) requires that we embrace contextually appropriate research tools and follow evermore innovative pathways to insight.

In this opening chapter, we are concerned with the manner in which we learn about growing old. Our intent is to reflect on the way in which we come to know about our elders. The global aging of populations and the economic, social, and cultural transformations attending this demographic transition make the beginning of the 21st century a ripe and ready time for expanding understanding of an aging world. The key to understanding older adults—acknowledging that they represent an increasingly diverse and complex group with each passing generation—lies in harnessing research methodologies capable of capturing this diversity and complexity. This necessitates the use of both quantitative and qualitative epistemologies; indeed, it requires that we employ the full arsenal of approaches to scholarship available to the scientific community. In this context, we do not intend to reiterate the tired debate on the relative merits of quantitative versus qualitative inquiry. Such issues have been articulated elsewhere (Hammersley, 1992; Rowles & Reinharz, 1988, pp. 13–16). Moreover, the boundaries and distinctions between qualitative and quantitative have become somewhat fuzzy (Berger & Berry, 1988). Rather, our goal is to provide a context for more adventurous and comprehensive study of aging as we pass beyond the adolescence of qualitative gerontology. Our hope in the essays presented in this volume is to present qualitative perspectives for the new century that enable scholars to approach the phenomenon of aging and its societal manifestations in dramatically different ways from those that characterized the childhood of the field.

There is a long tradition of qualitative research in the study of complex or processional phenomena and in revealing the richness and diversity of people's lives (Denzin & Lincoln, 1994, 2000). Gerontology also supports a growing tradition of qualitative research (Gubrium & Sankar, 1994; Poole & Feldman, 1999; Ramsey & Blieszner, 1999). In the first edition of *Qualitative Gerontology,* a rationale for the development of the field was presented and exemplars were provided of different styles of qualitative research. Qualitative gerontology was defined as concerned with:

> . . . describing patterns of behavior and processes of interaction, as well as revealing the meanings, values and intentionalities that pervade elderly people's experience or the experience of others in relation to old age. In addition, qualitative gerontology seeks to identify patterns that underlie the lifeworlds of individuals, social groups, and larger systems as they relate to old age. A primary focus is on understanding and conveying experience in "lived" form with as little *a priori* structuring as possible. Qualitative gerontology attempts to tap the *meaning* of experienced reality by presenting analyses based on empirically and theoretically grounded descriptions (Rowles & Reinharz, 1988, p. 6).

The heritage of research grounded in such definition that has developed over the past 12 years, coupled with the emergence of postmodern, critical, and feminist perspectives, allows us to build on and transcend the limitations of such a definition.

## Ontological Perspective: On the Nature of Being

Developing an ever-more sophisticated perspective on growing old involves refining assumptions on the nature of being, and internalizing
a series of overlapping beliefs reflecting hitherto unexpressed dimensions of the aging experience. An important first step in this process
is to develop receptivity toward and humble acceptance of the complexity of life (Peirce, 1995; Waldrop, 1992; see also Gubrium & Holstein,
chapter 8 in this volume). We must learn to celebrate, rather than
rue, the richness and diversity of the aging experience. A fundamental
conflict arises between such acceptance and celebration and the premise
of most scholarship to seek understanding of a phenomenon in a manner that will enable us to capture its essence. Invariably this involves
simplifying, or in positivist terms, reducing reality to manageable constructs and themes that represent the core features of a phenomenon.
This reduction of reality undoubtedly has its utility; it allows us to
explain, to predict, and, in some cases, to understand aspects of a
phenomenon. Indeed, such essentialism is the core of the science and
technology paradigm that underlies modern civilization. However, the
process of representation necessarily transforms phenomena, simplifying the complex and making transparent the opaque.

The sloughing off, or, at least, the reconsideration of assumptions
that problematize aging has been the preoccupation of a modest but
growing number of critical gerontologists (Arber & Ginn, 1991; Cole,
1993; Minkler & Estes, 1991). Those engaged in critical gerontology,
including participants in the feminist, political economy, and humanistic movements, attempt to creatively and deliberately dismantle embedded assumptions and reductionist notions about the uniformity of the
aging experience. Many of these scholars, like feminist symbolic interac-
tionist scholar Virginia Olesen, laud the shift away from essentialism
and toward deconstructism, noting that such orientations "encourage
provocative and productive unpacking of taken-for-granted ideas about
women in specific material, historical and cultural context" (2000, p.
215). Such critical perspectives not only reject reductionist notions, but
their scholarship also provides opportunities to "examine social issues
in ways that challenge dominant or mainstream thinking, and reveal
underlying ideological justifications of existing structural arrangements
and resource distributions that affect health and aging" (Estes & Linkins,
2000, p. 154).

To truly capture the complexity of experience and the structural
arrangements that shape the aging experience, it is important to adopt
strategies that replace the stark, sharp, and ordered contrasts of the

intellectually definitive with the fuzziness of shades of ambiguity. This is not easy for a science and ethos of scholarship that historically has been premised on control and prediction. Beyond this, it is necessary to grapple with the often-inchoate brilliance and variation of a world of color. Deep understanding necessitates abandoning the quest for control and predictability and allowing the phenomena and experiences we study to simply *be*, to exist in and of themselves. Such a quest for illumination has the potential to transform scholarship into a vibrant, descriptive, interpretive act of appreciation and wonderment.

A second and related ontological direction is the assimilation of a commitment to reveal and to investigate with a sense of the mystery of life, to appreciate the often unrecognized "horizons of meaning" (Gubrium, 1993) that all too often remain implicit in the life experience of individual elders (Albom, 1997; Ramsey & Blieszner, 1999). This entails recognizing levels of being in the world—an almost mystical presence—of which contemporary science is uncomprehending. In his conversations with a dying Morrie Schwartz, journalist Mitch Albom is able to reveal integrative aspects of his friend and mentor's life, a sense of the lifelong, lingering pain of childhood loss, of "how to give out love, and let it come in" (p. 52), of the importance of a kind of "spiritual security" within family (p. 92), and of making *a sense* of life in preparation for death that transcend the limits of conversation and capture unique aspects of his being in the world during his final weeks (see also Pope, 1999).

## *Epistemological Perspective: On the Nature of Knowing*

Qualitative gerontology in the new century is also likely to be tied to a broadening of epistemological perspective. In the quest for deeper understanding, there will be increasing need for the celebration of outliers. In the second edition of his *Dictionary of Statistics and Methodology*, W. Paul Vogt defines measure of central tendency as "any of several statistical summaries that, in a single number, represent the typical number in a group of several numbers" (1999, p. 38). To illustrate this definition, Vogt provides the example of baseball batting averages and scholastic grade point averages that are often expressed as means, modes, and medians. Computing the central tendency of a batting average is helpful, as such information can clarify the expectations for most baseball players and may identify a particularly outstanding athlete. Similarly, determining a student's grade point average may provide important information on academic strengths and may even predict a professional aptitude. In these cases, applying measures of central tendency is not only fruitful and appropriate, but it is also feasible. Computing the mean (or mode or median) of these activities is viable by applying simple mathematical formulae.

Less fruitful, appropriate, and feasible is the application of central tendencies toward understanding the complexities, inconsistencies, and variations inherent in human nature, activities, and perceptions. Certainly, there are many topical areas that warrant ascertaining "the typical number" (Vogt, 1999, p. 38), but we must ask ourselves: what are limitations of distilling or reducing the complexity of human experience to a few Arabic or Greek symbols? What is sacrificed in our attempt to adhere to rigid traditions that eschew interpretation and complexity in favor of central tendency? Furthermore, what are the problems inherent in labeling certain behaviors, attitudes, and, indeed, individuals as "outliers" and thereby excluding them from closer investigation? Conversely, what do we stand to gain from examining and interpreting data that appear to deviate from the norm? And what does such deviation (as well as our labeling and "othering" a phenomenon as such) imply about the norm?

These manifold questions are not offered as a critique of nonqualitative orientations nor are they meant as rhetorical devices to justify qualitative approaches. Indeed, we consider such critiques and justifications as redundant and distracting from one of the central foci of this volume and of a qualitative mandate: the respectful examination of life circumstances, lifeworlds, perceptions, meanings, values, and intentionalities that may not conform to preconceptions of the "mean" or "norm."

Nearly everyday, the careful observer is struck by images that appear to run counter to the norm. A geographically isolated octogenarian "surfs the web" for the latest information about the AIDS virus. A male teenager described as "impossible" and "antisocial" makes weekly visits to a nursing home where he has no family simply to listen to, as he describes them, "the stories that these people have to tell." A 78-year-old African American woman, formerly employed as a fieldhand and domestic, dons spandex tights and drives 30 miles a day to attend a step aerobics class with 20 young White women. And one of the oldest members of a religious congregation attends services twice a week, not to see his old friends (most of whom no longer come), but instead to revel in the noise and chaos of the congregation's young children.

What do these images tell us about individual capacities, social relationships, the dynamism of the human condition, and the process of history? What are we overlooking by dismissing these as outliers or *deviations* from the norm? How much is our vision obscured when these images are construed as anecdotal, idiosyncratic, or inexplicable, rather than collected, analyzed, interpreted, and celebrated for their value in drawing attention to and representing essential qualities of lived experience? It is instructive to note that most of the major breakthroughs in science and many of the social movements that have transformed civilizations were initiated by individuals and social movements at first viewed with skeptical gaze as outliers.

A second and related epistemological focus crucial to the continued development of qualitative gerontology is an increased acceptance of inconsistency. A rage for order sometimes blinds us to the fact that there may be no underlying explanations for inconsistencies in people's experience. Some aspects of life can only be adequately appreciated by acknowledging their very subjectivity and incomprehensibility (Murphy & Longino, 1996). Why do some frail elders cling to residence in a home that has been their dwelling since childhood, whereas others in the same community with similar lengths of residence and similar vulnerabilities eagerly desire to move to more supportive environments? Why do answers to similar, if not identical, questions posed at the beginning and the end of a questionnaire (to assess "reliability") elicit starkly differing responses, even when respondents acknowledge such inconsistent responses? How do we explain a brain autopsy clearly revealing that a recently deceased centenarian had an advanced stage of Alzheimer's disease, yet revealed no behavioral or cognitive symptoms during her life (Snowdon, 1997)? Why are most lives so full of contradictions? Extending this argument, perhaps if we stand ready to acknowledge and accept the inconsistencies and ambiguities we know exist in our own lives, we will develop the capacity to gain a deeper understanding of the lives of others.

It is our anticipation that the qualitative gerontology of the new century will be firmly grounded in the recognition of science as mirror of society. Despite endless and well-known examples of how values, orientations, and norms specific to a society are implicit in its science, some scholars continue to claim their craft as value-free. Paul Broca's "objective" approach to human ethnology consisted of measuring brain size to reveal "natural" skills and talents. His findings mirrored the values and preconceptions of the day,

> A prognathous (forward-jutting) face, more or less black color of the skin, woolly hair and intellectual and social inferiority are often associated, while more or less white skin, straight hair and an orthognathous (straight) face are the ordinary equipment of the highest groups in the human series. . . . A group with black skin, woolly hair and a prognathous face has never been

able to raise itself spontaneously to civilization (as quoted in Gould, 1981, pp. 83–84).

As evolutionary biologist Stephen Jay Gould concludes from Broca's laboratory efforts, "The human body can be measured in a thousand ways. Any investigator, convinced beforehand of a group's inferiority, can select a small set of measures to illustrate its greater affinity with apes" (1981, p. 88). The social mirror that was reflected in that cutting edge science of its day was the linear ranking of groups of people in terms of superiority and inferiority (see also the work of environmental determinists, such as Semple, 1911).

Has science, and those who undertake it, advanced so much that our scholarship no longer reflects current social norms and assumptions? Gerontology itself provides striking evidence of continuation of the tradition of science as a social mirror. Critical gerontologists maintain that long-accepted (although currently out of favor) constructs, such as disengagement and activity theories, are based on biased and often inaccurate ageist assumptions. Not surprisingly, with this problematizing and medicalizing of aging,

> . . . the aging process is viewed and assessed in terms of the biological break-down of the individual, or in terms of the individual personality and process, and the presumed concomitant dependency, loss and requisite adjustment to these states of being (Estes & Linkins, 2000, p. 157).

If our image of aging consists of decrepitude, malaise, isolation, and constant, painful decline, our scientific mandate will reflect these perceptions. Even the selection of topics deemed worthy of study will reflect such social norms and values. As Jon Hendricks wittily notes, "We measure what we treasure" (Gerontological Society of America meetings, 1999).

In his classic work, *The Structure of Scientific Revolutions* (1970), Kuhn argued that because of such treasuring, there is no objectively "good science"; rather, what is judged as good or even excellent is a direct reflection of the temporal and cultural expectations and constraints of the era. While contemporary scientists may scoff at what "passed for scientific" in previous centuries and contemporarily among so-called "primitive" peoples, Kuhn reminds us that the "good" science of today may suffer the same fate as its at-the-time illustrious ancestors. As De Munck and Sobo conclude in their essay, "The Forest of Methods," "Scientific truths are grounded in human (that is, subjective) consensus (that is, culture) about what is true and what is false rather than in some objective truth outside the human purview" (1998, p. 22).

Acknowledging that science tends to mirror society and evolves in tandem with societal change is not only a necessary constraint; it also provides an opportunity. Inasmuch as a scholar mirrors his or her society, so too does each of his or her subjects. Each of us is a product of our milieu. Consequently, it can be argued that we can learn much about society through study of the individual. Many of the most useful insights developed from qualitative research have arisen from biographical studies of individuals who exemplify, although not put forth to represent, the essence of their culture (Gubrium, 1993; Koch, 1990; Thomas, 1997). Sharon Kaufman's essay in this volume (chapter 4) provides an excellent exemplar of the manner in which a sensitive and perceptive case study of an individual can provide telling insight into the culture of aging and death in American society.

Throughout the ages, many scientific thinkers have maintained a sense that their theories, methods, and findings express an ever-closer approximation to an absolute, objective truth. Relatively few have had the humility, veracity, and vision to consider their conclusions relativistic and subject to paradigm shifts (Kuhn, 1970). Contemporary scholars, including those who embrace and practice qualitative approaches, would do well to acknowledge the foundation of their values, implicit or explicit. Such an orientation will imbue them with a freshness and honesty that has the potential to strengthen, rather than dilute, scientific rigor.

Recent cohorts of qualitative scholars have recognized that their approaches to defining problems, methods of analysis, and conclusions are shaped by both time and place and by their own presence and values. Ethnographers, for example, often make use of personal pronouns confirming that the researcher was, indeed, part of the scientific process. On occasion, such pronouns are used to divulge the authorship of a hunch, as Project AGE researchers describe in their cross-cultural comparisons of aging:

> On the basis of what we already knew about !Kung culture, we expected that it would offer both advantages and disadvantages for older people. We expected that as older people living in a technologically simple society with limited material resources, the !Kung would be disadvantaged compared to elders in societies with more material abundance (Keith et al., 1994, p. 4).

One of the most poignant and honest self-disclosures of the place of the researcher in scholarly activities is Barbara Myerhoff's ethnography about older Jews living in California. In her first chapter of *Number Our Days* (1987), she painstakingly recounts her unintentional involvement with studying "her own people" and its implication for her research. Speaking about participant observation, Myerhoff reveals,

> This assumption of the natives' viewpoint, so to speak, is a means of knowing others through oneself, a professional technique that can be mastered fairly easily in the study of very different peoples. Working within one's own society, and more specifically, those of one's own ethnic and familial heritage, is perilous, and much more difficult. Yet it has a certain validity and value not available in other circumstances. . . . Identifying with what one is now and will be someday is quite a different process (1987, p. 18).

Intimately connected with contemporary values as underpinnings of research and with the influence of the researcher's lens is acknowledgement and acceptance of the humanity of researchers. The research endeavor draws strength from embracing passion and caring as key elements of knowing, although such an endeavor invariably engenders debate about the legitimate role of the researcher in any investigation. For proponents of contemporary positivism, passion is often considered an anathema. Indeed, the logical corollary of value-free scientific objectivity is the notion of a passion-free science (excepting a passion for "the truth"). In contrast, passion and intuition are often viewed as fundamental attributes of qualitative researchers seeking to gain meaningful insight.

Clifford Geertz phrases this tension as, "A scientific worry about being insufficiently detached and a humanistic worry about being insufficiently engaged" (1988, p. 15). While most researchers struggle with the role of their emotions and the insertion of self in the research process, it is characteristic of many qualitative researchers to "have a sustained relationship with the interviewee" and to "regard themselves as part of the research instrumentation— . . . aware of the fact that their own personal style and interests will have an impact on the nature of the data collected" (Keith et al., 1994, p. 109). Consistent with this orientation, in his 1991 ethnography, Alan Peshkin notes that "The subjectivity that originally I had taken as an affliction . . . could . . . be taken as 'virtuous.' My subjectivity is the basis for the story that I am able to tell. It is a strength on which I build. It makes me who I am as a person and as a researcher" (p. 104).

Qualitative researchers often ground their interest and work in such a personal passion born of their own life experience, an imperative to probe for deeper levels of meaning than can be achieved through more traditional approaches. Indeed, to invest the hundreds of hours of participant observation, content analysis, or ethnographic exploration generally required to elicit meaningful data is difficult to accomplish without a resilient and pervasive sense of commitment. What may at first sight be misconstrued as a weakness—the volatility of a passion and commitment that begets tenacity—might be reconsidered to constitute a fundamental strength if it is able to reveal hitherto obscured or latent dimensions of human experience. William Tierney (2000, p. 549) has written that, in addition to the voice of the cerebral academic,

> . . . there also ought to be a place where my voice is vulnerable and passionate. As we enter the new century, for example, I am only too aware of how many friends I have lost to AIDS; such loss has unalterably tinged my life—all of it, personal, political, academic. At times in our work such vulnerability also needs to be heard, for without it we hold on to a unified voice that is power laden and dominant.

Ceding power through recognition of our vulnerabilities may be a prerequisite of enlightened epistemology.

Passion and caring fit comfortably with and merge seamlessly into a commitment to change, an imperative to undertake research that makes a difference. While scholarship solely for the advancement of knowledge may have its place in the academy, there is increasing recognition of the critical role that qualitative gerontology can and should play in changing societal images, exposing prejudice, providing practical insight, and making contributions to policy.

Transforming inaccurate, unflattering, and reductionist societal images is a goal common to feminist, critical gerontological, and to many other scholars who seek to "realize social justice . . . or present new ideas . . . for destabilizing knowledges about oppressive situations" (Olesen, 2000, p. 216). Most qualitative approaches assume the validity inherent in "personal knowledge and experience" (Ray, 1999, p. 175), with researchers employing various paths toward eliciting these perspectives. The importance of providing a speaking platform for the expression of personal knowledge, experiences, and perspectives is undeniably great. Congressional testimonies by survivors of weapon assaults or by families who have lost loved ones to drunk drivers have shaped the U.S. national and political consciousness. Similarly, qualitative researchers may provide a speaking platform for traditionally unheard individuals, amplifying these voices until they are audible in corridors of power.

Qualitative gerontology has rich potential to be constructively politically subversive (Wenger, 1999, p. 372). The rising popularity of action research and the demand for consideration of the practical implications of scholarship represent increased commitment to social involvement and the improvement of practice among qualitative researchers

(Kemmis & McTaggart, 2000). Murphy and Longino (1996) have eloquently advocated for an understanding of subjective meaning as a precursor of enhanced practice in applied gerontology. Reinharz (1994) has clearly articulated the importance of qualitative perspectives in program evaluation. We suspect that such applied orientations and an enhanced sense of societal responsibility will become increasingly important in the new century (Greenwood & Levin, 2000; Fine, Weis, Weseen, & Wong, 2000). Indeed, there is a growing tradition of intervention and action-oriented qualitative studies that have been utilized in the creation of aging programs and the formulation of policy (Cohen & Sokolovsky, 1989; Netting & Williams, 1999).

So where does this leave us with respect to emerging epistemologies of qualitative gerontology? The celebration of outliers, acceptance of inconsistency, acknowledgement of science as the mirror of an ever-changing society, a penchant for passion and caring, and a commitment to change all contribute to a vibrant, highly variegated, and ever-evolving collage of ways of coming to know about the process of growing old. Enhancing the likelihood of success of varied ways of knowing is the growing rapprochement among alternative styles of inquiry. An increasing openness to multiple new voices implicit in such rapprochement will not necessarily or inevitably require violation of the fundamental assumptions of any single approach (Lincoln & Guba, 2000). Rather, we envisage a growing pragmatism premised on the search for insight that is useful rather than true in any absolute sense.

## Methodological Perspective: On Ways of Finding Out

Emerging ontological and epistemological trends are reflected in a proliferation of methods of data gathering and interpretation. These have included but are not limited to: ethnography, participant observation, phenomenological narrative, grounded theory, text analysis, literary interpretation, in-depth interviewing, photography, life history, autobiography, focus groups, and case study analysis.

Since publication of the first edition of *Qualitative Gerontology*, there has been growing acknowledgement of the value of mixed methods, a blending of approaches, oftentimes qualitative and quantitative methods, to enhance triangulation (Flick, 1998, p. 229; Brannen, 1995; Tashakkori & Teddlie, 1998). Such blending also has become widely accepted in gerontology (Chappell & Kuehne, 1998; Travis & McAuley, 1998). Lisa Groger and Jane K. Straker (chapter 9) provide a critical interpretation of this trend in gerontology. It is important to consider the merits and limitations of such an approach, particularly in view of the increasing use of computers in qualitative research.

While increased appreciation for the use of qualitative approaches in mixed method research designs is a laudable development, we are concerned about the "sanitizing" or quantification of qualitative research. These concerns are apt to arise with an ill-considered or inappropriately intentioned use of increasingly popular qualitative data analysis programs, such as The Ethnograph and NUD*IST (Weitzman, 2000; Weitzman & Miles, 1995; Fielding & Lee, 1998). Grounded in the fear of a kind of "cheap grace," the legitimization of qualitative studies stems from the co-option of such research within the framework of reductionist methodologies. To what extent do such strategies squeeze the meaning out of qualitative data? How do quantitative methods administer protocols that accommodate intuition? Is the use of computer analysis merely a convenient way of handling large quantities of data or does it affect a substantive and invidious transformation of these data and represent another device for the privileging of quantification? All are questions that will become increasingly pertinent as qualitative gerontology matures and grows evermore accommodating of multiple approaches to inquiry. It is our hope that this maturation will entail a thoughtful and sensitive employment of new information-processing technologies within the rubric of an explicit acknowledgement of the need to preserve the integrity of qualitative insight.

A second methodological trend that has intensified over the past 12 years has been acceptance of the critical role of environmental context in the quest for deep understanding. All experience occurs in space and in time, the domains of geography and history. With respect to geography, there has been increasing recognition of the role of spatial relationship and place (both our contemporary physical setting and the places of our past) in conditioning the aging experience (Altman & Lowe, 1992; Rowles & Ravdal, in press; Wheeler, 1995). It matters where we grow old as is strongly evidenced by research on the meaning of home and current societal-policy emphasis on the desirability of aging-in-place (Kontos, 1998; Tilson, 1990; Rowles, 1993). As life-history and life-course perspectives have flourished, gerontologists have internalized the crucial role of both personal and social history beyond simply distinguishing among age, period, and cohort effects (Birren et al., 1996; Hendricks, 1995; Rybarczyk & Bellg, 1997). It matters when we grow old. Of course, time and place are intimately and inextricably interrelated in the experience of aging. Both are integral to developing deep understanding of each elder's being in the world.

Social contextual issues, albeit narrowly defined and often unidimensional, also have been a mainstay of gerontologists. Prolific scholarship has examined the association between social support and nursing home admissions or the association between religiosity and depression in later life. Less common to gerontological scholarship are inquiries that invite a grounded and holistic understanding of an elder's social universe. Such research necessarily goes beyond "controlling for" and instead relinquishes control to the elder to define and explain parameters of social meaning (see Rubinstein, chapter 7, and Gubrium & Holstein, chapter 8). Rarer still are those inquiries that squarely and explicitly situate improvement of life circumstances in the forefront of the academic enterprise. Thus, while it is important to document the higher degree of nutritional risk among African American elders than their White counterparts, we would enrich our understanding by focusing on the social, cultural, and historical contexts embedded in and the political and economic structures that shape eating patterns. Offering critical interpretations of contextual and structural influences on eating practices provides a deeper level of understanding and presents a springboard for social change.

A third methodological trend has been the almost universal acceptance and increasing sophistication of our understanding of the roles of reactivity and reflexivity in qualitative gerontology, the high level of researcher involvement in the data-gathering process that is both an inevitable and desirable component of research. Qualitative research is as much a methodological attitude as it is an array of procedures. The identity of the researcher as an agent of change and as a contributor to the creation of meaning, in the very process of collecting information, is increasingly accepted both in qualitative research in general (Ellis & Bochner, 2000; Fine et al., 2000; Lincoln & Guba, 2000) and in a maturing gerontology (Kaufman, 1994). Reinharz (1997), for example, has noted the need to acknowledge the role of multiple selves in the ongoing creation of meaning: the selves we bring into the field that represent our historically created viewpoints; our research-based selves (the identity we assume as investigators); and situationally created selves that are expressed within each specific field circumstance we encounter. Each of these selves must be reconciled as components both of the data we collect and the manner in which these data are represented and interpreted.

With the acknowledgment of the inherently reflexive nature of qualitative research methods comes responsibility toward the people within whose lives we insert ourselves. Benefits do not necessarily accrue to older people simply because research has become more inclusive of elders. Indeed, "the aging enterprise" (Estes, 1979) that has been so enriching to the health care industry and academy alike often has perpetuated the problematizing of aging and has justified existing social, economic, and political arrangements (Estes & Linkins, 2000). Rather, as in her discussion of the capabilities of feminist theoretical discussions and qualitative methods to "set the stage for other research, other actions, and policies that transcend and transform," Olesen advocates for research "for rather than merely about women" (2000, p. 215).

A sense of commitment to effecting positive change through genuine caring becomes more than merely an acknowledgement of our agency; it reinforces and intensifies our ethical obligation. The past decade has witnessed growing concern with an array of complex ethical issues in the conduct of qualitative research (Christians, 2000). Such issues are especially significant in qualitative gerontology when the focus of concern is elders who may be cognitively impaired, physically frail, or otherwise vulnerable (Kayser-Jones & Koenig, 1994).

## *Roads Traversed: "Back to . . . "*

At the time of the publication of the first edition of *Qualitative Gerontology*, it was possible to summarize the bulk of research in qualitative gerontology within the rubric of three broad approaches: interpretive content analysis; in-depth interviewing; and ethnography (including participant observation) (Rowles & Reinharz, 1988, pp. 16–19). While subsequent methodological innovations have dramatically increased the ways in which qualitative scholars examine aging, work in each of these domains also has continued to expand our knowledge of the aging experience.

Interpretive content analyses have included analysis of images of aging conveyed in advertisements, popular literature, poetry, and mass media. Multiyear media analyses have revealed the "graying" of models employed in *Modern Maturity* (Roberts & Zhou, 1997), the selection of progressively older *Playboy* centerfold models in parallel with the aging of the consumer population (Harris, Fine, & Hood, 1992), and the demeaning presentation or complete omission of older women from the mass media in Australia (Ellison, 1999).

Content analyses have also focused on artistic endeavors and the aging experience as revealed in the poetry of Richard Eberhart and an entire special issue of the *Journal of Aging Studies* devoted to the journal and poetry of Claire Philip (Berman, 1995; Cole, 1995; Philip, 1995; Smith, 1989, 1995; Wyatt-Brown, 1995). Deeper understanding of attitudes toward filial piety in parent care and the parent-child relationship has resulted from content analysis of the written stories of 931 Koreans (Sung, 1998).

In-depth interviewing has provided important insight into the gendered lifeworlds and spirituality of both older men (Cohen & Sokolovsky, 1989; Quinnan, 1997; Thomas, 1997) and older women (Porter, 1998; Ramsey & Blieszner, 1999; Shenk, 1998). We have gained deeper insight into patterns of decision-making and the experience of life in nursing facilities (Gubrium, 1993; High & Rowles, 1995; Rowles & High, 1996). In-depth interviews have been used to reveal important dimensions of aging in rural settings, including the pathways leading toward and self-management of nutritional risk (Quandt, Arcury, & Bell, 1998; Schoenberg, 2000). Particularly significant are recent efforts to widen the employment of in-depth interviewing in order to hear the voices of persons often considered beyond the purview of interactive social research. The work of Usita, Hyman, and Herman (1998) in eliciting narrative life stories from persons with Alzheimer's disease provides an exemplar of both the challenges and rewards of such methodological innovation. Finally, and especially critical to a discipline criticized for being data rich and theory poor, it is important to acknowledge recent use of in-depth interviewing to facilitate the elaboration of gerontological theory (Tornstam, 1997).

Using ethnography and participant observation, gerontology has been enriched by a growing genre of nursing home studies that are providing a deeper understanding of the many ramifications of nursing home life for residents, families, and staff (Diamond, 1992; Foner, 1994; Henderson & Vesperi, 1995; Rowles, Concotelli, & High, 1996; Savishinsky, 1991). We have learned more about the experience of both rural and urban community-dwelling elders as they grapple with the constraints of growing old in each of these settings (Cohen & Sokolovsky, 1989; Shenk, 1998).

## *Roads Ahead: " . . . the Future"*

The past decade has also heralded expanded and more sophisticated use of approaches that are relatively new to qualitative gerontology. Several examples of these new directions are provided in this volume. Major strides are being made through increased employment of biographical approaches, variously defined, undertaken, and articulated as narrative gerontology (Kenyon et al., 1999), life stories (Wallace, 1994), life-course analyses (Hockey & James, 1993), guided autobiography (Kenyon & Randall, 1997), and phenomenological narrative (Hasselkus & LaBelle, 1998). Each of these approaches enables us to explicitly incorporate the crucial temporal and social contextual domains in analyses of the aging experience. Contributions by Gary M. Kenyon (chapter 2) and by Johannes J. F. Schroots and James E. Birren (chapter 3) reveal both the richness and the subtlety of insight that can be gleaned from this increasingly popular cluster of methodologies.

The increasing use of focus groups provides a reflexive shared-interview context that enables elders to articulate and share what might otherwise remain as hidden and taken-for-granted dimensions of their experience. As Madriz (2000, p. 835) has noted:

> . . . focus groups allow access to research participants who may find one-on-one, face-to-face interaction "scary" or "intimidating." By creating multiple lines of communication, the group interview offers participants . . . a safe environment where they can share ideas, beliefs, and attitudes in the company of people from the same socioeconomic, ethnic, and gender backgrounds.

The outcome has been a broadening perspective on the voices of populations that might otherwise fall beyond our gaze or whose voices become more audible in a group setting. For example, Hennessey and John's (1996) focus group study of American Indian families has revealed important cross-cultural differences in the meaning of caregiving. Adler, McGraw, and McKinlay (1998) have explored assertiveness and empowerment in the patient-physician relationship as revealed by focus groups of ethnically diverse older women with breast cancer. In this volume, David Morgan's study of factors influencing caregivers' decisions to seek diagnosis for dementia (chapter 11) provides a clear illustration of the need to view such decisions in a broader "family" rather than more conventionally accepted "primary" caregiver context.

In addition to the increasing use of these approaches, qualitative studies are being implemented in diverse and flexible arrangements. There is a trend toward multiresearcher qualitative studies, such as the Project Age research of Keith and her colleagues that explored the meaning of aging in multiple countries (Keith et al., 1994), the Kayser-Jones' series of team-oriented studies of acute illness and nutrition in nursing facilities (Kayser-Jones, 1995, 1996), and the Rowles and High's team-oriented qualitative research on family involvement in decision making in multiple nursing homes (High & Rowles, 1995; Rowles & High, 1996). In this volume, Kevin Eckert and Sheryl Zimmerman (chapter 10) reveal how a multisite, multiresearcher study obtained unique and confirmatory insights into the quality of care at long-term care facilities. Although they generate a set of new epistemological and methodological challenges (including development of shared language, comparability in styles of interaction with research subjects, and reaching consensus among team members on matters of interpretation), such multi-researcher team studies are enabling gerontologists to participate in large-scale comparative research that transcends data limitations of single-researcher investigations.

Increasingly, qualitative gerontology is embracing more creative options, including the critical interpretation of poetry and literature (Smith, 1989; Stoller & Gibson, 2000), analysis of mass media (Ellison, 1999), and the use of photography (Shenk & Schmid, 1993) to reveal different facets of life experience and to foster enhanced appreciation of subtle meanings, emotionally evocative experiences, and nuances in the lives of elders (see Shenk & Schmid, chapter 12, and Vesperi, chapter 13). Well-suited for exploration and innovation, qualitative scholars have turned a curious and critical eye to the increasing presence of technology and virtual communities in the lives of elders (see Perkinson, chapter 6).

Each of these trends represents a broadening and a deepening of qualitative methodologies within an environment of increasing sophistication. Each portends new horizons for developing a truly meaningful understanding of the aging experience. With a goal of reinforcing such trends, in this book we have assembled a set of contributions from both current leaders and emergent scholars in the rapidly expanding field of qualitative gerontology. It is our hope that each chapter will reveal to the reader this promise and potential, the lingering dilemmas, and the new opportunities that epitomize contemporary qualitative gerontology. It also is our hope that, in the following pages, we can convey to you, the reader, something of the creative vigor of a burgeoning subfield in gerontology.

This volume is not a traditional methodological text or an ongoing justification for the use of qualitative methods. Each author was invited to submit an original manuscript in which he or she explored some aspect of an approach to qualitative gerontology in a spirit of demonstration and substantive illustration rather than merely proselytization. We recognized that such an invitation would lead to a diversity of contributions. Moreover, we anticipated that some chapters would focus on philosophical themes, others on substantive topical research and findings, and yet others would provide an abundance of epistemological context and background. Our task as editors was to weave together these diverse contributions in a manner that would accomplish three objectives: illustrate a diverse and ever-expanding array of contemporary qualitative methodologies; demonstrate the substantive richness of qualitative gerontology and its potential to contribute to enhancing the quality of elders' lives; and provide a template, a jumping-off point, for the next phase in the development of qualitative gerontology.

At the same time, we wanted to compile a volume with a degree of coherence and comprehensiveness. To achieve these ends, individual clusters of chapters are prefaced with contextual material from the editors designed to "fill the gaps" and orient the reader to the broad domains of qualitative inquiry in which the individual contributions are epistemologically located. Each section preface also serves to provide a brief orientation to the approach employed. The intent is to provide the reader with access to core themes and issues and reference to classic works in each methodological content area without disrupting the integrity of individual chapters by forcing authors to elaborate on material that is increasingly available in a plethora of "how to" qualitative texts.

In Part 2, we have grouped a set of chapters reflecting contributions to the burgeoning domain of life stories, life histories, personal narratives, guided autobiographies, and life-course analyses, one of the most vibrant areas in contemporary qualitative gerontology. Part 3, introduced with prefatory material by one of our contributors (Sharon Kaufman), comprises chapters employing ethnography and participant observation. Part 4 consists of contributions on various aspects of in-depth interviewing. There follows, in Part 5, three chapters that address the contentious and increasingly popular use of complementary methods. In Part 6, the focus turns to examples of the use of alternative, and we would argue, underemployed sources of qualitative insight. Exemplars include chapters on the use of photography and on literary interpretation. In a final chapter (Part 7), we provide concluding thoughts on the manner in which the field of qualitative gerontology may move forward in the new century.

## On the Threshold

It would be arrogant and foolish to suggest that this volume captures the full array of possible approaches to qualitative inquiry in gerontology. Indeed, we have merely scratched the surface at a time when we stand on the threshold, not only calendar-wise, of a new era in embracing many ways of understanding. We believe that qualitative gerontology is distinctive, not in its use of specific qualitative methods—methods that are common to most domains of the social and behavioral sciences—but rather in its potential to sensitively and ethically employ these methods in a manner that will unveil features of elders' being in the world that heretofore we have been barely able to imagine. We are at the dawn of a new era in which the value of qualitative work in gerontology is unquestioned, an era where we have both the freedom and obligation to be innovative and to cast off tired assumptions, an era when limits to the depth of our insight into the aging experience will be set only by the limits of our ingenuity.

In the pages that follow, we invite you to join us as, with a group of our intellectual colleagues, we continue our quest for a deeper understanding of later life.

## REFERENCES

Achenbaum, W. A. (1983). *Shades of gray.* Boston: Little, Brown & Co.

Achenbaum, W. A. (1995). *Crossing frontiers: Gerontology emerges as a science.* Cambridge, MA: Cambridge University Press.

Adler, S. R., McGraw, S. A., & McKinlay, J. B. (1998). Patient assertiveness in ethnically diverse older women with breast cancer: Challenging stereotypes of the elderly. *Journal of Aging Studies, 12*(4), 331–350.

Albom, M. (1997). *Tuesdays with Morrie.* New York: Doubleday.

Altman, I., & Low, S. M. (Eds.). (1992). *Place attachment.* New York: Plenum Press.

Arber, S., & Ginn, J. (1991). *Gender and later life.* London: Sage Publications, Inc.

Atchley, R. C. (1999). *Continuity and adaptation in aging.* Baltimore: Johns Hopkins University Press.

Bengtson, V. L., & Schaie, K. W. (1999). *Handbook of theories of aging.* New York: Springer Publishing Company.

Berger, J. O., & Berry, D. A. (1988). Statistical analysis and the illusion of objectivity. *American Scientist, 76,* 159–165.

Berman, H. J. (1995). Claire Philip's journal: From life to text, from text to life. *Journal of Aging Studies, 9*(4), 335–342.

Birren, J. E., & Deutchman, D. (1991). *Guiding autobiography groups for older adults: Exploring the fabric of life.* Baltimore: Johns Hopkins University Press.

Birren, J. E., Kenyon, G. M., Ruth, J. E., Schroots, J. J. F., & Svensson, T. (Eds.). (1996). *Aging and biography: Explorations in adult development.* New York: Springer Publishing Company.

Brannen, J. (Ed.). (1995). *Mixing methods: Qualitative and quantitative research.* Aldershot, UK: Avebury.

Carstensen, L. L. (1991). Selectivity theory: Social activity in lifespan context. *Annual Review of Gerontology and Geriatrics, 11,* 195–217.

Chappell, N. L., & Kuehne, V. K. (1998). Congruence among husband and wife caregivers. *Journal of Aging Studies, 12*(3), 239–254.

Christians, C. G. (2000). Ethics and politics in qualitative research. In N. K. Denzin & Y. S. Lincoln (Eds.), *Handbook of qualitative research* (2nd ed., pp. 133–155). Thousand Oaks, CA: Sage Publications, Inc.

Cohen, C. I., & Sokolovsky, J. (1989). *Old men of the Bowery: Strategies for survival among the homeless.* New York: Guilford Publications, Inc.

Cole, T. R. (1992). *The journey of life: A cultural history of aging in America.* Cambridge, MA: Cambridge University Press.

Cole, T. R. (1993). Preface. In T. R. Cole, W. A. Achenbaum, P. L. Jakobi, & R. Kastenbaum (Eds.), *Voices and visions of aging: Toward a critical gerontology* (pp. xii–xi). New York: Springer Publishing Company.

Cole, T. R. (1995). Gaining and losing a friend I never knew: Reading Claire Philip's journal and poetry. *Journal of Aging Studies, 9*(4), 329–334.

Cumming, E., & Henry, W. E. (1961). *Growing old: The process of disengagement.* New York: Basic Books.

De Munck, V. C., & Sobo, E. J. (1998). The forest of methods. In E. J. Sobo & V. C. DeMunck (Eds.), *Using methods in the field* (pp. 13–38). Walnut Creek, CA: Alta Mira Press.

Denzin, N. K., & Lincoln, Y. S. (1994). *Handbook of qualitative research.* Thousand Oaks, CA: Sage Publications, Inc.

Denzin, N. K., & Lincoln, Y. S. (2000). *Handbook of qualitative research.* (2nd ed.). Thousand Oaks, CA: Sage Publications, Inc.

Diamond, T. (1992). *Making gray gold: Narratives of nursing home care.* Chicago: University of Chicago Press.

Ellis, C., & Bochner, A. P. (2000). Autoethnography, personal narrative, reflexivity. In N. K. Denzin & Y. S. Lincoln (Eds.), *Handbook of qualitative research* (2nd ed., pp. 733–768). Thousand Oaks, CA: Sage Publications, Inc.

Ellison, A. (1999). Policy's black box: Mass media, women and aging. In M. Poole & S. Feldman (Eds.), *A certain age: Woman growing older* (pp. 17–35). St. Leonards, Australia: Allen & Unwin.

Erikson, E. H., Erikson, J. M., & Kivnick, H. Q. (1986). *Vital involvement in old age.* New York: Norton.

Estes, C. L. (1979). *The aging enterprise.* San Francisco: Jossey Bass.

Estes, C. L., & Linkins, K. W. (2000). Critical perspectives on health and aging. In G. L. Albrecht, R. Fitzpatrick, & S. C. Scrimshaw (Eds.), *The handbook of social studies in health & medicine* (pp. 154–172). Thousand Oaks, CA: Sage Publications, Inc.

Fielding, N. G., & Lee, R. M. (1998). *Computer analysis and qualitative research.* London: Sage Publications, Inc.

Fine, M., Weis, L., Weseen, S., & Wong, L. (2000). Qualitative research, representations, and social responsibilities. In N. K. Denzin & Y. S. Lincoln (Eds.), *Handbook of qualitative research* (2nd ed., pp. 107–131). Thousand Oaks, CA: Sage Publications, Inc.

Flick, U. (1998). *An introduction to qualitative research.* Thousand Oaks, CA: Sage Publications, Inc.

Foner, N. (1994). *The caregiving dilemma: Work in an American nursing home.* Berkeley, CA: University of California Press.

Geertz C. (1988). *Works and lives: The anthropologist as author.* Cambridge, MA: Polity Press.

Gould, S. J. (1981). *The mismeasure of man.* New York: W. W. Norton & Company.

Greenwood, D. J., & Levin, M. (2000). Reconstructing the relationships between universities and society through action research. In N. K. Denzin & Y. S. Lincoln (Eds.), *Handbook of qualitative research* (2nd ed., pp. 85–106). Thousand Oaks, CA: Sage Publications, Inc.

Gubrium, J. F. (1993). *Speaking of life: Horizons of meaning for nursing home residents.* New York: Aldine de Gruyter.

Gubrium, J. F., & Sankar, A. (1994). *Qualitative methods in aging research.* Thousand Oaks, CA: Sage Publications, Inc.

Haber, C. (1983). *Beyond sixty-five: The dilemma of old age in America's past.* New York: Cambridge University Press.

Hagestad, G. O. (1990). Social perspectives on the life course. In R. H. Binstock & L. K. George (Eds.), *Handbook of aging and the social sciences* (3rd ed.). New York: Academic Press.

Hammersley, M. (1992). Deconstructing the qualitative—quantitative divide. In J. Brannen (Ed.), *Mixing methods: Qualitative and quantitative research* (pp. 39–55). Aldershot, UK: Avebury.

Harris, D. K., Fine, G. A., & Hood, T. C. (1992). The aging of desire: Playboy centerfolds and the graying of America: A research note. *Journal of Aging Studies, 6*(4), 301–306.

Hasselkus, B. R., & LaBelle, A. (1998). Dementia day care endings: The uncertain limits of care. *Journal of Applied Gerontology, 17*(1), 3–24.

Henderson, J. N., & Vesperi, M. D. (Eds.). (1995). *The culture of long term care: Nursing home ethnography.* Westport, CT: Bergin & Garvey.

Hendricks, J. (1995). *The meaning of reminiscence and life review.* Amityville, NY: Baywood Publishing Company.

Hendricks, J. (1999, November). *Paradox of successful aging: A critical look at neglected dimensions.* Paper presented at the annual meeting of the Gerontological Society of America, San Francisco, CA.

Hennessey, C. H., & John, R. (1996). American Indian family caregivers' perceptions of burden and needed support services. *Journal of Applied Gerontology, 15*(3), 275–293.

High, D. M., & Rowles, G. D. (1995). Nursing home residents, families and decision making: Toward a theory of progressive surrogacy. *Journal of Aging Studies, 9*(2), 101–117.

Hockey, J., & James, A. (1993). *Growing up and growing old.* London: Sage Publications, Inc.

Katz, S. (1996). *Disciplining old age: The formation of gerontological knowledge.* Charlottesville, VA: University Press of Virginia.

Kaufman, S. R. (1986). *The ageless self: Sources of meaning in later life.* Madison, WI: The University of Wisconsin Press.

Kaufman, S. R. (1994). In-depth interviewing. In J. F. Gubrium & A. Sankar (Eds.), *Qualitative methods in aging research* (pp. 123–136). Thousand Oaks, CA: Sage Publications, Inc.

Kayser-Jones, J. S. (1995). Decision making in the treatment of acute illness in nursing homes: Framing the decision problem, treatment plan and outcome. *Medical Anthropology Quarterly, 92,* 236–256.

Kayser-Jones, J. S. (1996). Mealtime in nursing homes: The importance of individualized care. *Journal of Gerontological Nursing, 22*(3), 26–31.

Kayser-Jones, J., & Koenig, B. A. (1994). Ethical issues. In J. F. Gubrium & A. Sankar (Eds.), *Qualitative methods in aging research* (pp. 15–32). Thousand Oaks, CA: Sage Publications, Inc.

Keith, J., Fry, C. L., Glascock, A. P., Ikels, C., Dickerson-Putman, J., Harpending, H. C., & Draper, P. (1994). *The aging experience: Diversity and commonality across cultures.* Thousand Oaks, CA: Sage Publications, Inc.

Kemmis, S., & McTaggart, R. (2000). Participatory action research. In N. K. Denzin & Y. S. Lincoln (Eds.), *Handbook of qualitative research* (2nd ed., pp. 567–605). Thousand Oaks, CA: Sage Publications, Inc.

Kenyon, G. M., & Randall, W. (1997). *Restorying our lives: Personal growth through autobiographical reflection.* Westport, CT: Praeger.

Kenyon, G. M., Ruth, J.-E., & Mader, W. (1999). Elements of a narrative gerontology. In V. L. Bengtson & K. W. Schaie (Eds.), *Handbook of theories of aging* (pp. 40–58). New York: Springer Publishing Co.

Koch, T. (1990). *Mirrored lives: Aging children and elderly parents.* New York: Praeger.

Kontos, P. C. (1998). Resisting institutionalization: Constructing old age and negotiating home. *Journal of Aging Studies, 12*(2), 167–184.

Kuhn, T. (1970). *The structure of scientific revolutions* (2nd ed.). Chicago: University of Chicago Press.

Levinson, D. J., Darrow, C. N., Klein, E. B., Levinson, M. H., & McKee, B. (1978). *Seasons of a man's life.* New York: Knopf.

Lincoln, Y. S., & Guba, E. G. (2000). Paradigmatic controversies, contradictions, and emerging confluences. In N. K. Denzin & Y. S. Lincoln (Eds.), *Handbook of qualitative research* (2nd ed., pp. 163–188). Thousand Oaks, CA: Sage Publications, Inc.

Longino, C. F., & Cart, C. S. (1982). Explicating activity theory: A formal replication. *Journal of Gerontology, 37,* 713–722.

Madriz, E. (2000). Focus groups in feminist research. In N. K. Denzin & Y. S. Lincoln (Eds.), *Handbook of qualitative research* (2nd ed., pp. 835–850). Thousand Oaks, CA: Sage Publications, Inc.

Markides, K. S., & Black, S. A. (1996). Race, ethnicity and aging: The impact of inequality. In R. H. Binstock & L. K. George (Eds.), *Handbook of aging and the social sciences* (4th ed., pp. 153–170). New York: Academic Press.

Minkler, M., & Estes, C. L. (1991). *Critical perspectives on aging.* Amityville, NY: Baywood.

Murphy, J. W., & Longino, C. F. (1996). Reason, the lifeworld, and appropriate intervention. *Journal of Applied Gerontology, 16*(2), 149–151.

Myerhoff, B. (1987). *Number our days.* New York: Dutton.

Netting, F. E., & Williams, F. G. (1999). Implementing a case management program designed to enhance primary care physician practice with older persons. *Journal of Applied Gerontology, 18*(1), 25–45.

Olesen, V. L. (2000). Feminisms and qualitative research: At and into the millennium. In N. K. Denzin & Y. S. Lincoln (Eds.), *Handbook of qualitative research* (2nd ed., pp. 215–277). Thousand Oaks, CA: Sage Publications, Inc.

Peirce, A. G. (1995). The complex nature of stress, coping and adaptation. *Nursing Leadership Forum, 1*(3), 84–89.

Peshkin, A. (1991). *The color of stranger, the color of friends: The play of ethnicity in school and community.* Chicago: University of Chicago Press.

Philip, C. E. (1995). Lifelines. *Journal of Aging Studies, 9*(4), 265–332.

Pope, S. L. (1999). The meaning of life among persons with advanced cancer. Doctoral Dissertation, University of Kentucky, College of Nursing, Lexington, Kentucky.

Poole, M., & Feldman, S. (Eds.). (1999). *A certain age: Woman growing older.* St. Leonards, Australia: Allen & Unwin.

Porter, E. J. (1998). "Staying close to shore": A context for older rural widows' use of health care. In B. J. McCulloch (Ed.), *Old, female, and rural* (pp. 25–39). New York: The Haworth Press Inc.

Quandt, S. A., Arcury, T. A., & Bell, R. A. (1998). Self-management of nutritional risk among older adults: A conceptual model and case studies from rural communities. *Journal of Aging Studies, 12*(4), 351–368.

Quinnan, E. J. (1997). Connection and autonomy in the lives of elderly male celibates: Degrees of disengagement. *Journal of Aging Studies, 11*(2), 115–130.

Ramsey, J. L., & Blieszner, R. (1999). *Spiritual resiliency in older women: Models of strength for challenges through the life span.* Thousand Oaks, CA: Sage Publications, Inc.

Ray, R. E. (1999). Researching to transgress: The need for critical feminism in gerontology. *Journal of Women & Aging, 11*(2/3), 171–184.

Reinharz, S. (1994). Qualitative evaluation and policy. In J. F. Gubrium & A. Sankar (Eds.), *Qualitative methods in aging research* (pp. 263–276). Thousand Oaks, CA: Sage Publications, Inc.

Reinharz, S. (1997). Who am I? The need for a variety of selves in the field. In R. Hertz (Ed.), *Reflexivity and voice* (pp. 3–20). Thousand Oaks, CA: Sage Publications, Inc.

Reinharz, S., & Rowles, G. D. (1988). *Qualitative gerontology.* New York: Springer Publishing Company.

Roberts, S. D., & Zhou, N. (1997). The 50 and older characters in the advertisements of *Modern Maturity:* Growing older, getting better? *Journal of Applied Gerontology, 16*(2), 208–220.

Rosow, I. (1967). *Social integration of the aged.* New York: Free Press.

Rowles, G. D. (1993). Evolving images of place in aging and "aging in place." *Generations, 17*(2), 65–70.

Rowles, G. D., & High, D. M. (1996). Individualizing care: Family roles in nursing home decision making. *Journal of Gerontological Nursing, 22*(3), 20–25.

Rowles, G. D., Concotelli, J. A., & High, D. M. (1996). Community integration of a rural nursing home. *Journal of Applied Gerontology, 15*(2), 188–201.

Rowles, G. D., & Ravdal, H. (in press). Aging, place and meaning in the face of changing circumstances. In S. A. Bass & R. Weiss (Eds.), *Challenges of the third age: Meaning and purpose in later life.* New York: Oxford University Press.

Rowles, G. D., & Reinharz, S. (1988). Qualitative gerontology: Themes and challenges. In S. Reinharz & G. D. Rowles (Eds.), *Qualitative gerontology* (pp. 3–33). New York: Springer Publishing Company.

Rybarczyk, B., & Bellg, A. (1997). *Listening to life stories: A new approach to stress intervention in health care.* New York: Springer Publishing Company.

Savishinsky, J. S. (1991). *The ends of time: Life and work in a nursing home.* New York: Bergin & Garvey.

Schick, F. L. (1986). *Statistical handbook on aging Americans.* Phoenix, AZ: Oryx Press.

Schoenberg, N. E. (2000). Patterns, factors and pathways contributing to nutritional risk among African-American elders. *Human Organization, 59*(2), 234–244.

Semple, E. C. (1911). *The influences of geographic environment.* New York: Henry Holt and Company.

Shenk, D. (1998). *Someone to lend a helping hand: Women growing old in rural America.* Amsterdam: Gordon and Breach Publishers.

Shenk, D., & Schmid, R. M. (1993). Visual images of aging women. In D. Shenk & W. A. Achenbaum (Eds.), *Changing perceptions of aging and the aged* (pp. 71–74). New York: Springer Publishing Company.

Smith, C. H. (1989). Richard Eberhart's poems on aging. *Journal of Aging Studies, 3*(1), 75–80.

Snowdon, D. A. (1997). Aging and Alzheimer's disease: Lessons from the Nun Study. *The Gerontologist, 37*(2), 150–156.

Stoller, E. P., & Gibson, R. C. (2000). *Worlds of difference: Inequality in the aging experience* (3rd ed.). Thousand Oaks, CA: Pine Forge Press.

Sung, K. (1998). An exploration of actions of filial piety. *Journal of Aging Studies, 12*(4), 369–386.

Tashakkori, A., & Teddlie, C. (1998). *Mixed methodology: Combining qualitative and quantitative approaches.* Thousand Oaks, CA: Sage Publications, Inc.

Thomas, L. E. (1997). Late-life effect of early mystical experiences: A cross-cultural comparison. *Journal of Aging Studie, 11*(2), 155–169.

Tierney, W. G. (2000). Undaunted courage: Life history and the postmodern challenge. In N. K. Denzin & Y. S. Lincoln (Eds.), *Handbook of qualitative research* (2nd ed., pp. 537–553). Thousand Oaks, CA: Sage Publications, Inc.

Tilson, D. (Ed.). (1990). *Aging in place: Supporting the frail elderly in residential environments.* Glenview, IL: Scott, Foresman & Company.

Tornstam, L. (1994). Gero-transcendence: A theoretical and empirical exploration. In L. E. Thomas & S. A. Eisenhandler (Eds.), *Aging and the religious dimension* (pp. 203–229). Westport, CT: Auburn House.

Tornstam, L. (1997). Gerotranscendence: The contemplative dimension of aging. *Journal of Aging Studies, 11*(2), 143–154.

Tout, K. (1989). *Aging in developing countries,* New York: Oxford University Press.

Travis, S. S., & McAuley, W. J. (1998). Searches for a nursing home: Personal and situational factors. *Journal of Applied Gerontology, 17*(3), 352–370.

Treas, J. (1995). Older Americans in the 1990s and beyond. *Population Bulletin,* Vol. 50, No. 2. Washington, DC: Population Reference Bureau.

Usita, P. M., Hyman, I. E., & Herman, K. C. (1998). Narrative intentions: Listening to life stories in Alzheimer's disease. *Journal of Aging Studies, 12*(2), 185–197.

Vogt, W. P. (1999). *Dictionary of statistics & methodology* (2nd ed.). Thousand Oaks, CA: Sage Publications, Inc.

Waldrop, M. M. (1992). *Complexity: The emerging science at the edge of chaos*. New York: Simon & Schuster.

Wallace, J. B. (1994). Life stories. In J. F. Gubrium & A. Sankar (Eds.), *Qualitative methods in aging research* (pp. 137–154). Thousand Oaks, CA: Sage Publications, Inc.

Weitzman, E. A. (2000). Software and qualitative research. In N. K. Denzin & Y. S. Lincoln (Eds.), *Handbook of qualitative research* (2nd ed., pp. 803–820). Thousand Oaks, CA: Sage Publications, Inc.

Weitzman, E. A., & Miles, M. B. (1995). *Computer programs for qualitative data analysis: A sourcebook*. Thousand Oaks, CA: Sage Publications, Inc.

Wenger, G. C. (1999). Advantages gained by combining qualitative and quantitative data in a longitudinal study. *Journal of Aging Studies, 4*, 369–376.

Wheeler, W. M. (1995). *Elderly residential experience: The evolution of places as residence*. New York: Garland Publishing, Inc.

Wyatt-Brown, A. M. (1995). Creativity in the face of death: Claire Philip's journal and poems. *Journal of Aging Studies, 9*(4), 263–264.

# PART II

# Telling Stories

# Introduction

## Hege Ravdal

As researchers of later life, we now encounter elders who have experienced the early part of the last century, as well as the beginning of the new millennium. These are elders who both experienced the Great Depression and witnessed the development of a global economy. They perhaps learned their letters in a one-room schoolhouse, whereas their grandchildren and they, themselves, for that matter, now routinely employ e-mail and use the Internet on powerful laptop computers that only decades ago would have taken up an entire room. How can we capture such vast leaps of time and transition that occurred during a single person's lifetime? How do we begin to understand the lived experience of these elders?

A lifecourse perspective on aging studies is particularly suitable for synthesizing and integrating the richness of the long lives of our informants. Within this rubric, the same can be said of the use of life histories, life stories, and life narratives: the longer the life, the richer the stories are likely to be. Our challenge is to find ways to capture such stories, think about their context and purpose, and apply them toward increasing our holistic and integrative understanding of aging persons and their experiences of growing old. Life histories and life story methods enable us to tap the common human tendency to reminisce and weave memories into stories. Using their integrative properties, we can piece together the many stories that actually make up a person's "life as-a-whole" (Bruner, 1999). Indeed, Eisner (1997) describes a well-crafted narrative as "a platform for seeing what might be called our 'actual worlds' more clearly."

The many names given to stories of life and the means by which they are gathered bear witness to diverse origins and evolution. Some speak of life stories, others of biographies and autobiographies. Yet others refer to life narratives or life histories. Such differing designations suggest that the stories involve temporal aspects and diverse forms. Telling and recording life stories is far from a standardized methodological procedure. Certainly, material gathered reflects the actors involved, intimating the range and contrast of angles and perspectives from which lives may be interpreted by storytellers, story writers, and listeners, and perhaps the degree of editing allowed by a particular form.

At the heart of the appeal of gathering life stories lies the innate human ability, and even need, to express ourselves through stories. Storytelling predates the written record and structured accounts; by presenting a life history, we acknowledge linkages with prehistory and the unique nature of temporal communion between members of different generations of our species.

Through life stories, we attempt to capture and convey time and the timelessness of the human experience. This complicated task requires us to consider many dimensions of time, including intraindividual differences, the dynamic nature of life stories, and the interdependence of yesterday, today, and tomorrow. To decide when to create or record a story, and then grapple with the individuality of temporal experience, are only two of our challenges. We also must consider the situational, environmental, and historical context in which narration and recording occur (Luborsky, 1993). Finally, we must ponder the outcome of our efforts. Life stories, especially as they pertain to gerontology, often outlast their protagonists. If published, such stories become a fixed and physical record, as well as the possession of all who read them. Considering the degree of personal revelation involved in creating life stories, it is important to acknowledge diverse and complex ethical issues that may arise from employing this genre of inquiry (Kenyon, 1996; Kenyon & Randall, 1997; Mills, 1998; Rich, 1996).

## Life Stories and the Place of the Researcher

If the creation and collection of life stories is a method, then our units of study are the lives of our informants. The conduit for transmission of information is reminiscence, drawing on the tendency of elders to try to make sense of their lives and of aging by looking back (Butler, 1963; Coleman, 1986; Hendricks, 1995). We, the listeners and researchers, view the account as something that has value beyond the immediate gratification of the storytelling act. Perhaps we see a bigger picture, a composite whole that may benefit others in the telling of this particular story, or may provide answers to more global questions about the aging experience.

In gerontology, our informants are generally people with long lives already lived that continue to be "in process." Life-story methods provide depth and detail as we explore these lives. As listeners or facilitators, and to the third-hand reader (our audience), life stories are akin to personally knowing someone and the intricacies of their life. The process of creating life-story documents entails a sharing of experience between the elder and the facilitator/researcher that can be emotionally powerful and cathartic to both, commonly exceeding the emotional involvement afforded through a less comprehensive, in-depth interview. To explore an entire life generally necessitates time-consuming interaction between a researcher and his or her subject. It requires that the researcher have superior skills in developing rapport and trust. The intimacy that often results from revelation of deep-seated and personal experiences demands an empathic and committed listener.

## Life Stories as Data?

Some might ask if these narratives comprise "data." According to Schroots and Birren (chapter 3), life stories and the means of transforming them into data belong to a new generation of qualitative methods that may defy previous ways of conceptualizing scholarly information. In the words of Gubrium and Holstein (1998), "As social research increasingly points to the narrative quality of lives, the personal story is being resuscitated as an important source of experiential data" (p. 163). However, we must keep in mind that "Individuals do not have their readily narrated life stories in their back pockets or the back of their minds, waiting for a researcher to collect them" (Alasuutari, 1997, p. 6). The act of telling is an experience with a function and with distinct consequences.

Kenyon (chapter 2) encourages us to see narratives and life stories as *more* than just data. Life storying is process, and therefore has inherent value in and of itself. Many scholars speak to the inseparability of the Self and the story, in that the Self is constructed using stories. " . . . Human beings not only *have* a life story, they *are* stories" (Kenyon, Ruth, & Mader, 1999, pp. 40–41. Moreover, the story is coauthored, a product of the mutually creative dialogue of the storyteller and others present. Stories exist at the nexus of the inner life of an individual and the same life as observed by outsiders. As the stories unfold, both spheres influence their creation and are influenced by them. Life stories are possibly the most personal documents that can be created in a research setting.

Beyond the view of life stories as simply sources of data, a plethora of opportunities are available through the many possible modes of presentation and representation of narratives and life-history materials. Presenting a life, or making the single case study, has gained popularity among qualitative scholars (Mandelbaum, 1973; Sandelowski, 1996; Sokolovsky, 1996). Others combine life stories of several individuals into a collective presentation. Still others may emphasize certain aspects of the stories to address a particular theory, topical issue, or concept (Parker, 1995; Webster, 1999). For example, life histories can illustrate the presence of historical and cultural forces in shaping lives, indicating ways in which race, ethnicity, class, and gender influence us through the lifecourse (Bennett & Detzner, 1997; Kamler, 1996; Ray, 1998).

Life stories and life-history methods merge a variety of disciplinary perspectives, including psychology, anthropology, sociology, history, and the humanities in creating an interdisciplinary vision of the aging experience. In the past decade, this vision has been articulated through the publication of several anthologies (Birren, Kenyon, Ruth, Schroots, & Svensson, 1996; Gubrium, 1993; Randall & Kenyon, 2000), and two special issues of journals on biographical and narrative methods in aging research (*Ageing and Society*, 16, 1996; *Journal of Aging Studies*, 13 (1), 1999).

## Applications of Life-Story Methods

Beyond the conceptual and existential aspects of life storying, there are numerous possible applications of life-story methods. The authors of the two chapters that follow present two perspectives on one approach, guided autobiography (Birren & Cochran, 2001), although they utilize significantly different ways, illustrating the openness of interpretation and function that exists within this group of methods. Schroots and Birren (chapter 3) view guided autobiography as a way for researchers to obtain information about "the inside views of their [subject's] lives" (p. 58). Kenyon (chapter 2) likewise sees guided autobiography as a way for participants "to express their inside stories" (p. 41), but prefers to dwell on the benefits to the storyteller rather than a researcher.

Although Kenyon prefers to distance his work with guided autobiography from direct therapeutic practice, both he and Schroots and Birren (chapter 3) acknowledge the therapeutic potential inherent in life stories and guided autobiography, noting that narrative gerontology has roots in narrative psychology and the practice of narrative therapy (see also Kenyon & Randall, 1997). Indeed, as early as the 1960s, Robert N.

Butler (1963) became a proponent of the therapeutic role of life histories through the process he termed "life review." Since Butler's original treatise, notions of the life review have evolved, but both scholars and practitioners continue to find merit in the therapeutic value of life histories and the *process* by which they are generated (Cohen & Taylor, 1998; de Vries, Birren, & Deutchman, 1990; Helterline & Nouri, 1994; Mills, 1998; O'Connor, 1994). Rybarczyk and Bellg (1997) believe that when a qualified person facilitates the process of life storying, reminiscence, or life review, it can have a distinct stress-coping effect on the individual concerned. The process can provide perspective on the individual's *whole* life, emphasize the remembrance of past coping successes and strengths, and thereby aid an older person through an adverse life experience. Indeed, in the health sciences there is emerging a unique alliance between clinical practice and qualitative methods (Becker, 1999; Burnside, 1996; Clark, 1996; Gergen, 1996; Haight, Michel, & Hendrix, 1998).

Our fascination with storytelling, and thus with knowing about the inner workings of the lives of others, has to do with the way it affects our own lives in profound ways. As a panhuman occurrence, aging concerns us all. We have a stake in continuing to unravel the phenomenon of aging, aspiring to better understand its diverse facets, and hoping that we may, thereby, improve quality of life. As we are discovering, the experience of aging as revealed through life stories is one very powerful way to begin to understand.

# REFERENCES

Alasuutari, P. (1997). The discursive construction of personality. In A. Lieblich & R. Josselson (Eds.), *The narrative study of lives* (pp. 1–20). Thousand Oaks, CA: Sage Publications, Inc.

Becker, B. (1999). Narratives of pain in later life and conventions of storytelling. *Journal of Aging Studies, 13*(1), 73–87.

Bennett, J. A., & Detzner, D. F. (1997). Loneliness in cultural context: A look at the life-history narratives of older Southeast Asian refugee women. In A. Lieblich & R. Josselson (Eds.), *The narrative study of lives* (pp. 113–146). Thousand Oaks, CA: Sage Publications, Inc.

Birren, J. E., Kenyon, G. M., Ruth, J.-E., Schroots, J. J. F., & Svensson, T. (Eds.). (1996). *Aging and biography: Explorations in adult development.* New York: Springer Publishing Company.

Birren, J. E., & Cochran, K. N. (2001). *Telling the stories of life through guided autobiography groups.* Baltimore, MD: Johns Hopkins University Press.

Bruner, J. (1999). Narratives of aging. *Journal of Aging Studies, 13*(1), 7–9.

Burnside, I. (1996). Life review and reminiscence in nursing practice. In J. E. Birren, G. M. Kenyon, J.-E. Ruth, J. J. F. Schroots, & T. Svensson (Eds.), *Aging and biography: Explorations in adult development*. New York: Springer Publishing Company.

Butler, R. N. (1963). The life review: An interpretation of reminiscence in the aged. *Psychiatry, 26,* 65–76.

Clark, P. G. (1996). Communication between provider and patient: Values, biography, and empowerment in clinical practice. [Special Issues on Ageing, Biography and Practice]. *Ageing and Society, 16,* 747–774.

Cohen, G., & Taylor, S. (1998). Reminiscence and ageing. *Ageing and Society, 18*(5), 601.

Coleman, P. G. (1986). *Ageing and reminiscence processes: Social and clinical implications.* New York: John Wiley & Sons.

de Vries, B., Birren, J. E., & Deutchman, D. E. (1990). Adult development through guided autobiography: The family context. *Family Relations, 39*(1), 3–7.

Eisner, E. W. (1997). The new frontier in qualitative research methodology. *Qualitative Inquiry, 3*(3), 259–274.

Gergen, K. J. (1996). Beyond life narratives in the therapeutic encounter. In J. E. Birren, G. M. Kenyon, J.-E. Ruth, J. J. F. Schroots, & T. Svensson (Eds.), *Aging and biography: Explorations in adult development* (pp. 205–223). New York: Springer Publishing Company.

Gubrium, J. F. (1993). *Speaking of life: Horizons of meaning for nursing home residents.* Hawthorne, NY: Aldine.

Gubrium, J. F., & Holstein, J. A. (1998). Narrative practice and the coherence of personal stories. *The Sociological Quarterly, 39*(1), 163–187.

Haight, B. K., Michel, Y., & Hendrix, S. (1998). Life review: Preventing despair in newly relocated nursing home residents—short- and long-term effects. *International Journal of Aging and Human Development, 47*(2), 119–142.

Helterline, M., & Nouri, M. (1994). Aging and gender: Values and continuity. *Journal of Women & Aging, 6*(3), 19–38.

Hendricks, J. (1995). *The meaning of reminiscence and life review.* Amityville, NY: Baywood.

Kamler, B. (1996). From autobiography to collective biography: Stories of ageing and loss. *Women and Language, 19*(1), 21–26.

Kenyon, G. M. (1996). Ethical issues in ageing and biography [Special Issue on Ageing, Biography and Practice]. *Ageing and Society, 16,* 659–675.

Kenyon, G. M., & Randall, W. L. (1997). *Restorying our lives: Personal growth through autobiographical reflection.* Westport, CT: Praeger.

Kenyon, G. M., Ruth, J.-E., & Mader, W. (1999). Elements of a narrative gerontology. In V. L. Bengtson & K. W. Schaie (Eds.), *Handbook of theories of aging.* New York: Springer Publishing Company.

Luborsky, M. R. (1993). The romance with personal meaning in gerontology: Cultural aspects of life themes. *The Gerontologist, 33*(4), 445–452.

Mandelbaum, D. L. (1973). The study of life history: Gandhi. *Current Anthropology, 14*(3), 177–206.

Mills, M. A. (1998). *Narrative identity and dementia.* Aldershot, UK: Ashgate.

O'Connor, P. (1994). Salient themes in the life review of a sample of frail elderly respondents in London. *The Gerontologist, 34*(2), 224–230.

Parker, R. G. (1995). Reminiscence: A continuity theory framework. *The Gerontologist, 36*(4), 515–525.

Randall, W. L., & Kenyon, G. M. (2000). *Ordinary wisdom: Biographical aging and the journey of life.* Westport, CT: Greenwood.

Ray, R. E. (1998). Feminist readings of older women's life stories. *Journal of Aging Studies, 12*(2), 117–127.

Rich, B. A. (1996). Values history: Restoring narrative identity to long-term care. *Journal of Ethics, Law, and Aging, 2*(2), 75–84.

Rybarczyk, B., & Bellg, A. (1997). *Listening to life stories: A new approach to stress intervention in health care.* New York: Springer Publishing Company.

Sandelowski, M. (1996). One is the liveliest number: The case orientation of qualitative research. *Research in Nursing and Health, 19,* 525–529.

Sokolovsky, M. (1996). Case study as a research method to study life histories of elderly people: Some ideas and a case study of a case study. *Journal of Aging Studies, 10*(4), 281–294.

Webster, J. D. (1999). World views and narrative gerontology: Situating reminiscence behavior within a lifespan perspective. *Journal of Aging Studies, 13*(1), 29–42.

# CHAPTER TWO

# Guided Autobiography: In Search of Ordinary Wisdom

## Gary M. Kenyon

### INTRODUCTION

I am grateful to the editors of this volume for providing an opportunity to explore and even wax philosophical about two areas of emphasis that form the core of my interest in gerontology. The first is guided autobiography, a particular approach to "restorying our lives" (Kenyon & Randall, 1997). Having originally participated in my first guided autobiography course with Jim Birren, its creator, at the University of Southern California, I have now been teaching and sharing this approach in workshops, seminars, and academic courses with students, researchers, and practitioners for almost 10 years.

The second area of interest is wisdom. Although by original training I am a philosopher, and, at least historically this might be an understandable inclination, it is through my experience with guided autobiography that I have come to realize that wisdom is not something to be reserved for "saints and swamis," and thus the term "ordinary wisdom" in the title of this work. An expanded treatment of this concept can be found in a volume by Randall and Kenyon (in press).

In what follows, I argue that wisdom is ordinary in the sense that it is contained within the stories we are. Nevertheless, it is important to note that this means that each of our lives is quite extraordinary. I will elaborate these insights by exploring two central themes. The first is the life as story metaphor and how life stories are accessible in guided autobiography, and the second is ordinary wisdom and wisdom stories, again, as they can be observed in guided autobiography.

## THE STORIES WE ARE

In a recent article, Jerome Bruner, one of the creators of narrative psychology and an inspiration for narrative gerontology (Kenyon, Ruth, & Mader, 1999; Kenyon, Clark, & de Vries, in press) states that telling stories is not just something we do, but rather it is the "very process by which we construct Self, the central figure in this work of art. No story, no self" (Bruner, 1999, p. 8). In agreement with this insight, narratives and life stories are more than simply another form of data. Further, it is not enough to say that we have a life story (or stories). Rather, there is an ontological dimension to the relationship between a person and his or her life story. As David Carr notes, "There is nothing below this narrative structure, at least nothing experienceable by us or comprehensible in experiential terms" (1986, p. 66). Further, it is important to note that we do not cease to live our story even if we become victims of such conditions as dementia (Holst, Edberg, & Hallberg, 1999).

Due to its ontological nature, the processes of storytelling and storylistening (Kenyon & Randall, 1997) take on a spiritual quality in the sense that our stories express what is meaning-ful (or meaning-less) to us in life. Narrative therapists, for example, use terms such as "curiosity" and "mystery" in describing a biographical encounter with a client (White, 1991). The holistic nature of the life as story metaphor is also evident in that stories involve not just ideas or cognitive aspects of human nature. They also contain emotions and influence action or behavior. That is, from this perspective, not only how we think, but how we feel and what we do is significantly a function of the story we tell ourselves and/or others.

Conceptually, life stories are made up of both facticity and possibility. Facticity, in contrast to "facts," refers to the story that we live at any point in time, our ongoing life story. It is what we take to be true about ourselves, other people, and the world. This facticity, as we will consider later, is not quite a story to us as yet, since we cannot read it. We are in the middle of our story; in one way, our story lives us. We cannot live it and read it at the same time. Nevertheless, it is not a case of the facts of a particular situation, but our own interpretation of events and experiences. Our facticity also includes the larger story that we live within, that is, among other things, our sociopolitical story, our gender, race, age, ethnic story, and our hereditary predisposition story (Kenyon & Randall, 1997). These stories we find ourselves in influence but do not determine our personal or inside story. Finally, facticity also includes our basic feeling tone, emotionality (Mader, 1996), or the genre of our life story (Randall, 1995).

Our facticity develops as experiences and events become fortified stories over time. Thus, depending on our unique storying style, we come to expect particular themes and genres to be dominant in our stories, we see the world according to a particular story line. On the one hand, examples of genres and story lines would be depressive, self-blaming, and tragic stories. On the other hand, they are hopeful, loving, wisdom, and adventure stories. Ruth and Oberg (1996), for example, identified dominant themes that they call ways of life in the life stories of a group of older Finnish people that included the Careerist, the Bitter life, the Sweet life, the Hurdle Race, and the Trapping Pit. These ways of life are very instructive in helping us understand the way in which we come to compose our life stories uniquely and yet according to generalizable themes (see also Gubrium, 1993, for another interesting example of this type of study). While each of our stories is made up of combinations of various types of plots, characters, themes, and genres, the expression of each story, the way that we each put the pieces together, is unique, personal, and unendingly creative. In other words, the journey is personal, but it has shared station-stops (Randall & Kenyon, in press). If we care to listen carefully to our own or another's story, we will find that no two facticities, no two life stories are ever exactly the same.

The second element of lives as stories is possibility, or, more precisely, our sense of possibility. It is this aspect of our life stories that enables us to restory our lives through our ability to imagine, fantasize, and symbolize. The crucial point here, and one of the basic assumptions of narrative gerontology, and the life as story metaphor, is that we can never assume that a particular person at any particular time is locked-in by some element of their facticity. In principle, there is no story that cannot be rewritten, recomposed, or "re-genre-ated" (Randall, 1995). It is always possible to trade-in and trade-up our personal images and metaphors. This, again, is possible because we are fundamentally our stories.

One other basic "life as story" issue that deserves attention in this section is time. It is often thought, and some theories of development including that of Sigmund Freud concur, that we are locked-in at an early age to our way of being in the world. Or, more generally, it is believed that the past cannot be altered in any way. For example, we often consider whether we are on-time or off-time in terms of our career, marriage, or other major life events. In addition, our social structure imposes constraints based on calendar time, such as mandatory retirement, voting age, and eligibility for various social programs.

However, from a life-as-story perspective, human beings experience different kinds of time. Just think of how different our experience of time is when we are in love, when we are waiting for a diagnosis, when we are in meditation, or contemplating nature. In addition to what was first described, clock time, which is linear, unidirectional, and has a certain finality to it, there is also story time (Kenyon & Randall, 1997). Story time refers to the notion that our stories exist primarily in the present. While they do come from somewhere, our past lives and stories are given meaning today, they are recreated continuously in the present as we gain new experiences. Similarly, our stories are going toward a possible future, but this possible future is also based on our present facticity and possibility.

From a story-time perspective, what we do with our life stories today can change the meaning of where we have been and where we are going. It is for this reason that time is a central concept in narrative gerontology (Kenyon et al., 1999), both from the point of view of the potential to change our story of time and as a research question concerning how people live time differently over the life span (for example, see de Vries, Blando, Southard, & Bubeck, in press).

It is important to note that restorying is by no means a facile or mechanical process. Restorying our lives is a truly existential project that involves new meaning and presupposes new thoughts, emotions, and actions. We can re-make ourselves, but we cannot make ourselves up at will by means of a "quick fix" technique, or by simply deciding that we will be another story. The power of our facticity should not be underestimated. Moreover, the process of restorying involves both effort and letting go, that is, unlearning our old story (Randall & Kenyon, in press).

Restorying can also be complicated due to the fact that we do not have total control over our stories for various reasons, including that we cannot see our whole story since we are in the middle of it. It is opaque. Further, although as individuals we have a personal, unique, inside story, we also live within the larger story indicated earlier. Thus, paradoxically, we are in essence interpersonal beings with a deeply personal aspect as well. This means that we are creating our stories as we are simultaneously created by other people as part of that larger story. When it comes to our stories, we are simultaneously narrator, editor, protagonist, reader, and not sole author, but coauthor. Some of these coauthoring dimensions would include such things as our gender story, our ethnic story, our family story, and our work story.

This situation leaves a great deal of room for new and improved versions of a life story, but it is not a case of just anything goes.

## GUIDED AUTOBIOGRAPHY AND THE STORIES WE ARE

The discussion of narrative concepts just undertaken is important as prolegomena to considering the particular insights associated with guided autobiography. Guided autobiography is a particular type of biographical intervention that, at least in its original form, is not intended as therapy. It is best described as an existential or learning form of intervention. There are important ethical issues associated with this last statement that I will consider later. At this point, I would like to outline the process of guided autobiography and describe some of the outcomes I have witnessed.

At a general level, guided autobiography allows us the opportunity to "get the story out." As we discussed, the story that we are currently living is not yet a story to us as we are too close to it. Guided autobiography creates an opportunity to gain some distance and detachment from our life story so that we can begin the process of restorying our lives by telling, reading, and retelling that story (Kenyon & Randall, 1997). Our story has to be told in order for it to change, whether the audience is ourself, another person, a fictional character, or some other actual or symbolic audience. I like to call this initial step the "storying moment," what Randall (in press) calls the "it" phenomenon. It is the point when someone comes to see and feel his or her life as a story and begins to express it. In the way that I utilize guided autobiography, this is the primary emphasis and magic of this approach. Guided autobiography focuses on establishing a nonjudgemental, accepting, and confidential environment wherein participants feel comfortable to begin to express their inside stories. There is a tremendous amount of release and healing that occurs from this storying moment alone.

More recently, guided autobiography has been adapted for other uses, such as therapy and research (see Shaw, in press; Kenyon et al., in press; Kenyon & Randall, 1999). However, my focus and primary interest in guided autobiography is to "not do anything with the stories." In this way, guided autobiography becomes almost totally a matter of storylistening, without judgement, without interpretation (at least publicly), and with acceptance. In my experience, this process of leaving things alone is often a challenging task, especially for professionals who are accustomed to doing something with a person's story. In other words, the challenge for the professional is to "leave their hat at the door" and become just another storyteller in the group. Again, the focus for me is on the magic in the storying moment itself. But what is this magic?

What I often observe in guided autobiography, in the storying moment, is a movement from facticity to possibility. It does not seem to matter whether the story is about divorce, exile, abuse, loss of a spouse, loss of a child, a serious illness, or loss of career, there is a discovery of meaning realized by most participants in guided autobiography. To provide just one illustration, a participant in a summer course in guided autobiography started as a very quiet and preoccupied group member. I wondered whether he was enjoying the course at all. However, during the session on death and dying, this preoccupation lifted and he became visibly happy. He told us that he felt a tremendous release in just getting the story out about how he grieved for the death of his grandfather. He said that sharing his story in a trusting atmosphere had helped him feel more hopeful and positive about this loss. He had not shared this story with anyone over a period of several years. I saw this participant a year after the course ended and he again thanked me for the opportunity to tell his story within the guided autobiography framework. While not all participants experience such powerful change, most do report that they find the guided autobiography experience pleasant and meaningful.

It is important to repeat that guided autobiography functions in a learning context, in contrast to a counseling or other therapy context. As such, it is not appropriate to those who are experiencing recent trauma. This is because a person who is in an acute stage of a major loss is usually living that story as the "only story in town." There is usually little room for their sense of possibility to emerge from the overwhelming facticity of the situation. Guided autobiography is not usually appropriate in this context because, as is outlined in the introductory section to this chapter, it is not designed to spend a great deal of time validating each person's story. Nevertheless, it has been demonstrated that guided autobiography can be adapted for therapy purposes (Brown-Shaw, Westwood, & de Vries, 1999).

While new applications of this approach are evolving in combination with other interventions, I call guided autobiography "therapy for the sane." Nevertheless, it is actually a strong indicator of our ability to restory our lives that we see such sharing and healing in this process. Whatever the experience is, there is a space between it and the story that we tell ourselves about that experience, the meaning that we place on that situation. Guided autobiography helps us to find a new and better story by first allowing us the possibility to read the story we have been living up to now about a particular life theme. But how does guided autobiography work?

The process and dynamics of guided autobiography could and will be the subject of many interesting future research projects. At this point, however, I would like to provide my own reflections on these aspects of guided autobiography. As Mader (1995) has shown, there are five elements of guided autobiography. It is the combination of these elements that constitute the particular effectiveness of guided autobiography. First, guided autobiography involves setting a period of time aside for personal reflection. This is an experience that is strangely often missing in our late 20th century lifestyle. Experiences such as silence and solitude are anathema to many people, but they are requisite to the process of restorying, to the enhancement of our sense of possibility, and to the emergence of ordinary wisdom. It is the personal reflection dimension that allows the space to arise between my life and my story. Second, guided autobiography highlights particular existential themes. Although it is a minimally guided process, there is a focus on aspects of human life that are commonly shared. That is, none of us can avoid developing a relationship with, among other things, money, significant others, death and dying, and work or career (Mader, 1995). The guided themes facilitate the process of "mining" important pieces of our stories.

Third, in guided autobiography, we do not restory alone. The themes that are initially contemplated in solitude are subsequently shared in a small group. This activity is indispensable in that, as we discussed earlier, we are coauthors of our stories; other people, for better or worse, are part of our very nature and identity (Kenyon, 1996a). This does not mean that other people determine who we are in a strict social constructionist sense, but it does mean that we discover who we are in an interpersonal environment. In guided autobiography, other people provide a supportive, nonjudgemental setting for us to feel free to let our stories out. Further, our stories change and can improve through the coauthoring process of listening to the stories of others as well. For example, as Jim Birren has pointed out, we feel that "other people are more like me than I thought" (Birren & Birren, 1996, p 291). This is an interesting observation since it suggests that some of the things that as individuals we think are unique to us ("No one can understand me") are shared by others. Such a realization can create an interpersonal bond of intimacy.

Fourth, the activity of writing our stories down, while not completely necessary, does provide us with something literally to read. As with journal writing or keeping a diary, we see how our story moves from being part of our facticity to being a story available to our sense of possibility. Finally, the fifth element of guided autobiography is its encouragement of the use of metaphors and other creative media. In the effort to create an environment that will let our stories out, we may utilize creative language, for example, describe our life as a branching tree or a flowing river, or find our own metaphor for our life. In my experience with guided autobiography, participants have characterized their lives as mobiles, cactus patches, pizzas, and a pine tree with the lower branches falling off as the person grows.

Guided autobiography also encourages the use of poetry, photos and other memorabilia, and sensual material like dried leaves, fruit, as well as music and art. As an anecdotal testimony to the effectiveness of this approach, one of my students encouraged autobiography with several dementing persons, using some of these materials. She had many very moving experiences, including one female nursing-home resident who spoke for the first time in 2 years. I am more convinced that as long as we are alive (and perhaps even longer), we still have and are our life story, and we still have a story to tell (see also Gubrium, 1993, and Haight & Webster, 1995, for a discussion of related insights and approaches).

## *In Search of Ordinary Wisdom*

Guided autobiography, employed in the manner that I am emphasizing here, that is, with the focus on the storying moment, is very effective because it sets up, borrowing from Meacham (1990), a wisdom environment. As such, it facilitates a process whereby we come to feel good in our skin and with others (Josso, 1998). As Meacham (1990, p. 209) points out, "It is through the supportive and sharing relationships within a wisdom atmosphere that one gains the courage to engage in confident and wise action even in the face of one's doubts." In this case, the confidence to engage in wise action is to be able to look at our life stories as a step in coming to value our lives more, whether we are young or old, frail or well. There are two examples of this valuing process that I have very often observed in guided autobiography sessions. First, many young participants begin the process by stating that they are too young to have a life story worth telling. However, after a few sessions they realize that they have survived much, and have interesting stories and lives. Second, often older female storytellers will begin by saying that they do not have much of a story to tell because they were "just housewives." Again, after a few sessions they discover, through their own reflection and in the small-group sharing, just how rich and valuable their lives are. Further, in this process they often become a new story, in thought, feeling, and action. In my view, this is ordinary wisdom (Randall & Kenyon, in press). It is a process of finding new personal meaning from inside our own story, or from our inside story.

It is important to indicate that a wisdom environment can only be offered, so to speak. Restorying and the discovery of ordinary wisdom cannot be forced. As mentioned earlier, they are not technical or mechanical processes. We do not know very much about why a particular person experiences the storying moment or becomes aware of their biographical imperative at a particular time. Depending on the perspective we adopt, we might say it is grace, karma, or chance. One person will arrive at this point through trauma or suffering, and others suffer but do not engage in restorying their lives.

In this regard, guided autobiography is effective because it invites us to tell and share our stories with no real purpose in mind except to share stories. Unlike therapy or support groups, guided autobiography has no set story line that all must follow. Each person decides each step of the way what he or she will disclose and how he or she will disclose it; he or she can change their minds at any time in the process. If successful, the atmosphere created in a guided autobiography session is akin to a group of friends having a coffee together.

There are five important features of being human associated with ordinary wisdom that I often observe in guided autobiography sessions. First, in storytelling and storylistening, we come to realize that there is strength in, and even through, diminishment. As unpleasant as it is, we very often find meaning in suffering, and there is wisdom in learning true acceptance of some things in life. It is important to emphasize that acceptance is a life-affirming process and should not be equated with resignation. Acceptance is giving-in, but not giving-up.

Second, through guided autobiography we also come to realize that we cannot see or read our story, the whole story, and nothing but the story. Our lives and our life stories are not transparent, they have a quality of opaqueness. In guided autobiography sessions, participants experience this insight by seeing that they are or were not to blame for such and such, that they now see that they could not have known the whole story. Naturally, there is tremendous release often associated with this experience. I often observe heavy loads lifting off a participant's shoulders, sometimes loads that they say they have been carrying for many years. These insights are sometimes small and sometimes large, but all are a part of our ordinary wisdom.

A third feature that relates to the second is that, in guided autobiography, we find that our stories are never complete in the sense that there is not just one life story that belongs to each life. We are many stories and different ones emerge depending on the audience, the purpose of telling the story, our mood, and our current life situation or larger story. For example, guided autobiography participants are sometimes surprised, and even disturbed, that a major life theme, such as a divorce, a marriage, or the loss of a significant other did not come up in this particular version of their story. In the case of unpleasant events, they sometimes say that time really does heal. A tragic story can be re-genreated into a satire, a comedy, or even an unimportant story. This does not mean that we have no continuous identity as a person as some postmodern theorists have claimed (Gergen, 1991). After all, we do have our facticity. However, these story transformations do mean that we are complex stories or journeys in progress and we need not, and probably cannot, tie up all the loose ends in order to create one well-formed "story of my life" (Kenyon & Randall, 1997).

Fourth, as mentioned earlier, guided autobiography assists us in seeing that we are not alone in the world. Much of life's experience separates people. Guided autobiography can and sometimes does provide the ordinary wisdom insight that we are all fellow travelers with interconnected destinies. Such an experience can make us feel more at home in our world. We can experience communion, as well as separation and alienation in life. This effective and healing outcome of guided autobiography is observed in the intensity and intimacy of many small groups. Participants often say that fellow group members feel like very close friends after only two or three sessions. They also often say that they are disclosing things that they have never told anyone before. In addition to this, some groups continue to meet for years after the session is completed. I have had this very special experience when I meet participants even years after a session. There is very often a special intimacy and trust that is created between people through this process. I believe there are, for whatever reasons, many similarities between this process and the characteristics of authentic friendship that merit further examination.

The fifth feature of ordinary wisdom that can emerge in guided autobiography is the realization that despite suffering, loss, mistakes, confusion, and the wrong road taken, life really does go on. As long as we are alive, our story and our journey continue, if we can only continue to see it that way.

## GUIDED AUTOBIOGRAPHY AND ETHICS

It is important to emphasize three main ethical issues in connection with the use of guided autobiography and any other form of biographical intervention (see also Kenyon, 1996b). The first has to do with when to story and when not to story. It has become evident that not everyone wishes to engage in restorying their life. Some of us do not engage in reminiscence activities at any time and some of us are not interested at certain times in our lives. It is unethical, and can be harmful, to coerce or otherwise force someone to engage in a biographical encounter that is not clearly of his or her choice. This issue can arise particularly with vulnerable groups, such as older persons who reside in sheltered housing arrangements.

In contrast, there are situations when providing an opportunity to someone to tell his or her story, and have it listened to, is indispensable and a person's right. In health-care and competency situations, as examples, it is unethical not to gain access to a person's story and really listen to it as part of a treatment plan or evaluation of a person's ability to live an autonomous life.

The second issue has to do with the purpose of the biographical encounter. As we have already mentioned, there is a major distinction between learning or existential interventions, and therapeutic ones. Although all forms of restorying might be considered to have a therapeutic outcome, there is a very different story line in operation between the two types. Guided autobiography, utilized as I have outlined in this discussion, does not require a clinically trained person. It requires someone who, ideally, has experienced the process as a participant and, if possible, as a small-group leader. Otherwise, a guided-autobiography session coordinator needs to be a sensitive, good listener. The crucial issue in guided autobiography is to set up the assumptions and guidelines at the very beginning of the session. In this way, the expectations and behaviors of the participants will facilitate the accepting and nonjudgemental environment that characterizes this particular biographical intervention.

If these guidelines are not established up front, then the entire process is at risk of failing and even causing harm to participants. I have never experienced any problems in this regard, due to careful attention paid to this ethical issue. Participants need to know, for example, that no one will spend a great deal of time validating their particular story, or providing answers or advice. This further step in restorying is more properly reserved for appropriately trained interveners, as there is a different purpose for that form of biographical encounter. This second ethical issue becomes even more important as guided autobiography is adapted to therapeutic contexts: The boundaries need to be carefully delineated (see, for example, Brown-Shaw et al., 1999).

The third ethical issue can be called the whose story is it issue. As we have discussed, a person's life story is probably their most intimate possession, and it is uniquely his or her own. Further, we can neither know our own entire story nor that of another. It follows that we need to storylisten with a truly open attitude. While intervention techniques and models are helpful heuristics, they should not be the exclusive filter through which we read another's story. In a biographical encounter, whether guided autobiography or another approach to restorying, we need to learn what is really both an art and a science, to storylisten effectively. There is no end to the learning process of becoming a good listener. We are constantly attempting to sort out the various stories that are at play in a biographical encounter. For example, there can be my personal story, my professional story, and your personal story, all of which are involved in an encounter. On the one hand, from a life-as-story perspective, we cannot gain an objective perspective on another person's story by means of any professional model or technique. On the other hand, biographical encounters are always fresh, always new, because every story is different.

## Conclusion

Sustained and increasing interest in qualitative gerontology over the past decade is very encouraging, since it expands the conceptual and methodological framework for understanding lifelong development. The emphasis on the inside of aging, or aging as it is experienced, constitutes the seminal contribution of qualitative gerontology. As perspectives such as qualitative and narrative gerontology evolve, it is interesting to note that it is not in the direction of setting numbers and statistics in one corner, and life stories and qualitative data in another, as was more the case 10 years ago. Rather, today it is a matter of matching a particular research question with the most appropriate method or approach, whether that method involves either one or the other approach or a combination of the two. In other words, qualitative gerontology is moving forward with its own set of assumptions and methodological issues, and it need not be engaged in defending itself against other scientific traditions.

In this chapter, I have outlined an example of what it is possible to see through the life-as-story lens in the field of aging. This particular qualitative perspective, the practice of guided autobiography, assists us in gaining preliminary insights into the time-honored but subtle and complex phenomenon of wisdom. More important, it enables us to contemplate the possibility that wisdom is an integral part of our human heritage and, in its ordinariness, a potential outcome of aging.

## REFERENCES

Birren, J., & Birren, B. (1996). Autobiography: Exploring the self and encouraging development. In J. Birren, G. Kenyon, J. E. Ruth, H. Schroots, & T. Svensson (Eds.), *Aging and biography: Explorations in adult development* (pp. 283–299). New York: Springer Publishing Company.

Brown-Shaw, M., Westwood, M., & de Vries, B. (1999). Integrating personal reflection and group-based enactments. *Journal of Aging Studies, 13*(1), 109–119.

Bruner, J. (1999). Narratives of aging. *Journal of Aging Studies, 13*(1), 7–9.

Carr, D. (1986). *Time, narrative, and history.* Bloomington, IN: Indiana University Press.

de Vries, B., Blando, J., Southard, P., & Bubeck, C. (2001). Time and the life story. In G. Kenyon, P. Clark, & B. de Vries (Eds.), *Narrative gerontology: Theory, research, and practice.* New York: Springer Publishing Company.

Gergen, K. (1991). *The saturated self.* New York: Basic Books.

Gubrium, J. F. (1993). *Speaking of life: Horizons of meaning for nursing home residents.* Hawthorne, NY: Aldine.

Haight, B., & Webster, J. (Eds.). (1995). *The art and science of reminiscing.* London: Taylor and Francis.

Holst, G., Edberg, A. K., & Hallberg, I. (1999). Nurses' narrations and reflections about caring for patients with severe dementia as revealed in systematic clinical supervision sessions. *Journal of Aging Studies, 13*(1), 89–107.

Josso, M. C. (1998). Histoire de vie et sagesse: La formation comme quete d'un art de vivre. [Life-history and wisdom: Development as a quest for an art of living]. In R. Barbier (Ed.), *Education et sagesse* [Education and wisdom]. Paris: Albin.

Kenyon, G. (1996a). The meaning-value of personal storytelling. In J. Birren, G. Kenyon, J. E. Ruth, J. Schroots, & T. Svensson (Eds.), *Aging and biography: Explorations in adult development.* (pp. 21–38). New York: Springer Publishing Company.

Kenyon, G. (1996b). Ethical issues in aging and biography. *Ageing and Society, 16*(6), 659–675.

Kenyon, G., Clark, P., & de Vries, B. (2001). *Narrative gerontology: Theory, research, and practice.* New York: Springer Publishing Company.

Kenyon, G., & Randall, W. (1997). *Restorying our lives: Personal growth through autobiographical reflection.* Westport, CT: Praeger.

Kenyon, G., & Randall, W. (Guest eds.). (1999). Narrative gerontology [Special issue]. *Journal of Aging Studies, 13*(1).

Kenyon, G., Ruth, J. E., & Mader, W. (1999). Elements of a narrative gerontology. In V. Bengtson & K. W. Schaie (Eds.), *Handbook of theories of aging* (pp. 40–58). New York: Springer Publishing Company.

Mader, W. (1995). Thematically guided autobiographical reconstruction: On theory and method of guided autobiography in adult education. In P. Alheit, A. Bron-Wojciechowska, E. Brugger, & P. Dominice (Eds.), *The biographical approach in adult education* (pp. 244–257). Vienna: Verband Wiener Volksbildung.

Mader, W. (1996). Emotionality and continuity in biographical contexts. In J. Birren, G. Kenyon, J. E. Ruth, J. Schroots, & T. Svensson (Eds.), *Aging and biography: Explorations in adult development* (pp. 39–60). New York: Springer Publishing Company.

Meacham, J. (1990). The loss of wisdom. In R. Sternberg (Ed.), *Wisdom: Its nature, origins, and development* (pp. 181–211). New York: Cambridge University Press.

Randall, W. (1995). *The stories we are.* Toronto, Canada: University of Toronto Press.

Randall, W. (2001). Storied worlds: A narrative perspective on aging and everyday life. In G. Kenyon, P. Clark, & B. de Vries (Eds.), *Narrative gerontology: Theory, research, and practice.* New York: Springer Publishing Company.

Randall, W., & Kenyon, G. (2001). *Ordinary wisdom: Biographical aging and the journey of life.* Westport, CT: Praeger.

Ruth, J. E., & Oberg, P. (1996). Ways of life: Old age in a life history perspective. In J. Birren, G. Kenyon, J. E. Ruth, J. Schroots, & T. Svensson (Eds.), *Aging and biography: Explorations in adult development* (pp. 167–186). New York: Springer Publishing Company.

Shaw, M. (2001). Guided autobiography: Bridging stories and social change. In G. Kenyon, P. Clark, & B. de Vries (Eds.), *Narrative gerontology: Theory, research, and practice.* New York: Springer Publishing Company.

White, M. (1991). Deconstruction and therapy. *Dulwich Centre Newsletter, 3,* 2–40.

# CHAPTER THREE

# The Study of Lives in Progress: Approaches to Research on Life Stories

## Johannes J. F. Schroots and James E. Birren

There has been a remarkable growth of interest in autobiographies. The public seems enthusiastic about recording their life stories for family, friends, and themselves. Newspaper articles discuss personal accounts of individuals who have had diverse and interesting life experiences. Why there is such contemporary interest in autobiographies is itself an interesting question. Partly it may reflect that modern life has squeezed out opportunities to share the personal contents of our lives. While societies continue the practice of ceremonial burial of physical remains and the marking of graves, there are few, if any, archives for depositing and accessing the life stories of the deceased. This inaccessibility to life stories seems paradoxical in the information age. Indeed, life storytelling has become an evermore popular activity because people are seeking to exchange their life stories. This exchange is due to the lack of encouragement and opportunity in the contemporary institutions of daily life to tell and record the details of their lives—their growing up and their growing old.

Scholars from diverse disciplines have been attracted to autobiography because of the lure of its personal content. The science of the 19th and 20th centuries encouraged an objective, external approach to subject matter. Increasingly, scholars are recognizing that not only has the "inside view" of life—how life is experienced and interpreted by an individual—been neglected, but also that an understanding of this view is crucial to comprehending the human experience. In fact, the degree of correspondence between the self views of the life as lived and the views of outside observers is itself an area for research.

Numerous researchers from widely different backgrounds (e.g., social work, nursing, psychology, sociology, and the arts) are encouraging, gathering, and beginning to interpret autobiographies or narrative life stories. This increased multidisciplinary involvement offers the promise of a fertile period ahead in the exploration of life stories, although the boundaries of methods and interpretations in this domain are likely to be confusing and rapidly changing. This chapter begins with the assumption that gerontology is opening its doors to exploring the inside of the life experience. With the recognition that quantitative gerontology is limited in its ability to deal with questions of meaning, affect, self, and quality of life, particularly within the purview of the views of individuals, many scholars are attracted to techniques like autobiography. Also, the wide range of individual differences among older persons belies a singular, standardized, methodological approach.

Multiple forms of biographical materials, including self-reports, subjective or guided autobiographies, thematic interviews, personal documents including diaries and letters, and archival data have been used for the study of lives. These various types of biographical material present methodological problems with respect to the quantification of essentially unstructured, qualitative data, but they offer an alternative pathway to insight. This chapter describes two approaches to generating individual life stories—the Lifeline Interview Method and Guided Autobiography.

## *Lifeline Interview Method*

The authors and their colleagues developed an approach combining both qualitative and quantitative methods for eliciting (auto)biographical information, the Lifeline Interview Method, or LIM. In this section, we describe both qualitative and quantitative aspects of the LIM, but first we examine its origin in metaphor.

*Metaphors of Life.* The LIM has been developed on the basis of several studies of metaphors of aging and the individual life course (Schroots, 1991; Schroots, Birren, & Kenyon, 1991). In exploring the metaphorical basis of science, we concluded that metaphor seems to be the key to understanding both the methodological and creative aspects of scientific discovery and progress. Metaphor is an important way by which we create new meanings and make sense where previously there was little or none. Metaphor is a means of entering the unknown through the gateway of the known; it allows us to map what we know onto what we vaguely know and gives rise to new hypotheses and integration.

Taking the "mapping" function of metaphors almost literally, the question arises as to which metaphors are most useful for the study of lives. One of the oldest metaphors of life in human history is the "tree of life," situated in the center of the earthly paradise, a symbol of the immortality of humankind. The tree as metaphor of life hardly needs explanation; in the literature, one can find numerous analogies between the annual cycle of growing, budding, blooming, shedding leaves, and dying on the one hand, and the individual life cycle on the other hand (see, for example, Erickson's *The Life Cycle Completed*, 1982).

At the turn of the century, psychology discovered this botanical metaphor for the description of mental processes. Gesell (1928), for example, described child development in terms of plant growth, giving rise to "kindergarten," a protective learning environment to be tended by a gardener or teacher, hence the concept of kindergarten. Since that time, the tree metaphor has found many applications in psychology and other fields, including the "decision tree" in modern cognitive psychology, which represents, via a series of branching points, the potential and/or actual choices a person makes or might make to reach a decision. The branching points symbolize the events, experiences, and happenings that significantly affect the direction of individual lives.

Although the tree as a metaphor of life is very powerful, there is one serious flaw: the tree is basically a spatial metaphor that only vaguely suggests temporality (Lakoff & Johnson, 1980). Therefore, the "flowing river" may represent a more useful metaphor of life, because flowing movement suggests time as well as change. Waddington (1957) has given some scientific prestige to this spatio-temporal metaphor by introducing the concept of 'chreode' (from Greek: the pathway of desire or necessity) or 'canalized pathway of change'. This concept refers to the developmental trajectory of a living system as it crosses the metaphorical "epigenetic landscape."

When older persons are asked to describe their lives, they frequently use metaphors like the 'river' or 'footpath' (see also Vischer, 1961). The river symbolizes the stream of life, and the footpath stands for the journey one makes from birth to death, when one traverses the mountains and valleys of life. While both metaphors express the temporal dimension of experience, the "footpath" metaphor can also be used to express the important dimension of affect in people's lives. For example, when people say "I'm feeling up" or "I'm really low these days," they are using a spatial metaphor (i.e., hilly country) to express the positive and negative feelings they had in life.

*Description of Method.*   The metaphor of the footpath, representing the journey of life from birth to death, provides an appropriate framework for the LIM. The graphical, two-dimensional representation of a foot-path—with time on the horizontal axis and affect on the vertical axis—symbolizes the course of human life. In a typical LIM session, the interviewer first introduces the general plan of the session by saying that he/she is interested in the ups and downs of the human life course. It is pointed out that these are completely different from one person to another. The interviewer then solicits the interviewee's perceptions of his or her life visually in a temporal framework by drawing a lifeline representing the time from birth to present age in an LIM grid (Figure 1).

As soon as the lifeline has been drawn, the interviewee is asked to label each peak and each dip by chronological age and to then explain what happened at certain moments on the trajectory or during an indicated period. At the same time, the interviewer records a verbatim report of what the interviewee sees as the most important events in his or her life.

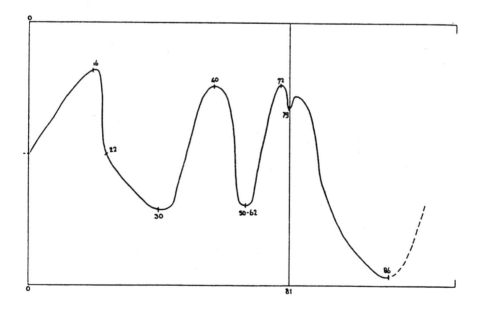

**FIGURE 1   LIM grid and lifeline of an 81-year-old woman.**

After the past has been visualized and described in detail, the future can be explored in the same manner. Starting from the point where the lifeline has stopped, the interviewee is asked to continue the line until the age of expected death is reached and to explain the anticipated future lifeline. Again, the interviewer records a verbatim report of what is said. The final result of the LIM session is a visual and verbal life history of the individual, including a visual and verbal representation of his or her expected future.

*Special Qualities.*  Central to development of the LIM was the idea that this method allowed a person to place perceptions of his or her life visually in a temporal framework. As has been shown in several studies (Schroots, 1984; Schroots & ten Kate, 1989), this turned out to be very important for several reasons. First, since most people (at least those from Western traditions) are familiar with the graphical representation of time by a straight line, they did not need much explanation or prompting before drawing their lifeline. However, most interviewees in our studies realized only after drawing the lifeline what they were revealing to the interviewer. Some of them even went so far as to try to 'correct' the original line. This is a positive sign of the LIM's ability to elicit (auto)biographical information at the cognitive-affective level of the behavioral organization of the individual's life. Another positive sign of the potential of this method to provide profound insight is that some persons become emotionally very upset because of the continual confrontation with their lifeline during the LIM process. Normally speaking, one can deny or just ignore what has been said a few minutes ago. Once the lifeline has been drawn, however, the sometimes-painful visualized 'truth' of an interviewee's life has been revealed on paper and is difficult to deny.

A second, special aspect of the LIM is its self-pacing quality. The lifeline is drawn and the life story is told at the person's own pace. The LIM allows each individual to set his or her own tempo, an advantage over standardized questionnaires. In addition, this nondirective atmosphere of the interview enhances disclosure of an individual's most sincere opinions, beliefs, and attitudes.

A final advantage of LIM is the quality of self-structuring. One of the unsolved problems with regard to the content analysis of open-interview transcripts concerns the meaningful categorization of unstructured interview data in such a way that they can be analyzed statistically. The flexibility of LIM enables the interviewee to categorize and structure the number of events, age at which the event occurred, and his or her affect at the time in a personally meaningful manner. This flexibility enhances validity by allowing the interviewee to represent his or her life as he or she sees it.

*Published Studies.*    The Dutch *Journal of Developmental Psychology* recently published the first results of empirical research on the LIM under the title: *LIM/Lifeline: A Comparative Study of Structure* (Schroots & Assink, 1998). Structural lifeline data on the LIM are reported for 33 men and 34 women, approximately equally divided among three age groups (young, middle-aged, and older adulthood). The LIM data are analyzed and compared with other published data, including the timeline approach to describing autobiographical memory (deVries & Watt, 1996); the life-drawing approach to elicit temporality (Whitbourne & Dannefer, 1985–1986), and the life-graph approach to capture typology (Back, 1982).

Generally, the distribution of life events on the LIM and timeline follows the same pattern. Individuals specified an average of 7.45 events (more affective-positive than affective-negative events), with the oldest group remembering a greater number of past events than the youngest group. The youngest group specified more affective-positive future events. Temporal dominance for LIM and the life-drawing approach varied across the life-span, from a dominance of present and future events in the youngest group to a greater dominance of past events among the oldest group. With regard to typology, the same four factors were extracted for LIM and for the life-graph approach—adolescence, early adulthood, late middle age, and old age. An additional factor, "experience," was extracted for the LIM only.

Content analysis provides the mechanism for examining lifeline or life-story data. Holsti (1968) defines content analysis as " . . . any technique for making inferences by systematically and objectively identifying specified characteristics of messages" (p. 601). Although widely used, Holsti's broad definition does not provide much guidance in selecting an appropriate technique for the qualitative analysis of LIM data. We suggest that analysis proceed in several steps. First, consistent with Kovach (1995), the unit of analysis must be identified. For LIM/Lifestory data, identification of the unit of analysis is rather simple: the life event is the basic unit of analysis. The second step, according to deVries and Watt (1996), consists of a thematic frequency analysis, that is, the life events are coded in terms of a limited number of life themes (e.g., school, career, or relationships), after which the relative frequencies (percentages) of the events per theme are determined. This type of content analysis generates a quantitative thematic description of the

LIM/Lifestory, which might be compared with the time line description (deVries & Watt, 1996; Assink & Schroots, 2000).

*Gerodynamics.*   As mentioned before, the LIM has been developed essentially on the basis of metaphors of life, particularly the tree, river, and footpath metaphors. Most metaphors of life have a basic pattern in common, the branching or bifurcation point. Such branching points, turning points, transitions or transformations may be defined as those changes in the life of the individual that direct the life path in a distinctive direction, and that are separated in time from each other by one or more affective or critical events or experiences (Birren & Deutchman, 1991). Thus defined, the LIM/Lifeline may be conceived of as a series of branching points from birth to death. The structure and content (LIM/Lifestory) of these changes can be analyzed at the more advanced level of gerodynamics, and branching theory (Schroots, 1995, 1996; Schroots & Birren, 1988; Schroots & Yates, 1999).

The notion of gerodynamics is based on general systems theory, notably the Second Law of Thermodynamics, and dynamic systems theory (chaos theory). The Second Law states that there is an increase of entropy or disorder with age in living systems, resulting in the system's death. Chaos theory postulates that internal or external fluctuations of dynamic, far-from-equilibrium systems can pass a critical point and create order out of disorder through a process of self-organization, that is, a process by which a structure or pattern of change emerges with the passage of time. From this metatheoretical viewpoint, the aging of living systems can be conceived as a nonlinear series of transformations into higher- and/or lower-order structures or processes, showing a progressive trend toward more disorder than order over the lifespan, and eventually resulting in the system's death.

Gerodynamics forms the basis of branching theory. The core of gerondynamics is the bifurcation or branching behavior of the individual at the biological, psychological, or social level of functioning. Metaphorically speaking, bifurcation means that the fluctuating individual passes a critical point—the bifurcation, branching, or transformation point—and can branch off into higher- and/or lower-order structures or processes. Higher- and lower-order structures can be translated in terms of mortality (probability of dying, life expectancy), morbidity (disease, disorder, disability, or dysfunction), and quality of life (well-being, life satisfaction). For example, traumatic life events and a healthy lifestyle may result in lower and higher order structures, respectively, and consequently in higher and lower probabilities of dying. It should be noted that lower-order bifurcations at the biological or psychological level of functioning (e.g., illness or divorce) do not always result in lower-order behavior (i.e., some people are strengthened by illness, and divorce may have a positive, rather than a negative, effect on mental health in terms of life expectancy and quality of life). An advanced-branching analysis of the LIM/Lifeline and life story needs to incorporate acknowledgement of this dynamic phenomenon. However, given the complexity of lifeline and life-story data, it remains to be seen how current research will lend support to the proposed branching analysis of individual lifelines utilizing this gerodynamic perspective.

## Guided Autobiography

The method of Guided Autobiography (GAB) began about 25 years ago as an outgrowth of psychology-of-aging graduate student seminars (see Birren & Deutchman, 1991). Graduate students prepared papers on the emergence of autobiography during the Renaissance and its growth during the rise of individualism as many physical threats to life diminished. During these 25 years, there has been a growth of interest in GAB that has encouraged research and scholarship on autobiography (Birren & Hedlund, 1987; Birren & Deutchman, 1991; Birren, Kenyon, Ruth, Schroots, & Svensson, 1996). Not only does GAB help individuals to organize and tell the stories of their lives, it offers an approach to accessing information on aging distinct from quantitative studies of mental abilities, personality, social roles, health, and physical capacities. Instead, GAB enables researchers to obtain information from individuals about the inside views of their lives. Also, GAB allows participants to relate their life stories in a group setting, potentially enriching recall by the priming provided by the life stories of others. The method not only provides a new source of information for scholars, it also appears to have a therapeutic effect. While not originally designed or intended to be therapeutic, it appears that involvement with the method often results in more positive attitudes toward life.

Since the initiation of the GAB approach, about 500 autobiographies have been gathered and placed on computer disks for later analysis. Only participants who are willing to have their life stories used for research purposes are included in the data archive. Interested participants sign human-subject agreements, and the information collected is stored anonymously with only demographic data attached to the narrative text.

*Description of Method.*   Typically, GAB groups meet once a week for 2 to 2.5 hours per session. Each session has three components: a) an introduction to the life theme of the week by the program leader, b) a sensitizing and memory-priming period of about 30 minutes in which the leader reviews the theme that participants will be writing about during the week, and c) small group sessions of five to six participants in which prepared, written pages are read to the group and participants provide their comments. Guided Autobiography involves a 10-session sequence. The usual topical sequence of the themes for the 10 weeks is:

1. The major branching points in my life
2. My family history
3. My major life's work or career
4. The history of my health and body
5. The role of money in my life
6. The history of loves and hates in my life
7. The history of my gender roles and identity
8. My experiences with death
9. The history of my aspirations and goals
10. The future and next steps

The use of memory-priming questions about major life themes in the groups tends to elicit many previously forgotten events. The group dynamic has a strong influence on prompting recall as the participants hear other persons recall events. The "Oh, yes, I remember something like that now," is a regular occurrence as participants share their recollections. The use of major life themes and questions elicits recollections of events that shaped a childhood, life in a particular household, or the spirit of community during particular eras. Participants are told not to approach the questions as something to be answered literally, but to determine if they prompt useful or interesting associations. They are told to ignore questions that seem unproductive or provoke no associations.

*Uses of the Method.*   There are many reasons for preparing one's autobiography, including the desire to publish a book, to bolster a sense of self, or to contribute to the history of an organization, community, or profession. Autobiography also is instrumental in allowing researchers and scholars a window on the inside of life not accessible through other methods. An external event may be described by other persons (e.g., an accident, birth, wedding, or death), but the event is subject to wide differences in interpretation and feelings by individuals. For example, individuals vary in their feelings about the significance and meaning of their health and illnesses. With similar physical conditions, they may regard themselves as either frail or hearty. How individuals experience and interpret their lives is most directly accessed through their own statements.

*Questions to Be Answered.* Many scholars have proposed schemes or theories for explaining the flow of lives. Appropriately, such theories are concerned with scientific generalizations or developmental theory about how most people grow up and grow old, rather than the examination of individual uniqueness or exception. Often, developmental theory involves the concept of stages through which individuals pass. Guided autobiography, on the other hand, does not require the use of stages. Rather, GAB may be used to explore the possibility of stages and the extent of their distribution in populations or to elicit unique interpretations of lives.

## Future Perspective and Unanswered Questions

The growth of interest in narrative information does not diminish the importance of research on aging from an objective or outside perspective. Exploring the inside of life—our personal feelings and views—supplements what we have learned from insights obtained in the more traditional mode of externally produced data. One may easily forecast that large-scale, longitudinal studies will obtain more information from the "inside" perspective of individuals, thus providing answers to a growing number of important questions about growing up and growing old.

While understanding how our internal view of life may influence our health, disabilities, activity level, and productivity is relatively untapped, it is reasonable to project that major research studies of aging in the future will include autobiographical information as a complement to externally gathered information. The way health is viewed subjectively may influence health outcomes as they are measured objectively. The way we view life and our values may, over time, affect our network of relationships that are important to the maintenance of well being in the later years.

Further exploration of the way life is experienced and viewed from the inside is warranted for practical, applied reasons, as well as for enhancing scholarship. Quality of life can be increased by improving health and extending active years, but it may also be improved by learning what older people seek and facilitating opportunities for them to meet their needs and aspirations (Burnside & Schmidt, 1994). Rachelle Dorfman (1994) explored the aspirations and values of older persons living in a continuing-care retirement community by talking to the residents, as well as living with them. It is almost startling to see her use of the word "aspirations" in the context of aging. Part of the stereotype of old age may be that aspirations and goals are no longer part of life, as though there was an implicit assumption that "You have lived your life, what more do you want or expect?" In addition, much of gerontology has focused on obtaining objective data that has squeezed out the subjective. She concluded her work by noting that

> Models of care will have to be developed that are flexible enough to insure that every elderly person cannot merely live, but live well—in a way that is in harmony with his or her own unique set of aspirations and values. . . . The elderly—like adults of any age—are equally responsible for the quality of their own lives. However, in order for the aged to assume that responsibility, the resources must be available to help them discover what is right for them and fulfill those aims (Dorfman, 1994, p. 173).

Knowing more about inside views of life may provide clues to help extend healthy life expectancy and may raise the quality of those additional years. Thus, the legitimacy of encouraging explorations of aspirations and the inner view of life, including the spiritual (McFadden, 1996), rests not solely on supplementing objective information, but is, in its own right, a very significant area of study.

The next steps in exploring the personal perceptions of life require the development of new topical foci and new methods of gathering and interpreting narrative material. Such methods include the study of narrative documents. One of the more tantalizing topical foci concerns how secular drift and epoch influence an individual's interpretations of life. It is impossible to reach back into earlier historical periods to assess such drifts since standard personal autobiographical documents are generally not available. However, for persons now living, one may begin to assay the carry-forward effects of past events in their lives (for example, the student revolts of the 1970s) on their current perceptions of life and their attribution of the importance of such events. The individual and cohort effects of major events, such as war, famine, natural disasters, and economic recessions, on views of life are a fertile area for longitudinal studies. Other questions amenable to rich narrative approaches include: How are men's and women's interpretations and perspectives on life similar and different? How do individuals attempt, over the course of their lives, to adapt to transitions and changes in occupation, economic and health status, family situation, and personal relationships? How do immigrants adapt and adjust to residence in a new country?

Autobiographies gathered by LIM and GAB may be used to gather longitudinal data over the lifespan. For example, the tensions of adolescence might be examined in an autobiography. Teen-aged tensions and ways of managing such tensions might be contrasted with transitional difficulties of persons in different decades of life. The general issue is that of clarifying the major transitions in life and the ways in which people manage themselves and adapt to change.

It may be useful to utilize both before and after GABs, since GAB itself appears to result in a reorganization of attitudes and feelings about life events and persons. This is not unlike the expectation that growing up changes the ways we view our adolescence, parents, and siblings. Aspects of memory and cognition may remain fixed, but our feelings about someone and some event can shift from negative to positive and humorous as we mature. Thus, the resented teacher may, in later life, come to be respected, and the disliked brother may become an intimate confidant, although the events that made such persons disliked may remain characterized in terms similar to those used in the past (e.g., she made me step out of the classroom and he always broke my toys).

Each day brings about change as an accompaniment of new experience. The measurement of such change has not been simple or easy. In particular, the changes purportedly brought about by psychotherapy have been elusive to pin down even after many years of attempting to change behavior (Kopata, Lueger, Saunders, & Howard, 1999). "We now know that psychotherapy is generally effective but we are uncertain as to why" (p. 461). The fact that such a statement can be made by senior persons in their field implies that the sources of change, the processes of change, and even the outcomes of change are not at all clear. In this context, the use of the LIM and autobiography may have value if used before and after psychotherapy or other change processes. They may help to describe the individual's views of the structure of his or her life and provide the bases for the measurement of the areas and magnitude of change attributable to development, aging, psychotherapy, or other suspected influences.

## Autobiography, Science, and Applications

There are at least two purposes in exploring life stories—to advance our knowledge and to improve lives. Using autobiographies for scientific advancement raises numerous important questions. How closely does our recall of early life events resemble the contemporary recordings of the same events and their context? Are the emotions and feelings about an event recalled with the same level of verity as the recall of the cognitive or concrete details about an event, such as its place, persons, time, and sequence? Can individuals report with some degree of verifiable reliability their feelings of an event at the time of occurrence and also their present and perhaps modified feelings (i.e., "answering the question how I felt about it then and now")?

Finally, what are the possible implications of the relative arbitrariness, if not purposeful distortion, of the recall and personal interpretation of events when reconstructing the past? These implications relate, among other things, to the training given to professionals and others engaged in eliciting life stories. At an extreme level, there is the issue of the extent to which one should encourage the deliberate reconstruction of events in the service of an acceptable, optimistic, or hedonistic outlook. The concept of life stories to some extent suggests arbitrariness in the way we express the basic plots of our lives. Stories in literature are written to serve the author and are designed to capture the attention of the reader. Randall (1995) has described lives in terms of the stories that people tell about themselves that are continually being revised.

For researchers, concern about verity may lead to a need for corroboration through the eyes of different participants, such as siblings, parents, and other persons who shared the same events. Growing out of this context is the question of the extent to which there are individual differences in the need to "tell it like it was" in contrast to telling it the way "it feels good" in the present. Future applications of autobiographies should explore the value of different ways of restructuring the stories of our lives.

The current wave of interest in life stories will result in a proliferation of insights, some of which will result from parallel and complementary research studies (e.g., Coleman, 1986). Further research should produce more knowledge and insight into patterns of growing up and growing old and individual differences in the experience of life and its interpretation that are differentiated by the diversity so characteristic in the older population (Runyan, 1984). Such knowledge should facilitate assisting individuals to maintain sound mental health, despite the rapidly changing employment, economic and social environments that complicate the aging experience.

Knowledge gained through the study of narrative material not only has potential for practical uses, but it can expand our understanding of the organization of behavior. The study of individuality, for example, is often neglected in favor of central tendencies (Tyler, 1978). Each person is a collection of unique experiences, contradictions in values, with some traits only minimally expressed and others not at all. Perhaps it is in the life stories of individuals that human uniqueness is most clearly expressed and may be most fruitfully studied.

## REFERENCES

Assink, M. H. J., & Schroots, J. J. F. (2000, June). *Life-line interview method: Signature of the self.* Poster presented at First International Conference on "The Dialogical Self." Nijmegen, The Netherlands.

Back, K. W. (1982). Types of life course and gerontology. *Academic Psychology Bulletin, 4,* 9–16.

Birren, J. E., & Deutchman, D. (1991). *Guiding autobiography groups for older adults: Exploring the fabric of life.* Baltimore: Johns Hopkins University Press.

Birren, J. E., & Feldman, L. (1987). *Where to go from here.* New York: Simon & Schuster.

Birren, J. E., & Hedlund, B. (1987). Contributions of autobiography to developmental psychology. In N. Eisenberg (Ed.), *Contemporary topics in developmental psychology* (pp. 394–415). New York: John Wiley.

Birren, J. E., Kenyon, G. M., Ruth, J-E., Schroots, J. J. F., & Svensson, T. (Eds.). (1996). *Aging and biography: Explorations in adult development.* New York: Springer Publishing Company.

Burnside, I., & Schmidt, M. G. (Eds.). (1994). *Working with older adults: Group process and techniques.* Boston: Jones & Bartlett.

Coleman, P. G. (1986). *Aging and reminiscence processes: Social and clinical implications.* New York: John Wiley.

deVries, B., & Watt, D. (1996). A lifetime of events: Age and gender variations in the life story. *International Journal of Aging and Human Development, 42,* 81–102.

Dorfman, R. A. (1994). *Aging into the 21st century: The exploration of aspirations and values.* New York: Brunner/Mazel.

Erickson, E. H. (1982). *The life cycle completed.* New York: Norton.

Gesell, A. (1928). *Infancy and human growth.* New York: Macmillan.

Holsti, O. R. (1968). Content analysis. In G. Lindsey & E. Aronson (Eds.), *The handbook of social psychology.* London: Addison-Wesley.

Kopata, S. M., Lueger, R. J., Saunders, S. M., & Howard, K. I. (1999). Individual psychotherapy outcome and process research: Challenges to greater turmoil or a positive transition? *Annual Review of Psychology, 50,* 441–469.

Kovach, C. R. (1995). A qualitative look at reminiscing: Using the autobiographical memory coding tool. In B. K. Haight & J. D. Webster (Eds.), *The art and science of reminiscing: Theory, research, methods, and applications* (pp. 103–122). Washington, DC: Taylor & Francis.

Lakoff, G., & Johnson, M. (1980). *Metaphors we live by.* Chicago: The University of Chicago Press.

McFadden, S. H. (1996). Religion, spirituality, and aging. In J. E. Birren & K. W. Schaie (Eds.), *Handbook of the psychology of aging* (pp. 162–177). San Diego, CA: Academic Press.

Randall, W. L. (1995). *The stories we are: An essay on self-creation.* Toronto, Canada: University of Toronto Press.

Runyan, W. M. (1984). *Life histories and psychobiography: Explorations in theory and method.* New York: Oxford University Press.

Schroots, J. J. F. (1984). The affective consequences of technological change for older persons. In P. K. Robinson, J. Livingston, & J. E. Birren (Eds.), *Aging and technological advances* (pp. 237–247). New York: Plenum Press.

Schroots, J. J. F. (1991). Metaphors of aging and complexity. In G. M. Kenyon, J. E. Birren, & J. J. F. Schroots (Eds.), *Metaphors of aging in science and the humanities* (pp. 219–243). New York: Springer Publishing Company.

Schroots, J. J. F. (1995). Gerodynamics: Toward a branching theory of aging. *Canadian Journal on Aging, 14,* 74–81.

Schroots, J. J. F. (1996). Theoretical developments in the psychology of aging. *The Gerontologist, 36,* 742–748.

Schroots, J. J. F., & Assink, M. (1998). LIM/Levenslijn: een vergelijkend structuuronderzoek (LIM/Life-line: a comparative analysis of structure). *Tijdschrift voor Ontwikkelingspsychologie, 24,* 1–23.

Schroots, J. J. F., & Birren, J. E. (1988). The nature of time: Implications for research on aging. *Comprehensive Gerontology C, 2,* 1–29.

Schroots, J. J. F., & ten Kate, C. A. (1989). Metaphors, aging and the Life-line Interview Method. In D. Unruh & G. Livings (Eds.), *Current perspectives on aging and the life cycle. Vol. 3: Personal history through the life course* (pp. 281–298). London: JAI Press.

Schroots, J. J. F., & Yates, F. E. (1999). On the dynamics of development and aging. In V. L. Bengtson & K. W. Schaie (Eds.), *Handbook of theories of aging* (pp. 417–433). New York: Springer Publishing Company.

Schroots, J. J. F., Birren, J. E., & Kenyon, G. M. (1991). Metaphors and aging: An overview. In G. M. Kenyon, J. E. Birren, & J. J. F. Schroots (Eds.), *Metaphors of aging in science and the humanities* (pp. 1–16). New York: Springer Publishing Company.

Tyler, L. E. (1978). *Individuality: Human possibilities and personal choice in the psychological development of men and women.* San Francisco: Jossey-Bass.

Vischer, A. L. (1961). *Seelische Wandlungen beim alternden Menschen.* Bazel/Stuttgart, Germany: Benno Schwabe.

Waddington, C. H. (1957). *The strategy of the genes.* London: Allen and Unwin.

Whitbourne, S. K., & Dannefer, W. D. (1985–1986). The "Life drawing" as a measure of time perspective in adulthood. *International Journal of Aging and Human Development, 22,* 147–155.

White, R. W. (Ed.). (1966). *The study of lives.* New York: Atherton.

# PART III

# Being There

# Introduction

## Sharon R. Kaufman

Ethnographers specialize in taking the "emic" or insider's view of a culture or social group, examining individuals' perspectives, experiences, and practices. They study small populations, observing and talking with people at length and in depth to discover the principles, events, and concepts that explain a given situation or process. With this ethnographic approach, the group or sample under investigation may not be widely representative, in a statistical sense, of a larger population, but the investigator is able to gain a deeper knowledge of meanings and practices in that group. This type of research does not test hypotheses nor does it present a causal model. Rather, the focus of ethnographic investigations is whether an object of study is exemplary of broader cultural processes and actual practices. Findings come not through explicit statements about specific, discrete variables, taken out of their context, but rather through concrete descriptions of everyday life and ordinary practices.

Ethnographic fieldwork is the process in which data is collected and through which a social world—of actors, actions, and moral positions—is understood. Because it is both a method and an analytic/interpretive perspective, it differs from other methodologies used in the social and behavioral sciences. It is the traditional technique of anthropology and distinguishes the anthropological approach to social analysis from that of other disciplines. Fieldwork is labor intensive. It is grounded in attention to the everyday and the ordinary, and its goal is an intimate knowledge of a community or group (Marcus, 1995). It usually involves full-time or extensive involvement over a long period of time with the group, individuals, or institutions being studied. Data are collected primarily in the form of field notes and are usually a mixture of diaries, observational notes, descriptions of settings and persons, theoretical and methodological musings, interviews and reflections on them, and explorations of what various things mean, both to the "natives" in the setting and to the ethnographer. Field notes may be supplemented by other data-gathering techniques, such as surveys, census data, and questionnaires. There is no single way to collect ethnographic data, no prescribed script or technique about how much or what is necessary and important.

Accident and serendipity shape the fieldwork experience and enterprise as much as planning. When one enters a particular setting to begin observations or after some time spent in a social world, certain events, processes, people, or questions emerge as more interesting than others; certain features of the fieldwork experience seem more central to the social problem that engages the ethnographer. Thus, the ethnographer must choose how to spend his or her time and which issues are worthy of detailed focus. One cannot know ahead of time which cultural logics or formations will emerge as interesting or which associations and connections should be pursued until one immerses oneself in a particular cultural milieu. (When I began fieldwork in an acute care hospital to study how death occurs there, I did not know that I would be spending about half my time observing activities in the intensive care unit. But after participating in the daily routine on many hospital wards, it became apparent to me that the dilemmas about prolonging life and the cultural conversation about the problem of death were most evident in that particular setting.) In addition, the ethnographer may leave the initial field site entirely to follow ideas or cultural patterns that emerged as important in one site, but that are located also in other arenas. (In my study, for example, I also pay attention to public debates represented in the news media and to grassroots organizations and movements that are responding to "the problem" of death. Paying attention to those debates and newer cultural forms takes me out of the hospital setting and into a more diffuse cultural world of end-of-life concerns, thus enriching the overall study.)

Ethnography joins the practice of fieldwork with the representation of a particular cultural world through written texts (Van Maanen, 1988). Many anthropologists have turned to the idea that "culture" is written, not factually portrayed. That consciousness raises its own set of problematics about the "science" of anthropology and the portrayal of social life. Ethnographies, the written reports, stories, and interpretations of what was observed and what happened in the field, are not the "truth" of a particular locale or process in any scientific or positivistic sense. Rather, they are representations of cultural formations, interpreted and filtered through the subjective and personal experiences of the ethnographer. Ethnographies are thus "partial truths" (Clifford & Mar-

cus, 1986), conceptually shaped and physically organized by the experience of the fieldworker and by the goals of the project.

Clifford Geertz has examined the tasks of 'knowing,' truth-making,
and representing the cultural Other and summarized the central tension
in contemporary anthropology created by the turn from fact-finding to
interpretation, from assuming some kind of 'objectivity' is possible to
articulating the impact of literary processes on the understanding of
cultural phenomena. Geertz notes the difficulty of "constructing texts
ostensibly scientific out of experiences broadly "biographical" (Geertz,
1988, p. 10): ethnography is a record of "being there" that aims both
to establish authority about the way things are and to acknowledge the
subjective terrain of the ethnographic encounter.

Ethnographies are also politically mediated and motivated. Feminist
scholars and anthropologists who have engaged the postcolonial experience stress in their writings that the ethnographer is always situated in
a relationship of power to the group being studied. Those relationships
influence the construction of ethnographic writing and the portrayal
of a group of people. The identity, ethnicity, age, and self-understand-
ings of the ethnographer also are brought to bear on fieldwork sites
and situations and play an important role in shaping how cultural worlds
and processes are seen by the ethnographer and revealed to various
audiences. Thus, the practice of ethnography is not a straightforward
matter. Cultural worlds and lives are experienced by a situated and
motivated ethnographer who decides what information to portray and
what to ignore, what to emphasize as important and what to de-empha-
size, which writing styles and conventions to employ, and where to
locate and how to express meaning. The term employed in recent years,
"experimental ethnography," refers to the heightened awareness of
these issues as anthropologists struggle to break away from historical
conventions of portraying culture as a static and bounded artifact, while
at the same time retaining certain concepts and approaches from the
ethnographic tradition.

## Narrative

Contemporary interest in narrative in fields outside of the traditional
humanities, for example, cultural anthropology and medicine, is a product of the "interpretive turn" in the social sciences and in trends in
intellectual reformulation more generally since the late 1960s and 1970s
(Rabinow & Sullivan, 1979). The various uses of narrative in ethnographic writing—and here I use the term in a restricted, yet well-recog-

nized sense: accounts from informants that portray their subjective experience, including a sense of intention, explanation, and emotion— are methodological and textual strategies employed by authors to grapple with how best to represent the cultural Other. The uses of narrative in the social sciences have been subjected to a great deal of scrutiny in recent years as many anthropologists attempt to deal in their writings with the pull between the kinds of truth represented by the idea of science on the one hand and by literature and the humanities on the other. Thus, there are many works that experiment with the portrayal of informants' voices and with authorial presence and that use narrative theory from philosophy, linguistics, history, and psychology to frame interpretive schemes.

In the great surge of experimental writing in anthropology (Clifford & Marcus, 1986; Marcus & Fischer, 1986), narrative forms of first-person accounts have sought to give voice to persons or communities who are low-status within a particular social world and system: the poor, the chronically or terminally ill, the elderly, and the disenfranchised. Narrative has been used to address questions of human agency, to explore the feelings, thoughts, and intentions of social actors. Narrative has been viewed as a useful expansive tool by scholars wishing to articulate, from details of the native's point of view, how individuals construct meaning and negotiate their worlds. Critics of the narrative approach suggest that it encourages blind spots in its reliance both on the experience of the ethnographer and the experiences of those persons whom it seeks to illuminate. Advocates of narrative in the social sciences argue that it captures and constitutes both lived morality and experience and the dynamics of social practice and convention, thus revealing an open, richer field of cultural understanding than allowed by objectivist perspectives. In medical anthropology and sociology specifically, the by-now large literature on illness and clinical narratives offers multiple ways to think about relationships among illness, medicine, culture, and experience. Narrative conceptualizations and representations of aging, illness, and dying, for example, provide a way to explore the multiple meanings, truths, and voices that are expressed during life-course transitions and liminal moments.

## REFERENCES

Clifford, J., & Marcus, G. E. (1986). *Writing culture.* Berkeley, CA: University of California Press.

Geertz, C. (1988). *Works and lives: The anthropologist as author.* Stanford, CT: Stanford University Press.

Marcus, G. E. (1995). Ethnography in/of the world system: The emergence of multi-sited ethnography. *Annual Reviews of Anthropology, 24,* 95–117.

Marcus, G. E., & Fischer, M. M. J. (1986). *Anthropology as cultural critique.* Chicago: University of Chicago Press.

Rabinow, P., & Sullivan, W. M. (1979). *Interpretive social science.* Berkeley, CA: University of California Press.

Van Maanen, J. (1988). *Tales of the field: On writing: ethnography.* Chicago: University of Chicago Press.

# CHAPTER FOUR

# Ethnography of the Particular: The Individual Case and the Culture of Death in America

## Sharon R. Kaufman

"In presenting culture as a subject for analysis and critique, the ethnographic perspective develops an interplay between making the familiar strange and the strange familiar. Home cultures can appear so normal to their members that their common sense seems to be based in universal human nature. Social descriptions by, of, and for members of a particular culture require a relative emphasis on defamiliarization, so they will appear—as they in fact are—humanly made, and not given in nature."

Renato Rosaldo, *Culture and Truth* (1989)

More than 50% of persons in the United States over age 65 die in acute care hospitals, and a frequent institutional response to the end of life is to forestall death with the most sophisticated technological means available (Institute of Medicine, 1997; The SUP-PORT Principal Investigators, 1995). Because of this phenomenon, a great many adult Americans have personally experienced—as patient, family member, friend, or health care provider—the "problem" of hospital deaths, that is, the seemingly insoluble tension between the desire for extending life by technological means and the value of allowing death to occur "naturally" or "with dignity," without artificial prolongation. The problem of death in the United States is now widely acknowledged both within and outside of medicine.

The conceptual goal of this chapter is to juxtapose the abstract and diffuse cultural conversation about "death with dignity" and "control over dying" against the unfolding of particular hospital practices in one instance to illustrate: first, the tensions, ambiguities, and care trajectories that are produced in the contemporary hospital setting; and second, how particular practices surrounding an individual case fuel the cultural need to solve the "problem of death." A case study written from an ethnographic perspective describes ordinary hospital activities and on-the-ground knowledge about those activities to illustrate the embeddedness of individual players and decisions within structural imperatives and how some "normal," although not desired, deaths occur. The in-depth story of one hospital-dying trajectory shows that the practice of dying is, in many cases, much more muddled than the cultural conversation claims. This particular story of a hospital death, while idiosyncratic in its precise details, is, I suggest, a cultural document. Readers, especially those who have experience with dying hospital patients, will be familiar with the interplay of institutional forces and individual sensibilities, the conflicts that arise, and the shape of the story.

The methodological goal is to employ an exemplar case study in order to problematize hospital practices that surround dying, to emphasize their strangeness despite their familiarity so that they are no longer perceived as "natural" or inevitable. Highlighting details of hospital practice and quandaries that emerge as the story unfolds enables the reader to question the seemingly inevitable, to ponder what is given in the world of the contemporary American hospital. The chapter is organized so that the case study appears between two cultural frames. First, I offer a brief discussion of the health care context and background that both defines the problem and provides and channels choices of action and means of understanding for all actors in the hospital setting. After the case study, I present a discussion of particular institutional forces at work that shape the practice of death in the hospital. My move from context (macro) to specific story (micro) to structural situation (macro) is deliberate. Tacking from cultural problem and background to detailed incident and then back again to broader issues of structure and power relations within the institution, we can critically examine the multiple ways in which individual choices are embedded in and produced by institutional and structural forces. This method allows for a broader and more grounded understanding of how work is conducted, rules are enacted, and expectations are defined as death is approached or staved off in U.S. hospitals at the end of the 20th century.

## The Ethnographic Study and Theoretical Framework

Data, story, and analysis reported here are part of a larger anthropological investigation of how dying and death are approached and understood by health professionals, patients, and families, and how dying and death occurs among older adults in one community hospital. The study is based on the collection of data by participant observation on the adult wards in one midsize acute care hospital and by conversations and interviews with physicians, nurses, social workers, chaplains, patients, and family members. Over a 12-month period, I observed the course of events surrounding hospitalization and death for 80 individuals aged 50 and older. Thirty-one of the 80 individuals I observed died in the intensive care unit (ICU). The case study presented here is selected from those cases. Based on statistics available from the medical records department of the hospital, 370 people aged 50 and older died during the year of my observations, one third of them in the ICU. In all, I observed activities surrounding about 20% of hospital deaths for older adults over a 1-year period.

This project is grounded in theory from medical anthropology, which suggests first, that medical practice is a social enterprise, rooted in and influenced by cultural knowledge and activities (Lindenbaum & Lock, 1993; Lock & Gordon, 1988), and second, that medicine's power both responds to and affects the older person through its construction of various meanings of "old age" and "dying" (Kaufman, 1994). For example, the "biomedicalization of aging" (Estes & Binney, 1989), the most recent characterization of medicine's power to define aging, is thought to result from, first, the dominance of scientific models for understanding the life course, and second, the use of proliferating biomedical technologies both for solving the problems of disease associated with advanced age and for staving off death in late life. Medicine, as institution, system of knowledge, and practice, has become a dominant framework for knowing and confronting the lifecourse of the elderly in the industrialized world (Cole, 1992; Hurwicz, 1995).

In its varied clinical and research activities, medicine is producing a discourse of senescence (Katz, 1996), that is, a way in which we, members of industrialized society, form understandings about medical progress and the uses of biomedical science, approach decline, frailty, terminal illness, and finitude, and value a range of dying practices. This discourse includes (among others) the following features relevant for my discussion: a) Progress, as an enduring feature of modern medicine, is enabled by science and manifest in technology, b) Social value is placed on the scientific search for extending the lifespan and prolonging or enhancing the biological attributes of youth, c) Death does not occur until and unless life-prolonging strategies are deliberately abandoned or rejected, and d) All persons have both a right to life-extending technologies regardless of cost and a right to manage their own deaths. The discourse of senescence is full of contradiction and controversy. Its impact on both understanding and dealing with the end of life is almost entirely unexplored in the field of gerontology.

## The Health Care Context: Defining a Problem

The largest and most recent study ever conducted on the process of dying in the hospital was carried out in five university hospitals across the United States over a 4-year period beginning in 1989 (The SUPPORT Principal Investigators, 1995). In the first 2-year phase of the project, 4,300 patients (median age, 65 years) diagnosed with life-threatening illnesses were enrolled in order to understand the character and quality of dying in the hospital. The SUPPORT investigators concluded that the dying process in the hospital was not satisfactory for patients or their families. For example, only 47% of physicians knew when their patients wanted to avoid cardio-pulmonary resuscitation (CPR); 38% of patients who died spent 10 or more days in an ICU preceding death; 46% of "Do Not Resuscitate" (DNR) orders were written within 2 days of death even though 79% of the patients had a DNR order; and for 50% of the conscious patients, families reported moderate-to-severe pain at least half the time in the 3 days preceding death. A second 2-year intervention phase involving approximately 5,000 different patients (about half in a control group, half in an intervention group) was intended to affect positively the perceived quality of hospital deaths by enhancing the flow of information between doctors and patients. The startling results were that interventions aimed at improving physician-patient communication and physician knowledge of prognoses and patients' end-of-life wishes did not change the practice of medicine regarding the use of ICU treatments, timing of DNR orders, avoidance of CPR, or provision of pain relief, nor did those interventions alter the quality of patient and family experience (The SUPPORT Principal Investigators, 1995; Moskowitz & Nelson, 1995). Even when a focused and concerted effort was made to reduce pain and to respect patient wishes regarding end-of-life care, no overall improvement in care or outcomes was made. Some observers have noted that the culture of the hospital—characterized by its press toward life-saving or life-prolonging action with the best technology available—is so powerful and compelling that it cannot allow for the wishes and voices of individual patients to be expressed (Lo, 1995).

In the years preceding that publication of the SUPPORT Study results and in the years since then, discussion about the problem of death in the United States has grown and now manifests itself in many institutions and arenas, including the U.S. Supreme Court's consideration of physician-assisted suicide in 1997; ballot initiatives in California, Oregon, and Washington to legalize euthanasia; newspaper editorials on the difficulty of dying without unwanted medical intervention; hospital ethics-committee deliberations; articles in medical, nursing, and bioethics journals and the popular press discussing end-of-life controversies; a comprehensive Institute of Medicine report on improving care for dying persons (1997); the emergence of private philanthropic foundation support for programs to change the ways in which death occurs; new medical school curricula to sensitize students to the inevitability and naturalness of death; and community movements and organizations whose goals include improved "comfort care" and control of the means, timing, and location of death. The cultural conversation about what is wrong with death in the United States and how it can be made better is now exceptionally widespread.

## The Cultural Background: Making Modern Death by Staving It Off

*No Dying Passage.*   An essential feature of the contemporary problem of death is a lack of clarity, among health professionals, patients, and families alike, about when dying begins. For all its diagnostic acumen at the end of the 20th century, medicine, as a system of knowledge and clinical practice, is seemingly unable to consider first, whether a particular medical crisis is the last one for an individual regardless of chronological age or extent of disease (Callahan, 1993), and second, whether a person is dying (Muller & Koenig, 1988; The SUPPORT Principal Investigators, 1995). Related to this is the claim that physicians are neither expert at predicting when patients are terminally ill nor when death will occur (Lo, Snyder, & Sox, 1999; Lynn, Teno, & Harrell, 1995). One common result of not knowing and not acknowledging when dying begins and not knowing when death is likely to occur is adherence to curative and restorative treatment regimens, sometimes almost to the moment of death (Stolberg, 1998; The SUPPORT Principal Investigators, 1995). Moreover, medicine generally does not allow a transition, a process, a passage between life and death except in the most perfunctory way. This is especially evident when biomedical technologies are being employed (Chambliss, 1996; Zussman, 1992). Thus, medicine's ideology cannot account for what that process might look like and what its range of variation is likely to be, and its practice cannot consider new forms of action appropriate to a "time for dying" (Glaser & Strauss, 1968).

*The Technological Imperative.* As medicine has become the dominant framework for understanding what to think about illness and old age and how to act as the end of life approaches, responsibility in medicine has been conceived through action, through continued treatment to the point of cure, stability of the condition, or death of the patient. That stance is held not only by health care practitioners, but it is widely shared by the public. As more technological and clinical innovations become available, there is more that can be done to postpone death. The technological imperative (Fuchs, 1974) in medicine—to order additional diagnostic tests, to perform procedures, to intervene with ventilators, medications, and surgery in order to prolong life or stave off death whenever there is an opportunity to do so—is the most important variable in contemporary medical practice. The notion of palliative care is gaining support and acceptance among health care practitioners and the public (Campbell & Frank, 1997; Institute of Medicine, 1997; Lo et al., 1999), but the press to control and conquer end-stage disease still strongly influences medical thought and action. Appropriate courses of intervention are determined by the immediacy of solving particular problems in specific situations with the best tools available.

A decade ago, anthropologist Koenig (1988) illustrated how the technological imperative is sustained through social processes of routinization in which new technologies quickly come to be considered standard or routine in clinical practice. Standard of care is embodied in the newest technologies, she argued, and "becomes a moral as well as a technical obligation" (1988, pp. 485–486). Ethnographic work carried out in various medical settings in the 1980s and 1990s also shows how the technological imperative is sustained through social practices and treatment settings in which choice is both constructed and limited by clinical realities that make the use of the newest technologies and procedures inevitable (Anspach, 1993; Bosk, 1992; Fox & Swazey, 1992; Franklin, 1997; Zussman, 1992).

The technological imperative shapes the field of actual practice for all players in the hospital, even though death without high-technology intervention is valued, in principle, by many. One survey of nurses and physicians revealed that health professionals would not want aggressive life-prolonging treatments for themselves, and many would decline aggressive care on the basis of age alone (Gillick, Hesse, & Mazzapica, 1993). In another study of end-of-life preferences conducted at five hospitals, approximately 50% of physicians and nurses interviewed stated they had acted contrary to their own values by providing overly aggressive treatment (Solomon et al., 1993).

*The Mechanical Ventilator.* By the early 1970s, the mechanical ventilator (also called artificial ventilator or respirator) or "breathing machine" was standard equipment in all tertiary medical centers and most community hospitals in the United States. Like many technologies before it, the mechanical ventilator was applauded for enabling new forms of treatment, such as coronary artery bypass graft surgery and for life prolongation of persons with neuromuscular diseases (Snider, 1982). Historian Rothman (1997) notes that this technology was implemented in hospitals as soon as it was available. The mechanical ventilator sparked the creation of the ICU and immediately was considered essential technology. Although its development was inspired by the desire to solve the problem of keeping patients alive through surgery or infection, it is also capable of staving off death for days or weeks among patients who are frail and elderly, have multiple chronic conditions, and have terminal disease.

It is the widespread, negative public reaction to the mechanical ventilator, more than to any other particular medical technology or procedure, that has sparked the "right to die" movement across the United States and inspired the cultural cry for "death with dignity." Yet elderly people who have pneumonia (once considered "the old man's friend" for hastening an inevitable death) or who go into cardiac or respiratory arrest and are resuscitated, easily can be, and sometimes are, placed on mechanical ventilators when they arrive at hospital emergency rooms. Unless there are written documents regarding the patient's wish not to be resuscitated or strong family advocates available, standard practice throughout the United States is to place the patient on mechanical ventilation if the patient would otherwise die immediately. The case study here embodies this technological imperative and the dilemmas it creates.

## One Story of the Practice of Dying

*Ethnographic Representation.* There is, of course, more than one way to tell a story, and more than one point of view or one lens through which it can be told. The creation of a story out of the flow of observed events is problematic for all textual analyses and has been discussed widely in the anthropological literature (Clifford & Marcus, 1986; Geertz, 1988; Jackson, 1996). I faced that problem in deciding how to represent individual patient cases from my lengthy notes written during rounds, informal discussions, formal interviews, and conferences. I was only a part-time witness to the cases I observed; my interpretation is dependent on what I saw and recorded. In addition, for each case, I gathered information from different players. In some instances, family members were my primary informants. In other cases, such as this one, one physician or another member of the hospital staff provided the dominant lens through which I "saw" and then reconstructed events. In addition, the position of my informants in the power/knowledge hierarchy of the hospital world influenced my understanding of the ways in which death occurred.

*Thinking With Narrative.*   A narrative-rendering of events is not to be confused with real events, facts, or objective recordings of what actually occurs in the flow of clinical work and everyday life. Following Bruner (1986) in analyzing narrative as a "mode of thought," Katharine Young (1997) points out that persons and their lives are constructed narratively "by being enclosed in a trajectory given a narrative shape by the ethnographer" (1997, p. 140). The resulting narrative selves, she points out, are not the same as the persons whose lives are represented through the narrative as text. Thus, writing about the Other "contracts the presentation of a person to its narratable aspect" (p. 141). This limitation of narrative is not always acknowledged by ethnographers, who, in their writing at least, sometimes blur the distinction between self and story, between person and identity created through narrative. The claim, Young notes, that narrative texts, scenes created in narrative writing, represent a cultural or phenomenological world "rides on the Aristotelian assumption that language imitates reality" (p. 141). The problem, of course, is that the realm of the Other is not known directly through ethnographic writing; rather, it is constituted by such writing (Clifford & Marcus, 1986). The constraints of narrative in anthropological writing, that it contracts and constitutes persons and events, are as important as the meanings it can express and generate.

Yet in spite of this methodological limitation, a narrative rendering and analysis of advanced age and dying provides a way to "examine clinical life as a series of existential negotiations between clinicians and patients" (Mattingly, 1994, p. 821), in which the moral worlds of various players are revealed and the background assumptions of cultural practice surrounding medical care for the old come into view. The following case study encapsulates the cultural discomfort created when the idea of "giving up" clashes with another kind of knowledge that the end of life is near and must be accepted. The clash of contradictory discourses plays an important role, I suggest, in the construction of the problematic.

*The Case of Mr. Thomas: Example of "The Problem."* I have selected a case considered problematic by the players I observed. Similar to 38% of cases followed by SUPPORT study investigators, Mr. Thomas remained unconscious and in the ICU for many days before he died. There are many variables that contribute to such dying trajectories: physician and health-care team decisions; family wishes; the fact that patients are rarely clear about their desire for artificial-life prolongation; the complex way in which hospital rules and practices become "facts" (Arney & Bergen, 1984); the role of technology; and the diffuse power of litigation that hangs over every hospital activity. It is impossible to cite one activity, procedure, policy, or player as responsible for unwanted and prolonged ICU deaths. In my observations over a 1-year period of ICU deaths considered problematic, family members and physicians, in equal proportion, wanted to pursue aggressive life-extending treatments in the hope that the patient would live. This story is one example of how the problem of death in the United States unfolds daily in hospitals across the nation.

*The Story of Mr. Thomas: "Dialysis Every Other Day, on a Ventilator, Unconscious."* The patient's long-term primary care doctor drew my attention to Mr. Thomas 4 days after he was hospitalized in the ICU. I learned from the physician that Mr. Thomas was 72-years-old and "the patriarch of a large family" that included three wives, seven children, and numerous siblings. The family members were on good terms and all were involved in his care, although his current wife of 25 years was the person primarily responsible for speaking on the patient's behalf and for articulating family consensus on treatment options. Mr. Thomas had end-stage renal disease, bad vascular disease, hypertension, diabetes, coronary artery disease, and lung disease. He had been receiving outpatient hemodialysis for 3 years. During the past week, while he was in the outpatient clinic on the dialysis machine, he had a cardiac arrest. The nurses there resuscitated him and he was then taken to the hospital emergency room where, according to his primary care doctor, he "arrested again, at least one, probably two more times, and had to be shocked a total of three times. And wound up in the intensive care unit in a coma." Mr. Thomas was receiving mechanical ventilation and would not survive without it.

The physician then told me that hospital protocol (similar in most places) is to wait 72 hours before making a decision to withdraw techno-

logical life support. That time period had just passed, and the physician
had called a family conference to review the patient's situation, discuss
the grim prognosis, and give his own advice about how to proceed.
The family of Mr. Thomas was close-knit and religious, the physician
reported, "They came from all over the country to be at the bedside."
He told the family that they should think about what the patient would
want. He said that Mr. Thomas was "deeply comatose, was not responsive
to anything, including deep pain. He had brain stem activity, his eyes
would wander, things were going on in his brain stem . . . he wasn't
brain dead, but he was unaware, as far as we could tell." The physician
then told them what he wanted—to remove the ventilator support and
let Mr. Thomas die. Specifically, he told the family he would like to:
a) make the patient a DNR (that is, do not institute cardiac resuscitation
if the patient should have another cardiac arrest), b) discontinue dialysis
treatments, c) "wean him off the vent" (that is, slowly reduce to nothing
the oxygen support enabling the patient to live), and d) take Mr.
Thomas out of the ICU and put him in a room where he could die
with his family present. The physician continued, "I actually thought
that they were pretty much in agreement with me that he probably
wouldn't want to continue and that he would want life support stopped,
and that's what we ought to do."

To this doctor's surprise, after the family discussed the situation
among themselves, they were "unanimous in wanting to continue all
life support, including CPR, if he should arrest. I was actually very
surprised after the long discussion we had about this. They wanted 'to
go for life,' as the wife said. . . . She, in particular, could not fathom
the idea of stopping any treatment that would hasten his death. And
that's exactly the way she sees it—as tantamount to euthanasia." The
physician continued, "We took opposite points of view about this letting
go. . . . In the end, I could just say, 'I respect your position. I think it's
your decision about what he would want, and I'll support it.' " The
physician told me, "I want to say, also, that I think that they are realistic
about the prognosis. There's only one relative who talks about miracles. . . . The wife understands that he is dying, knows that that may
happen any time, is not expecting miracles, but just cannot affirmatively
take that step to end his life."

Other members of the medical and hospital staff, however, thought
the family's judgment was wrong, and thought that dialysis treatments
and ventilator support should be withdrawn from the patient immediately. "Some people put it in moral terms," I was told by Mr. Thomas's
doctor, "that it was immoral what we were doing to him. Just like the
moral terms the wife used when she said it was immoral to stop."

The fifth day of Mr. Thomas's hospitalization, I accompanied the medical team on their morning rounds of the ICU and saw Mr. Thomas for the first time. He was very slender and frail looking. The intensive care specialist, cardiologist, and renal specialist voiced their agreement that Mr. Thomas should not be receiving dialysis. A consulting neurologist wrote in the medical chart: "I would recommend to continue following the patient over the next 24–48 hours in order to determine whether indeed his progress continues to be poor, and if so, suggest making recommendations to the family to discontinue support. . . . " The primary care doctor said, "He'll probably 'code' [undergo CPR following a cardiac arrest], and it won't be successful, and he'll die." The cardiologist replied, "But he could code tomorrow and he could code two years from now." He confided to me that he did not know the hospital policy, did not know how to act, when medical staff are unanimous in wanting to stop treatment and family members want to continue. Later in the day, the pulmonologist clarified the situation: If the patient is determined by standard tests to be 'brain dead,' doctors can withdraw support, regardless of what the family wants. If the patient is in a coma or persistent vegetative state, as was Mr. Thomas, the hospital cannot withdraw support unless the family (or a previously written document by the patient) gives permission to do so.

Two weeks later, the patient was still in the ICU. Mr. Thomas's primary care doctor brought together several members of the hospital ethics committee, some of the treatment physicians, and several family members in the hopes that an open discussion would lead to resolution of the "problem." That is, he hoped first, that the family could be persuaded now to stop life-prolonging treatment. If that was not possible, he hoped that the medical team could, through learning the family's perspective of the situation, feel more comfortable providing care to a permanently comatose patient. Neither of those hopes was realized. After that meeting, the doctor wrote in Mr. Thomas's medical chart: "All about the same. Unresponsive but with posturing of arms (spontaneous), head and eye movements. Assess: no change. Ethics committee discussion with physicians, family, social worker, committee members— the meeting was to allow all parties a chance to express opinions/beliefs about continued treatment of Mr. Thomas. All present agreed that the family has the right to make the decision, that they were doing so conscientiously/in good faith; although not all present agreed that the decision was the 'right' one. Plan is to continue all tx [treatment]. We will continue to revisit code status."

Three weeks into the hospitalization, that doctor said to me, "I vacillate between appreciating the family's position and wanting to support them, and thinking that in fact it is their decision to make, on the one hand, and on the other hand when I go to examine this person, this person who was a person, it's uncomfortable to see what we're doing, keeping him alive in this state. It doesn't quite feel right. My sense is that, you know, a lot of it is projection, that I wouldn't want to be kept alive in an intensive care unit like this, dialysis every other day, on a ventilator, unconscious."

The social worker assigned to the case informed me that the primary care doctor had called in a gastroenterologist who had refused to insert a feeding tube in the patient's stomach, saying that that would be a "futile" act, and, in good conscience, he could not do it. The specialist also felt the patient should not have his life and his dying prolonged. Another gastrointestinal specialist had agreed to insert the tube, but not for another 2 weeks, as he wanted to wait and see if the patient's condition changed for the better or worse. The social worker was perplexed about these developments and their implication for discharge of the patient. She pondered aloud, does the second gastrointestinal specialist want to wait to let the patient die? If the patient had a stomach tube inserted now, she could discharge him to a long-term facility that cares for comatose, ventilator-dependent patients. Without the feeding tube, "They were in a discharge limbo." She also noted that the practice of 'aggressive treatment' was murky in this case. The patient was receiving antibiotics, along with nutritional support, through a nasogastric tube. This was very inefficient she informed me, like a 'slow code' [in which the medical team, in order to allow a patient to die rather than attempt to prolong life, goes through the motions, but slowly and without commitment, of cardiopulmonary resuscitation]. She noted that a much better way to deliver antibiotics is directly through an intravenous line. So, she asked rhetorically, what is going on here?

The pulmonologist also discussed the situation with me. He said he had known the patient when he was hospitalized about a year before with a gangrenous foot. Mr. Thomas informed him then that he did not want his foot removed, did not want that done to his body, and if his time was up, it was up. The pulmonologist asked, so how can the family, knowing that Mr. Thomas did not want life-extending treatments a year ago, prolong his comatose condition now? That physician felt that the treatments were futile and were probably causing the patient to suffer.

One month and 4 days after he was admitted, Mr. Thomas died. I learned from an ICU nurse that he was having cardiac problems while on dialysis the day before and treatment was 30 minutes shorter than usual. At that point, the renal specialist did not want to treat him any longer. The next day, Mr. Thomas had a cardiac arrest. The nurse told me that "he was coded for a very long time. They shocked him ten times . . . usually they shock a person maybe three times" [through cardiopulmonary resuscitation]. The family was not at the bedside at the time of the CPR or death. They were called when the code was over, very early in the morning. They came and sat by the bedside with the hospital chaplain and prayed together. Then they left the hospital.

The primary care doctor gave me his version of the final moments: "Mr. Thomas died after a longish CPR—truly a 'full code.' Not a peaceful death. But clearly the death his loved ones chose for him by requiring that all efforts be made to keep him alive. Of all the procedures we put him through, this was the worst, something I wanted to prevent from happening. The family, particularly his wife, knew my wishes. She and they considered them, I think, but couldn't let go even that much—to have a DNR order written. I spoke with the wife just after she arrived in the ICU after Mr. Thomas died. She was tearful and appreciative of everything I/we had done to help keep him alive. She knew we had tried our best. She and her family have to live with what happened, and it appears that giving 'life' our best shot is some consolation to them. Even though I wish his death could have been other than it was—more 'peaceful,' 'better,'—I don't regret acceding to his family's wishes."

## Social Processes: Shaping the Practice of Dying

A case study such as this illuminates sociocultural processes and specific institutional forces at work 'on the ground' in the clinical setting. Our next step is to look at the case of Mr. Thomas in the context of the structure and ideology of the hospital world. Such a contextualization allows us to view relationships among culture, structure, and particular practices, and to understand the social embeddedness of particular decisions, actions, and explanations. Viewing individual cases in various contexts shows that there are no easy or unilateral solutions to the problem of death. While better communication, greater use of written advance directives, and patient and family education are all worthy goals that have been discussed widely, none of those specific approaches alone can eradicate the problem of death, as the SUPPORT study and countless other personal and professional testimonials since then have shown. A discussion of three phenomena central to the culture and structure of the hospital, each embodied in the story of Mr. Thomas, illustrates the complexity of the problem.

First, the issue of 'code status'—determining whether a patient wishes to have CPR attempted in the event of cardiac arrest—looms large in hospital policy and practice. All seriously ill patients must have a code status designated in their hospital chart. The default designation, policy, and practice assumes that all patients will be resuscitated from a cardiac or respiratory arrest unless someone (patient or family) specifies otherwise. This policy and procedure is also the source of deep concern among elderly people, their family members, and the broader public who claim they do not want heroic measures automatically performed on them when the end of life is near. In addition, the topic of code status generates a great deal of debate in medical journals, popular magazines, newspaper editorials, and opinion pieces.

It was brought to my attention that hospital policy regarding the matter of DNR orders is not clear-cut and is under periodic discussion at the hospital I observed by professional staff. Actual policy on this matter is, in fact, a fuzzy and protean matter. The ethics committee at that hospital frequently reviews its policy in an attempt to offer a clear guideline for physician action. But in general, a well-articulated family decision regarding code status trumps physician opinion, as was the case in this particular story. Similarly, hospital policy regarding the withholding or withdrawing of mechanical ventilation or other life-supporting measures does not allow physicians or others to act against a patient's or family member's wishes. While I learned from hospital staff that they did not believe the treatment of Mr. Thomas was appropriate because it could not enable meaningful recovery, did not preserve the patient's dignity, and did not make good use of hospital resources, I also learned that the hospital administration would not condone or support physician action that opposed family desires.

I learned from observing and talking with many families that hospital rules, especially those regarding the need to designate a code status, are usually outside their world of experience. Most families I encountered had never conceptualized, let alone discussed with their relative, the notion of choice surrounding a resuscitation attempt. Very few families had discussed the possibility of or desire for resuscitation or intubation, specifically, with their relative before hospitalization. Most people confront such decisions, for the first time, either immediately after a relative has been resuscitated and is already on life support, or in an emergency context when families are told that the patient needs these measures immediately or he or she will die. While this particular case was problematic for hospital staff because the family wanted indefinite mechanical ventilation and insisted on CPR if the patient's heart stopped beating, other cases are problematic for families when physicians do not write DNR orders or they place the patient on a ventilator without discussing alternatives with family members beforehand.

Various observers have noted the lack of clarity about medical goals at the end of life (Brody, 1992; Callahan, 1993). The conflicts produced by the coexistence of the broad value of patient and family autonomy and patient- and family-centered care, hospital policies and practices about the use of resuscitation and mechanical ventilation, and the legally based need for patients and families to be the decision makers regarding withdrawal of life support all contribute first, to an uneasiness about relationships among institutional priorities, medical goals, and cultural values surrounding the extensive use of life-supporting technologies, and second, to discomfort on-the-ground about how the dying process is handled.

Second, the use of CPR is not unusual in dying trajectories in American hospitals. Two recent qualitative studies of the nature of cardiac resuscitation as a cultural artifact make the point that resuscitation efforts have become a default measure used in practically all cases of cardiac failure that occur in the American hospital, even though survival rates for patients with multiple illnesses are poor, a fact that has been known by health professionals for more than a decade (Bains, 1998; Mello & Jenkinson, 1998). Initially associated only with the relatively young surgical heart patient who was otherwise healthy, and performed first in the operating room, cardiac resuscitation has, during the past 30 years, spread beyond the confines of surgery and is now widely applied to dying persons with diseased hearts, within or beyond hospital walls (Bains, 1998; Eisenberg, Bergner, & Hallstrom, 1984). A variety of studies note that, depending on the type of cardiac problem, age, comorbid conditions, and other characteristics, only 8% to 15% of hospitalized patients survive CPR to be discharged (Hilberman, Kutner, Parsons, & Murphy, 1997; Schultz, Cullinane, Pasquale, Magnant, & Evans, 1996; So, Buckley, & Oh, 1994; Von Gunten, 1991). In one recent study of CPR in an intensive care unit, only 3% of ICU patients survived the procedure (Karetzky, Zubair, & Parikh, 1995). In a study of CPR in dialysis patients, 95% were on mechanical ventilation in an intensive care unit at the time of death (Moss, Holley, & Upton, 1992). Despite many studies of poor outcome, respect for patient and family decision making as we saw in this case renders physicians without ultimate authority to call a halt to what they consider the inappropriate use of CPR (Mello & Jenkinson, 1998).

Third, we must pay attention to the language used by actors in the story about the interpretation of events because that language reveals how "facts" about death and life are constituted. In their volume, *Lan-*

*guage and the Politics of Emotion*, Abu-Lughod and Lutz (1990) note (following Foucault, 1972) that language does not merely reflect thought or experience. Rather, talk is "productive of experience and constitutive of the realities in which we live and the truths with which we work. . . . " (1990, p. 10). The productive nature of language became evident to me as I listened to various actors describe what happened. No one said to me that Mr. Thomas "died" as I was trying to understand the story of his hospitalization and treatment. The language used, first by the primary care doctor and later by the intensive care nurses, to describe the patient's condition was the medical language of diagnosis and physiologic emergency and the institutional language of appropriate response strategy. It was not the humanistic language of existential knowledge about the end of life. Thus, the medical crisis began for the patient when, according to the primary care doctor, he "arrested" in the dialysis clinic, and then "arrested again, at least once, probably two more times, and had to be shocked a total of three times. . . . " The initial "cardiac arrest" was not framed as either cause or indication of Mr. Thomas's death. If it had been framed as death, the month of ICU treatments would not have occurred and the medical staff would not have been placed in a prolonged ethical dilemma. But in the clinic setting, death was framed as a catastrophic medical event that constituted the starting point for the CPR procedure. After the procedure, the patient was stabilized on mechanical ventilation. At that point, the family assumed or hoped he could recover and they spoke of wanting "to go for life." The story did not end until a month later, when the patient "was coded for a very long time. . . . " The primary care doctor explained that Mr. Thomas "*died after* a longish CPR—truly a full code." He was not considered dead until the resuscitation procedure ended. While that final cardiac arrest was probably listed in the medical record as the cause of death, the prolonged and unsuccessful resuscitation effort was the actual passage point between life and death. In the end, the dramatic and extraordinary resuscitation effort *sanctioned and legitimated* (Bains, 1998) Mr. Thomas's death. Thus, CPR has a symbolic aspect. It makes death acceptable and legitimate for some because it graphically demonstrates that death has been fought up to (and perhaps beyond) the last moment.

### Conclusion: Back to Method

In her article, "Writing against culture," Abu-Lughod (1991) makes a strong case for writing "ethnographies of the particular." Responding both to feminist critiques of an absence of reflexive positionality in traditional anthropology and to postcolonial critiques of anthropology as making essential cultural "Others," she notes that the culture concept, in its assumption of boundedness, timelessness, and coherence, may have outlived its usefulness. The process of generalization inherent in the representation of culture tends to flatten difference and contradiction. It minimizes or ignores ambiguous circumstances, changing opinions, and problematic categorizations. Local accounts with their particular strategies, innovations, and struggles are de-emphasized in the interest of articulating broad patterns, rules, and shared values and behaviors. Abu-Lughod suggests that social scientists treat generalization with suspicion, and states:

> "When one generalizes from experiences and conversations with a number of specific people in a community, one tends to flatten out differences among them and to homogenize them. The appearance of an absence of internal differentiation makes it easier to conceive of a group of people as a discrete, bounded entity . . . who do this or that and believe such-and-such. The effort to produce general ethnographic descriptions of people's beliefs or actions tends to smooth over contradictions, conflicts of interest, and doubts and arguments, not to mention changing motivations and circumstances" (1991, p. 152).

The homogenization inherent in "writing culture" tends to gloss the complex ways in which social life actually proceeds (see also Rosaldo, 1989). Focusing on particular individuals and telling specific stories allows for a more nuanced portrayal of contradictory discourses, as well as descriptions of practices that are not easily categorized.

Yet the argument for "ethnographies of the particular" is not a justification for privileging micro processes and de-emphasizing macro processes. Instead, this form of analysis attempts to illustrate the very human concerns, actions, and feelings that occur in local situations, while at the same time showing how everyday particular lives and practices are informed and constituted by larger effects and dynamics. Broader social forces remain inexact concepts when reified or portrayed only as generalizations (Abu-Lughod, 1991; Kaufman, 1993). The connection of social forces, such as pervasive biomedical ideologies and rules of institutional health care delivery, to particular lives and events, such as an ICU dying trajectory, reveals the tenaciousness of certain medical dilemmas and the ambivalence surrounding the creation of solutions to the problem of death.

It is hoped that this ethnography of the particular highlights the importance of making connections between the micro and the macro, between the particular scenario with its individual drama and anguish and the structural circumstances and cultural world that produces and enables it. Paying attention to the articulations between specific people, activities, feelings, and strategies on the one hand, and broader structures, politics, and medicocultural discourses on the other hand shows, in this case at least, that the locus of responsibility for the problem of end-of-life medical care does not reside solely in individual decision making, but rather must be conceived in the structural features and priorities of medical institutions and in cultural knowledge about the lifecourse and the benefits and limits to technology use. This strategy of connections works well to expose the reasons why death in the hospital is considered a problem. Such a strategy also shows how the 'normal' (hospital activities) and 'natural' (ways in which events unfold) are humanly made, constructed and enacted through on-the-ground interpretations of ideology and social processes by a variety of specific individuals.

## ACKNOWLEDGMENTS

The studies on which this chapter is based were funded by the National Institute on Aging, Grant No. AG13636, and the National Institute on Nursing Research, Grant No. NR05109, to Sharon R. Kaufman, Principal Investigator. I am deeply indebted to the hospital staff, patients, and families who participated in this project. Many thanks go to Co-P.I. Guy Micco for his insights about hospital practice, policy, and ethical issues in end of life care. Additional thanks go to project assistants Karen Van Leuven and Chris Wood.

## REFERENCES

Abu-Lughod, L. (1991). Writing against culture. In R. G. Fox (Ed.), *Recapturing anthropology: Working in the present* (pp. 137–162). Santa Fe, NM: School of American Research Press.

Abu-Lughod, L., & Lutz, C. A. (Eds.). (1990). *Language and the politics of emotion.* Cambridge, MA: Cambridge University Press.

Anspach, R. (1993). *Deciding who lives.* Berkeley, CA: University of California Press.

Arney, W. R., & Bergen, B. J. (1984). *Medicine and the management of living.* Chicago: University of Chicago Press.

Bains, J. (1998). From reviving the living to raising the dead: The making of cardiac resuscitation. *Social Science and Medicine, 47,* 1341–1349.

Bosk, C. (1992). *All God's mistakes.* Chicago: University of Chicago Press.

Brody, H. (1992). *The healer's power.* New Haven, CT: Yale University Press.

Bruner, J. (1986). *Actual minds, possible worlds.* Cambridge, MA: Harvard University Press.

Callahan, D. (1993). *The troubled dream of life.* New York: Simon and Schuster.

Campbell, M. L., & Frank, R. R. (1997). Experience with end of life practice at a university hospital. *Critical Care Medicine, 25,* 197–202.

Chambliss, D. F. (1996). *Beyond caring: Hospitals, nurses, and the social organization of ethics.* Chicago: University of Chicago Press.

Clifford, J., & Marcus, G. E. (1986). *Writing culture.* Berkeley, CA: University of California Press.

Cole, T. (1992). *The journey of life.* Cambridge, UK: Cambridge University Press.

Eisenberg, M. S., Bergner, L., & Hallstrom A. (1984). Survivors of out-of-hospital cardiac arrest. *American Journal of Emergency Medicine, 2,* 189–192.

Estes, C., & Binney, E. A. (1989). The biomedicalization of aging. *The Gerontologist, 29,* 587–596.

Foucault, M. (1972). *The archeology of knowledge and the discourse on language.* New York: Pantheon.

Fox, R. C., & Swazey, J. P. (1992). *Spare parts.* New York: Oxford University Press.

Franklin, S. (1997). *Embodied progress: A cultural account of assisted conception.* London and New York: Routledge.

Fuchs, V. R. (1974). *Who shall live?* New York: Basic Books.

Geertz, C. (1988). *Works and lives: The anthropologist as author.* Stanford, CT: Stanford University Press.

Gillick, M., Hesse, K., & Mazzapica, N. (1993). Medical technology at the end of life: What would physicians and nurses want for themselves? *Archives of Internal Medicine, 153,* 2542–2547.

Glaser, B., & Strauss, A. (1968). *Time for dying.* New York: Aldine.

Hilberman, M., Kutner, J., Parsons, D., & Murphy, D. J. (1997). Marginally effective medical care: Ethical analysis of issues in cardiopulmonary resuscitation. *Journal of Medical Ethics, 23,* 361–367.

Hurwicz, M. (Ed.). (1995). Cultural contexts of aging and health [Special issue]. *Medical Anthropology Quarterly, 9,* 143–283.

Institute of Medicine. (1997). *Approaching death: Improving care at the end of life.* Washington, DC: National Academy Press.

Jackson, M. (Ed.). (1996). *Things as they are: New directions in phenomenological anthropology.* Bloomington, IN: University of Indiana Press.

Karetzky, M., Zubair, M., & Parikh, J. (1995). Cardiopulmonary resuscitation in intensive care unit and non-intensive care unit patients. *Archives of Internal Medicine, 155,* 1277–1280.

Katz, S. (1996). *Disciplining old age: The formation of gerontological knowledge.* Richmond, VA: University of Virginia Press.

Kaufman, S. R. (1993). *The healer's tale.* Madison, WI: University of Wisconsin Press.

Kaufman, S. R. (1994). Old age, disease, and the discourse on risk: Geriatric assessment in U.S. health care. *Medical Anthropology Quarterly, 8,* 76–93.

Koenig, B. (1988). The technological imperative in medical practice: The social creation of a "routine" practice. In M. Lock & D. Gordon (Eds.), *Biomedicine examined* (pp. 465–496). Boston: Kluwer.

Lindenbaum, S., & Lock, M. (Eds.). (1993). *Knowledge, power and practice: The anthropology of medicine and everyday life.* Berkeley, CA: University of California Press.

Lo, B. (1995). Improving care near the end of life. *Journal of the American Medical Association, 274,* 1634–1635.

Lo, B., Snyder, L., & Sox, H. C. (1999). Care at the end of life: Guiding practice where there are no easy answers. *Annals of Internal Medicine, 130,* 772–773.

Lock, M., & Gordon, D. (Eds.). (1988). *Biomedicine examined.* Boston: Kluwer.

Lynn, J., Teno, J., & Harrell, F. E. (1995). Accurate prognostications of death. *Western Journal of Medicine, 163,* 250–257.

Mattingly, C. (1994). The concept of therapeutic 'emplotment.' *Social Science & Medicine, 38,* 811–822.

Mello, M., & Jenkinson, C. (1998). Comparison of medical and nursing attitudes to resuscitation and patient autonomy between a British and an American teaching hospital. *Social Science & Medicine, 46,* 415–424.

Moskowitz, E. H., & Nelson, J. L. (Eds.). (1995). *Hastings Center Report, November–December* (Special Suppl.), S2–S36.

Moss, A. H., Holley, J. L., & Upton, M. B. (1992). Outcomes of cardiopulmonary resuscitation in dialysis patients. *Journal of the American Society of Nephrology, 3,* 1238–1243.

Muller, J. H., & Koenig, B. (1988). On the boundary of life and death: The definition of dying by medical residents. In M. Lock & D. Gordon (Eds.), *Biomedicine examined* (pp. 351–374). Boston: Kluwer.

Rosaldo, R. (1989). *Culture and truth.* Boston: Beacon

Rothman, D. J. (1997). *Beginnings count: The technological imperative in American health care.* New York: Oxford University Press.

Schultz, S. C., Cullinane, D. C., Pasquale, M. D., Magnant, C., & Evans, S. R. (1996). Predicting in-hospital mortality during cardiopulmonary resuscitation. *Resuscitation, 33,* 13–17.

Snider, G. L. (1982). Historical perspective on mechanical ventilation: From simple life support to ethical dilemma. *American Review of Respiratory Disease, 140,* S4–S5.

So, H. Y., Buckley, T. A., & Oh, T. E. (1994). Factors affecting outcome following cardiopulmonary resuscitation. *Anesthesiology Intensive Care, 22,* 647–658.

Solomon, M., et al. (1993). Decisions near the end of life: Professional views on life-sustaining treatments. *American Journal of Public Health, 83,* 14–23.

Stolberg, S. G. (1998). As life ebbs, so does time to elect comforts of hospice. *New York Times,* p. A1, March 4.

The SUPPORT Principal Investigators. (1995). A controlled trial to improve care for seriously ill hospitalized patients. *Journal of the American Medical Association, 274,* 1591–1634.

Von Gunten, C. F. (1991). CPR in hospitalized patients: When is it futile? *American Family Physician, 44,* 2130–2134.

Young, K. (1997). *Presence in the flesh.* Cambridge, MA: Harvard University Press.

Zussman, R. (1992). *Intensive care.* Chicago: University of Chicago Press.

# CHAPTER FIVE

# Participant Observations of a Participant Observer

## Juliet M. Corbin

There are times when I am envious of my colleagues after watching them use psychometrically sound questionnaires and listening to them talk about their sophisticated statistical programs. Here I am, spending long days out in the field observing, talking to people, or examining documents. I can discuss the stories that people tell me, but I cannot quote impressive numbers. Instead, my task is to make sense out of all that qualitative data. At these times, I cannot help but wonder: why do participant observation anyway?

This chapter, an exploratory essay, examines the meaning and value of participant observation. I commence with a general analysis of participant observation as an epistemology, then move to consideration of several methodological issues pertinent to the use of participant observation as a methodology for revealing the lives of elders.

There are many answers to my rhetorical question—why do participant observation? Some researchers suggest that participant observation fits with their personalities, their humanistic view of the world. Others say that the approach enables them to become familiar with worlds that they would not otherwise experience. And yet others emphasize that participant observation enables the researcher to get close to the people he or she studies, to enter into their experiences, and to observe them in their natural settings. While I myself have given all of these responses, such answers seem rhetorical and lack sophistication. I find myself wanting more in-depth responses to questions such as: What does it mean to "enter into experience?" What can I learn using participant observation that could not be gleaned using other research methods?

In pondering these questions, I am drawn to my experience working in a community of elders. I did not initially enter this community as a participant observer or to collect data. Rather, I became a participant observer quite by accident, first entering the lives of elders in my capacity as a nurse-clinician and only later as a trained field worker who for more than 20 years has been conducting qualitative research. Though my primary function in the community of elders was as a clinician, I could not separate the researcher from the nurse. The two aspects of self are intertwined in a very complex relationship in which I was collecting data, although I was not aware I was doing so at the time.

I refer to myself as a "participant observer *of sorts.*" To explain the qualifier, I turn to the classic article written by Gold (1959), which identifies four types of participant observers. As is the case with many typologies, I do not fit neatly into any of these profiles. The "participant-as-observer" role denotes that both the observed and the observer are aware that data is being collected. I was not doing research, in fact, at the time, I was not even aware of the images of the community forming in my mind. I was not a "complete participant" because I did not live in the community and fully participate as a resident. Nor was I an "observer as participant," conducting one-visit interviews. Finally, I was not a "complete observer" because I was not entirely removed from the situation. I did interact with participants. Upon reflection, I was a participant in the community because, in my role as a nurse, I was part of the lifeworld of the setting. I was an observer because of my sociological training. A wise teacher once told me, "Remember everything is data and you'll have a use for it." It seems he was correct. While I will never directly publish what I know about this place in the form of research findings, I am using the information I have accrued over the years to do an interpretive analysis of participant observation. The analysis is not so much a report on a specific community of elders as an examination of the process of participant observation itself.

## The Clinical Facility

I entered the place where I was to become a participant observer "of sorts" when I was assigned to a residential setting for elders as a clinical instructor in a nursing program. The facility is a medium-sized complex of 130 apartments where my students and I provide a wide range of health care services both in the resident's homes and in a drop-in clinic. The facility consists of two residential towers. One tower comprises apartments priced at market value. The other is Housing and Urban Development (HUD)-supported housing. The two towers share common rooms located between them. To live in this facility, residents must be able to function independently. Those who cannot care for themselves must have a care provider, either a family member or hired help, as there is no full-time nursing staff. One meal a day is served in the evening. There are no in-house transportation services, but "Outreach," a form of public transportation for the elderly, is available for a small fee. The facility provides a variety of activities for residents, including religious services, exercise classes, and leisure opportunities such as Saturday afternoons at the movies. On-call staff is available 24 hours a day to handle emergencies.

Because I have been working at this facility for about 7 years, I appear to be accepted as an "insider," and my presence hardly raises an eyebrow. I care deeply about these "old people" and have immersed myself in their lives, sharing in their joys and sorrows. For several years, I was at the facility twice a week, but the nursing program reduced the hours students spend in the community setting and, consequently, has reduced my clinical presence to 1 full day a week. This has drawbacks for providing continuity of care, but provides the opportunity to gain some "distance" and to recharge my "emotional batteries."

## What Have I Learned as a Participant Observer?

My first response is to say that I have developed a "feel" for the community. But, this does not say much. A better answer might be that I have come to understand the meaning of the facility to those who live there and how the structural features of the environment support that meaning. This requires some elaboration and documentation.

*A Housing Complex Becomes "Home."* One concept that emerges from my participation and observation at the facility is a distinctive reconceptualizing of the idea of "home" (Altman & Werner, 1985; Boschetti, 1990; Maloney, 1997; Rubinstein, 1989). Transplants from all over the country, most residents come to this place for security and convenience. Some move to the facility by choice, others come at the urging of their children or other relatives. For most, the move represents a major life transition; it forces an admission that they can no longer manage completely on their own, that they need to be closer to their children, in a place where there is always someone "on call." Entering such a facility often means leaving a home behind, the house and community where they lived for most of their adult lives, to live with a group of people brought together by the shared dimension of age and functional ability (Rowles & Ravdal, in press; Young, 1998).

Significant symbolism is often attached to home (Eliade, 1959; Fogel, 1992). Moving away entails letting go of old symbols. Creating a new home necessitates fashioning new symbols out of new interests, objects, spaces, and relationships (Hartwigsen, 1987; McHugh & Mings, 1996; Rowles & Ravdal, in press). Not every elderly person accommodates easily to the new residence: a place to live, it will never be home. There is a refusal to abandon spaces, objects, and relationships left behind. Such residents often complain about trifling issues; they live on the periphery, never fully engaging in the life of the community. After a time, if they are able, some move out to search for a place more like the "old home." In sharp contrast, some elders quickly make the transition to a new life without much effort. Most persons fall somewhere between the two extremes, needing time to grieve the loss of the past, but nevertheless adjusting to their new life. The process is eased when older persons have families and friends who lend emotional support and help to maintain links with their past, as well as providing assistance in forging a pathway to the present.

Creating a sense of "home" is more than just arranging and rearranging furniture. It involves developing a sense of attachment both to a new place and to other persons who live and share in this place. It also means establishing new routines for daily living. Setting up new routines helps to reestablish a sense of orientation as the resident finds an acceptable hairdresser, becomes familiar with the local grocery store, identifies a new, caring doctor, and joins a religious congregation where he or she feels comfortable.

*Creating "Home" Through Cultivating Community.* Engaging in community activities facilitates becoming acquainted with other elders, forming new relationships, and developing a sense of community belonging. New acquaintances cannot replace life-long friendships, but they can provide contacts for occasionally going out for a shared dinner, talking over concerns, or "calling on" in an emergency. Residents tend to become most closely affiliated with persons they share a table with in the dining room or with whom they discover a common interest, such as in playing Scrabble® or cards. They may also develop strong relationships with neighbors on the same floor or in the same wing of the building. When significant birthdays come along, such as the 85th or 90th, it is these new friends who are invited to share in their family celebration. Residents who are immigrants seek out other immigrants, especially those who speak the same language: it seems more like home when there is some meaningful part of the past to share. Persons with an interest in gardening volunteer to care for the plants and the flowers outside on the grounds. Some elders plant small personal gardens in designated spaces, sharing the flowers or vegetables they grow with their neighbors. Those with leadership interests run for office in the tenant's council or volunteer to serve as coordinators for special events like the monthly birthday parties or a spring luncheon. Those who are mobile extend the notion of home to the surrounding community and volunteer in the library of the nearby hospital, the local zoo, or one of the homeless shelters.

Informal and formal communication networks help to establish a sense of familiarity. There are plenty of opportunities for information sharing or gossip while waiting by the mailboxes. If someone becomes ill or goes to the hospital, a card is passed around for everyone to sign. Receiving one of these cards contributes to the sense that one is part of a community. As one gentleman told me, "Look at all those signatures. I can see that they really care about me." More formally, there is a quarterly newsletter put out by residents. The newsletter reports on major events, introduces newcomers, and notes special accomplishments of residents or their families. A monthly calendar of events keeps everyone informed of upcoming activities. Monthly meetings of the Tenant's Council are open to all residents. At these meetings, issues pertaining to the operation of the facility are discussed and upcoming events are planned, giving all persons in attendance a voice in shaping the daily life of the community.

The spatial order of the facility contributes to the feeling that this place is home. Apartments are personalized with residents' belongings. However, home extends beyond the apartment and includes the common rooms, the grounds, and the surrounding area. Residents take pride in the appearance of these areas, use them as communal interaction areas, and gain a sense of ownership of these spaces. Some residents would rather sit in common areas than in their living rooms and can be found in the entry area much of the day. They sit and watch everything that goes on. If anyone wants to know who passed by on a certain day or time, where someone is, or what's happening, the "lobby sitters" are able to provide that information. If a resident violates the sense of common space by sprawling out on one of the couches with his or her feet up, they are chastised by other residents because of shared concern about what visitors to "their home" might think if they see someone messing up the "living room." In the winter, a fireplace in the lobby area is lit and chairs are arranged around it so that people can sit and talk. Conversations may be about something happening at the facility that day, but mostly there is a sharing of personal lives, the trip to the doctor, a trip to the children's home, or a visit to a friend. Achievements and travels of children and grandchildren are reported with pride. In warm weather, chairs are placed near the windows and garden, opening the inside to the outdoors, while retaining the intimacy of a "talk area." There is a well-worn path to the coffeepot and a nearby table serves as a meeting place in the morning and early afternoon. An hour or so before dinner, the normally quiet lobby comes to life. Residents, dressed for dinner, gather to socialize. When the doors of the dining room swing open at 5:00, activity shifts inside as residents move to assigned tables. The lobby is once again still. After dinner, some residents sit around and talk. Others make their way back to their own or a friend's apartment to watch television or to play a game of Scrabble®.

How far residents venture into the surrounding neighborhood varies depending upon physical ability, access to a car, or willingness to take a bus or taxi. Residents often like to shop at the K-mart® across the street. Even residents with mobility restrictions have a direct path to the store. They risk crossing a busy street using walkers or electric carts so that they can shop, eat lunch, or just get out of their apartments. Many residents walk to a grocery store located about a mile away for the exercise. Others walk in the surrounding neighborhood or sit outside enjoying a little sunshine.

The shared sense of community is striking. There is a pervasive sense of caring about others, even those who are not close friends. There is sadness when someone dies. Many residents attend the memorial service, even if they did not know the individual very well. There is respect for the religious rights of others and everyone joins in events, such as decorating the Christmas tree and the rituals of a Seder (the Jewish celebration of Passover). Persons less able to care for themselves are watched over by others. If someone forgets to come to dinner, that person is either called or someone brings dinner up to him or her. Residents who are forgetful and found wandering in the neighborhood are brought back to the facility by other residents. The general attitude among residents is that we need to look out for one another. In the end, the new home becomes not unlike the old—a place where a person can feel safe and cared about. This feeling can be summed up in the words of one woman who said to me recently, "You know we really are a family!"

## An Analysis of Participant Observation

What makes participant observation different from other methods of data collection? I believe that it is not so much just being in a place and observing, but the sustained connections with people that one makes in the participant's own environment. Participants are not just subjects to be counted, but interacting human beings with thoughts, feelings, emotions, and stories to tell. The researcher listens, shares in important events, and experiences the sadnesses and joys that are part of the everyday lives of participants. Recently, I bid a final goodbye to one elderly woman. I cried with the family and was as much comforted by them as they were by me. While in many ways I feel connected to these elderly persons, I also know that I remain an outsider. I speak at the memorials, celebrate birthdays, and participate in the Seder. But I have not reached the age of Social Security. I do not yet live there, although in my mind, I often project ahead to a time when I might. Scholars have discussed the particular perspectives derived from being an insider versus being an outsider (Keith, 1986; Myerhoff, 1978; Phoenix, 1994). Seemingly apparent advantages, such as familiarity with language, certain customs, and a presumed higher comfort level on the part of both the interviewer and the interviewee may be balanced by not-so-obvious disadvantages. These potential disadvantages include a dangerous assumption of values or behaviors that may silence the voice of informants in favor of the presumed knowledge of the interviewer and role transference (see Rubinstein, chapter 7). Does it matter as a participant observer that I remain somewhat an outsider? That is a matter of debate, but I do not think so. I do know that I can put distance between the residents and myself when necessary (Agar, 1986). I can step back and ask: "What is going on here?" Stepping back is essential because what is transpiring often is not obvious to those immersed in a situation. It takes an outside gaze to grasp the significance of seemingly unrelated events and connect them to form a whole. Participants, concerned with the immediacy of what is happening to them, are not always cued into the subtleties of mood and the nuances of action and interaction. A participant observer is likely to view the larger picture, observe and interpret events as they unfold and integrate the perspectives of all involved (Muller, 1995). Furthermore, a participant observer is often able to locate actions in context, to note structural conditions operating as events transpire.

This ability to observe and understand varying actor's viewpoints derives from being sufficiently "outside" to adopt rather neutral perspectives while at the same time having achieved an insider's understanding. One of the most interesting events that occurred recently in the apartment complex was the response of residents when a person with a psychiatric condition moved in. Edward, as I shall call him, was actively psychotic, but was not on any form of medication. He could often be found in the lobby staring into space, following people around, or just talking nonsense. Residents were afraid to come into the lobby at night, especially if they were alone, because Edward was always sitting there. Sometimes he would sit down by a group of elders talking in the lobby and sit and stare, but not partake in the conversation. Feeling uncomfortable, the group would close their circle or move away. Everyone moved away from Edward in the dining room because he smelled bad and lacked table manners. Residents began to talk among themselves. Fears were magnified by talk of what might potentially happen. "He might become violent." "He might rape someone." Furthermore, Edward did not fit the profile of the type of person with whom they should be living. He was not old. He behaved strangely, quite unlike those persons they were used to with dementia, a little forgetful and sometimes cranky but not "strange." They worried about what their family or friends would think if they saw Edward sitting in the lobby, or worse yet, if he happened to follow them out to their car at night. Residents took their concerns to the facility manager and the Board of Directors. They were told that nothing could be done because Edward was admitted to the facility on the HUD side and had as much right to live there as anyone. This made the residents angry. In addition, the facility manager accused officers in the Tenant's Council of not demonstrating appropriate leadership. From the manager's perspective, it was up to them to gain Edward's acceptance by the other residents. Everyone was on edge waiting for something to happen. Eventually, Edward was asked to stop following visitors to their cars. He became agitated. The police were called and he was taken to the hospital where he was placed on a 72-hour hold. The residents were not informed of why the police took Edward away, but there were many rumors, most of them false. When Edward returned from the hospital, his family took him on an extended vacation, much to the relief of the residents.

Throughout this incident there was fear, anger, and resentment on the part of all involved. Residents were reactive, responding not so much to fact as to potential. The manager was concerned about Edward as an individual, his right to live there, and the obligation he had to uphold the regulations stipulated by HUD. I was able to view the situation from all perspectives. I tried to ease the discord by translating the perspective of each side to the other. In doing so, I realize now that I was fusing my roles of nurse and researcher. The message I sent was: we need to do something to make residents feel safe, for this is their home and a major reason why they came to live here. They are reacting because they feel threatened and vulnerable. At the same time, I argued for the protection of Edward's rights.

Although participant observation is time consuming, it has the potential to reveal processes, structures, interactions, and outcomes. At the same time, the researcher cannot hide behind standardized measurement protocols. He or she must "connect" with the persons being studied, even though it may be difficult to witness and cope with the expression of strong emotions, such as anger or fear. In this context, it may be necessary for the researcher to confront and deal with his or her own personal emotions, acknowledging that these are often an integral part of an empathic research process.

Finally, participant observation begets creativity. Life events often cannot be predicted or anticipated. Each research situation is unique and contingent on local circumstances. Consequently, methods must be adjusted to meet the evolving demands of the research situation. Certain types of persons, often those with a high tolerance for ambiguity, flexibility, and a willingness to listen, are attracted to fieldwork. Effective participant observers tend to be curious about life, sensitive to nuances of interaction and, most of all, willing and able to enter the experience of the people to be studied.

What does it mean to "enter into another's experience"? One cannot be that person in that place. But, for a short time, one can symbolically take on the role of the other. One can dialogue with the other, insert oneself in their place, and try to capture the essence of what one sees, hears, and feels. Like an Impressionist painter, one can translate the images formed into a picture. For the scholar, the images are created, not of paint, but of words. The goal is not photographic accuracy. Rather, it is the ability to recreate the conceptual essence of the multiple realities of persons, at some time, in some space, as interpreted through the researcher's lens. The picture formed is biased, created by the researcher in partnership with the participants. Nevertheless, it presents a view of the world that might otherwise have remained inaccessible.

## Researcher in the Research

Participant observation brings multiple aspects of the self to the research situation. I cannot separate the clinician from the researcher; the two are fused to create the fabric of my being. Although my primary role at the facility was that of clinician, the researcher part of me was active in the background. These selves and the influence of status, power, gender, and clinical roles on the research process have been discussed extensively in the literature (Cartwright & Limandri, 1997; Punch, 1986; Warren, 1988). For example, Hamberg and Johansson (1999), two female physicians from Sweden, conducted a grounded-theory study on their patients. The focus of their study was the problem faced by women seeking help for medically undefined, long-term, musculoskeletal pain. Discussions of the research with other investigators raised the issue of bias. How could two physicians interviewing their own patients expect to obtain an unbiased picture? The two researchers decided to scrutinize their data for evidence of how their own reactions, values, and interpretations of events affected the stories told by the participants. Focusing on interview passages where there were signs of tension, contradictions, or conflicting codes, their analysis revealed that at these times, the investigators were acting primarily from one of three positions: as physicians, as women, and as researchers. Although they tried to elicit the perspective of their patients, it was evident that the participants in their research did not always feel able to express themselves fully. At times, the physician or woman selves unwittingly entered into the research persona of the investigators, setting up subtle contexts of power and conflict, and cutting off full disclosure.

My roles and status as a woman, health professional, back-door sociologist, teacher, and researcher have all influenced the nature of the data I have collected, my reactions to varying circumstances, and my interpretation of these data. I have not always been aware of how much these aspects of my self have determined what I heard, said, or did, or how others responded to me. Being a woman, a nurse, and a teacher have, at various times, helped me gain access to populations and to sites, to understand events, and to feel comfortable in diverse situations. I have also found that being a participant observer has greatly influenced how I practice as a clinician (Schein, 1987). Before I began conducting interviews and observing chronic illness, I accepted the medical model of illness and its management. What an awakening I had after talking to people; only then did I begin to discover the multiple dimensions of aging and health.

## Keeping It All in Perspective

There are divergent opinions about maintaining a balance between reflexivity and objectivity when analyzing fieldwork experiences. On the one hand, reflexivity is necessary for intellectual honesty and clarity of thought. On the other, sooner or later one must get down to the nuts and bolts work of data analysis. The balance between finding a way to combine reflexivity with common sense logic requires a dose of craft.

Common sense is important because it helps us to maintain a sense of balance about research. There are multiple realities, many ways of seeing and interpreting (Denzin, 1994). There are also multiple roles for researchers in the field, determined by training, perspective, and inclination. Adler and Adler (1987) describe three such roles, each denoting varying degrees of active researcher involvement in a group: the peripheral member, the active member, and the complete member. A peripheral member seeks an insider's perspective, but refrains from engaging in activities that stand at the core of group membership. Active members take on core activities of the group, but only to the extent that these are defined and agreed upon by the group. In complete membership, the researcher becomes one of the group, sharing in its common vision, goals, and experiences. Each role has advantages and disadvantages for data collection. For some researchers, and for some studies, being a complete member may be essential. Lieberman (1999) believed it necessary to live among a group of aboriginal people in Southern Australia for a year in order to truly experience life in the desert in intense heat. Having a chronic illness may make one more sensitive to what it is like to live with an ongoing and, perhaps, even life-threatening disease. Instead of situating myself in circumstances that are identical to those of my participants, in my research I have relied on other ways to enter into such an experience. These have included: living with family members and having friends who are chronically ill; undertaking extensive field observations; carefully listening to what persons are telling me about their illnesses; and working with the chronically ill to help them manage their conditions. Many variables enter into a research situation. Some arise from the researcher, others from the situation to be researched. No one role, technique, or approach is necessarily better than another. Only the person doing the research can judge what is right for him or her. As Atkinson and Hammersley (1998, p. 119) state: "Above all: we must not be misled into assuming that we are faced merely with a choice between dogmatism and relativism, between a single oppressive conception of science and some uniquely liberating alternative."

While reflexivity is inevitable and necessary, the burden is on the researcher to determine how much, at what point, and by what means. Too much and one is paralyzed. Not enough and one runs the risk of unduly influencing the research and misrepresenting the participants. Although researchers are not always as reflective as they should be, it must be acknowledged that participants are not always insightful about what is going on either (Denzin, 1992). There are times when participants are more reactive than thoughtfully active. Although an outsider's perspective is only one vision of "reality," and objectivity is never fully realized, an outsider has the potential to view a situation from all angles and present a picture of multiple views (Agar, 1986). There are some strategies that researchers can use to increase reflexivity. Keeping a journal record of one's emotions, responses, and difficulties while gathering data can increase self-awareness. Critically examining transcriptions for points of discordance, as did Hamberg and Johansson (1999), is also helpful. Bringing researchers' interpretations to participants for critical review and comment is often enlightening. Actively involving participants in the research process as in some forms of action research is another way of enhancing reflexivity (King, 1995; Neysmith, 1995; Reason, 1998). Also helpful during analysis are techniques designed to break through researcher-biased perspectives, such as those described in Dey (1993), Miles and Huberman (1994), Morse (1994), Strauss and Corbin (1998), and Wolcott (1994).

The acknowledgement and use of reflexivity and common sense alone cannot make up for a lack of craft. Craft here has two separate meanings. The first is technique. There was a time when technique was learned through apprenticeship, a junior scientist working, sometimes for years, under the guidance of a more senior mentor. The danger was that the more-experienced researcher was able to pass on false assumptions, biases, and bad habits, along with more-helpful insight. While apprenticeship is still possible, it is more difficult to obtain because of growing constraints of time, money, and the sheer numbers of students needing direction in most academic institutions.

The second meaning of craft refers to being "open," flexible, and responsive to what Lieberman (1999) calls the "contingencies" or the emergent issues, concerns, and social conventions that are central to those one is studying. This is in contrast to stubborn and oblivious adherence to predefined research agenda, despite the twists and turns taken by the research. Having craft in this sense calls for redirecting one's orientations, methods, and approaches when issues emerge that are important to the participants. Responding to contingencies is the basis for research ethics:

> Because each research situation poses its unique contingencies, qualitative sociological research is a craft and not merely technology. But this craft is always and inextricably fused with ethics of our relations with the people we study (Lieberman, 1999, p. 59).

Ethics goes beyond accurate representation of research participants. It involves "exchange" or a giving back to respondents for, in the short term, the intrusion into their lives (Lieberman, 1999) and, in the long term, the enhancement of knowledge to improve lives. My experience has been that interviews take place on two levels (at least). On one level, the person is telling a story and I am listening. At another level, the participant wants something from me. While I am listening, I am trying to figure out just what that is. Sometimes, it is a desire to have his or her voice heard; participation in research provides a means to this end. At other times, participants want reassurance, information, a sympathetic ear, or temporary respite from loneliness. At my work, older persons often come to me and say, "Come sit with me and talk awhile. I'll give you a cup of coffee and a cookie." It is not nursing care that they want, but to connect with a caring person for a time.

Russell (1999) points out that the control of an interview is not necessarily in the hands of the researcher as is sometimes believed. The vulnerability of older research participants is often a construction of the researcher, a fable rather than reality. In many cases, respondents are very much in control of the research situation: confiding what they feel safe telling, sometimes telling deliberate falsehoods, steering conversation in directions they deem important, detaining the researcher much longer than he or she had intended, and stopping talking only when they feel physically or emotionally ready. Self-deprecating or embarrassing information may be communicated, but unless coerced, such revelation is their choice. These revelations are a way for respondents to gain power, keeping me there by piquing my curiosity.

Of course, there are exceptions to the degree of respondent power and autonomy, raising ethical questions about data gathering (Brandriet, 1994). When collecting data from persons who are not fully cognizant, persons who are "trapped" in nursing facilities, or who are in other circumstances where there is an implicit culture of consent to being researched, the balance of power tilts in favor of the researcher. Mitchell and Koch (1997) suggest two strategies for enhancing the voice of the vulnerable under such circumstances: allowing significant others to speak on behalf of persons with dementia and reading fragments of resident-interview transcriptions to staff so that their voices and concerns can be heard. Researching vulnerable persons often means that the questions, as well as the answers become very complicated (Russell, 1996; Schuster, 1996). As Russell (1999, p. 415) expresses the dilemma:

> I would suggest that by asking if it is ethical to interview vulnerable people at all if one can do nothing for them, we run the risk not only of paralyzing our own research efforts but of excluding from the public domain those very voices that otherwise remain muted.

## Conclusion

Is it complete objectivity that we seek or a canvas that resonates with the essence of some experience brought forth through dialogue and active participation in a social research setting? Does participant-observation research paint pictures that provide new understandings and glimpses into worlds often obscured by their very ordinariness? Participant observers inevitably miss some things, prevent other things from being said or done, misinterpret, and over interpret. However, if they are able to put aside their own agendas and let the emergent social practices and concerns of respondents reveal themselves, power is shared in an ethical manner. Reflection, a little bit of common sense, and large doses of craft, make it possible to create images that embrace multiple realities, including those of the researcher. Researchers are "participants" in participant observation in even more profound ways than originally dreamed of by Gold (1997). Participant observation provides a lens that clarifies and mutes, reveals and obscures, but in the end adds one more layer to our understanding of the world around us.

> The challenge remains to think about the work and how we do it, but above all, still to do the work of understanding and presenting various life worlds and their important participants. Just as surely as everyday-life participants negotiate and resolve their uncertainties about their own knowledge and criteria of knowing, so, too, can ethnographers reflect on our purpose at hand and celebrate one of our meaningful activities, that of clarifying the nature, context, process, significance, and consequences of the ways in which human beings define their situation (Altheide & Johnson, 1998, p. 309).

## REFERENCES

Adler, P. A., & Adler, P. (1987). *Membership roles in field research.* Newbury Park, CA: Sage Publications, Inc.

Agar, M. H. (1986). *Speaking of ethnography.* Beverly Hills, CA: Sage Publications, Inc.

Altheide, D. L., & Johnson, J. M. (1998). Criteria for assessing interpretive validity in qualitative research. In N. K. Denzin & Y. S. Lincoln (Eds.), *Collecting and interpreting qualitative materials* (pp. 283–312). Thousand Oaks, CA: Sage Publications, Inc.

Altman, I., & Werner, C. M. (Eds.). (1985). *Home environments.* New York: Plenum.

Atkinson, P., & Hammersley, M. (1998). Ethnography and participant observation. In N. K. Denzin & Y. S. Lincoln (Eds.), *Strategies of qualitative inquiry* (pp. 110–136). Thousand Oaks, CA: Sage Publications, Inc.

Boschetti, M. A. (1990). Reflections on home: Implications for housing design for elderly persons. *Housing and Society, 17*(3), 57–65.

Brandriet, L. M. (1994). Gerontological nursing application of ethnography and grounded theory. *Journal of Gerontological Nursing, 20*(7), 33–40.

Cartwright, J., & Limandri, B. (1997). The challenge of multiple roles in the qualitative clinician researcher-participant client relationship. *Qualitative Health Research, 7*(2), 223–235.

Dey, I. (1993). *Qualitative data analysis.* London: Routledge.

Denzin, N. K. (1992). Whose Cornerville is it anyway? *Journal of Contemporary Ethnography, 21*(1), 120–131.

Denzin, N. K. (1994). The art and politics of interpretation. In N. Denzin & Y. S. Lincoln (Eds.), *Handbook of qualitative research* (pp. 500–515). Thousand Oaks, CA: Sage Publications, Inc.

Eliade, M. (1959). *The sacred and the profane.* New York: Harcourt, Brace & World.

Fogel, B. S. (1992). Psychological aspects of staying at home. *Generations, 16*(2), 15–19.

Gold, R. L. (1959). Sociological field observations. *Social Forces, 36,* 217–223.

Gold, R. L. (1997). The ethnographic method in sociology. *Qualitative Inquiry, 3*(4), 388–402.

Hamberg, K., & Johansson, E. E. (1999). Practitioner, researcher, and gender conflict in a qualitative study. *Qualitative Health Research, 9*(4), 455–467.

Hartwigsen, G. (1987). Older widows and the transference of home. *International Journal of Aging and Human Development, 24*(3), 195–207.

Keith, J. (1986). Participant observation. In C. L. Fry & J. Keith (Eds.), *New methods for old age research* (pp. 8–26). South Hadley, MA: Bergin & Garvey.

King, J. A. (1995). Bringing research to life through action research methods. *Canadian Journal on Ageing, 14*(1), 165–176.

Lieberman, K. (1999). From walkabout to meditation: Craft and ethics in field inquiry. *Qualitative Inquiry, 5*(1), 47–63.

Maloney, M. F. (1997). The meanings of home in the stories of older women. *Western Journal of Nursing Research, 19*(2), 166–176.

McHugh, K. E., & Mings, R. C. (1996). The circle of migration: Attachment to place in aging. *Annals of the Association of American Geographers, 86*(3), 530–550.

Miles M., & Huberman, M. (1994). *Qualitative data analysis* (2nd ed.). Thousand Oaks, CA: Sage Publications, Inc.

Mitchell, P., & Koch, T. (1997). Attempt to give nursing home residents a voice in the quality improvement process: The challenge of frailty. *Journal of Clinical Nursing, 6*(6), 453–461.

Morse, J. M. (1994). *Qualitative research methods.* Thousand Oaks, CA: Sage Publications, Inc.

Muller, J. H. (1995). Care of the dying by physicians-in-training: An example of participant observation research. *Research on Aging, 17*(1), 65–88.

Myerhoff, B. (1978). *Number our days.* New York: Touchstone.

Neysmith, S. M. (1995). Feminist methodologies: A consideration of principles and practice for research in gerontology. *Canadian Journal on Ageing, 14*(1), 100–118.

Phoenix, A. (1994). Practicing feminist research: The interaction of gender and "race" in the research process. In M. Maynard & J. Purvis (Eds.), *Researching women's lives from a feminist perspective* (pp. 35–45). London: Taylor & Francis.

Punch, M. (1986). *The politics and ethics of fieldwork.* Beverly Hills, CA: Sage Publications, Inc.

Reason, P. (1998). Three approaches to participatory inquiry. In N. K. Denzin & Y. S. Lincoln (Eds.), *Strategies of qualitative inquiry* (pp. 261–291). Thousand Oaks, CA: Sage Publications, Inc.

Rowles, G. D., & Ravdal, H. (in press). Aging, place and meaning in the face of changing circumstances. In R. S. Weiss & S. A. Bass (Eds.), *Challenges of the third age: Meaning and purpose in later life.* New York: Oxford University Press.

Rubinstein, R. L. (1989). The home environments of older people: A description of the psychosocial processes linking person to place. *Journals of Gerontology, 44,* S45–S53.

Russell, C. (1999). Interviewing vulnerable old people: Ethical and methodological implications of imagining our subjects. *Journal of Aging Studies, 13*(4), 403–417.

Russell, C. K. (1996). Passion and heretics: Meaning in life and quality of life of persons with dementia. *Journal of the American Geriatrics Society, 44*(11), 1400–1402.

Schein, E. H. (1987). *The clinical perspective in fieldwork.* Newbury Park, CA: Sage Publications, Inc.

Strauss, A. L., & Corbin, J. M. (1998). *Basics of qualitative research.* Thousand Oaks, CA: Sage Publications, Inc.

Schuster, E. (1996). Ethical considerations when conducting ethnographic research in a nursing home setting. *Journal of Aging Studies, 10*(1), 57–67.

Warren, C. A. B. (1988). *Gender issues in field research.* Newbury Park, CA: Sage Publications, Inc.

Wolcott, H. F. (1994). *Transforming qualitative data.* Thousand Oaks, CA: Sage Publications, Inc.

Young, H. M. (1998). Moving to congregate housing: The last chosen home. *Journal of Aging Studies, 12*(2), 149–165.

# CHAPTER SIX

# Online Ethnography: Studying Group Dynamics of a Virtual Community of Dementia Caregivers

## Margaret A. Perkinson[1]

Recent innovations in technology, especially computer technology, portend significant social change. Some have compared the impact of the Information Revolution with that of the Industrial Revolution in terms of the potential to change social structure, cultural norms, and basic social interaction (Meyrowitz, 1997; Wixon, Furlong, Poole, & Rossman, 1998). How will these changes affect older adults? Will advances in electronic technology further marginalize older adults and their caregivers or break down present barriers? Recent research indicates thousands of older adults have joined online communities (Wixon et al., 1998). These communities represent potentially significant sources of information, support, and friendship. How do these groups develop into communities, and what can they contribute to older populations, especially persons with dementia and their caregivers? How can we maximize their positive effects?

Electronic communities, in which group processes and identities are sustained solely through interactions via computer, are relatively new phenomena (Correll, 1995; Escobar, 1994). Nevertheless, the rapid proliferation of various web sites directed toward specific interest groups indicates that these communities are serving significant functions for growing numbers of site participants. What happens to the individuals who connect with each other through these sites? How do these groups develop and change over time? How do group processes within such electronic communities differ from traditional face-to-face groups?

Anthropologists have traditionally concerned themselves with the impact of technology and technological innovations on social structures and cultural change (Harris, 1968). A growing number of cultural anthropologists are examining the influence of recent trends in modern technology, including advances in computers and information technology, on the nature of contemporary social life (Escobar, 1994; Downey, Dumit, & Williams, 1995; Haraway, 1991; Pfaffenberger, 1992; Hess & Layne, 1992; Turkle, 1984; Rice-Lively, 1994; Rheingold, 1993; Shedletsky, 1993). Methods that were initially developed to describe and understand remote and exotic cultural groups and more recently modified to study subgroups in contemporary modern societies would seem well-suited to investigate the new social phenomena of electronic communities and cyberculture, as evidenced by many recent calls for online anthropological fieldwork (Escobar, 1994; Hakken, 1990, 1999; Ito, 1996; Jacobsen, 1996; Lea & Spears, 1995; Parks & Floyd, 1996; Walther, 1996). What can we learn about group processes and cultural practices of computer-mediated communities using ethnographic methods? Are these social processes and cultural phenomena significantly different from those occurring in traditional, face-to-face groups? What are the implications of these differences, especially for older adults and their caregivers?

## Computer-Mediated Communication

Proponents of medium theory suggest that media represent social contexts that foster different forms of interaction and social identity (Meyrowitz, 1997). Some have noted that social processes have undergone such fundamental changes within the expanded social environment of cyberculture that basic concepts, such as social interaction, social ties, identity, and experience must be re-examined and redefined (Cerulo, 1997; Escobar, 1994).

How does the electronic medium affect group processes and the nature of communication? What aspects of computer-mediated communication lead to basic changes in the nature of social interaction? A brief overview of various characteristics of computer-mediated communication will provide insight into these questions and suggest the special relevance of this mode of interaction for family caregivers of persons with dementia.

Online communication is convenient. It offers a vast potential for interactions with large numbers and diverse types of individuals for persons who are unable to get out. This is especially relevant for caregivers of persons with dementia who are themselves frequently homebound and socially isolated because they cannot leave their relative unattended.

Asynchronous communications, the fact that messages are not exchanged in real time, allow a busy caregiver to participate regardless of her or his schedule. In addition to offering valuable information on dementia and aspects of caregiving, online communities can provide respite and contact with the outside world for these family caregivers.

The nature of interaction within online communities differs from face-to-face interactions in ways that are distinctly advantageous for dementia caregivers. Since one has as much time as necessary to compose a posting, a participant can carefully craft his or her "presentation of self" (Correll, 1995; Goffman, 1959). One has greater control over the "front" that one presents, compared with face-to-face interactions. A participant can also exert greater control over the level or extent of interaction, and can choose to "lurk" or observe interactions without "coming out" or identifying him or herself as a member of the group. This is especially relevant for individuals who may perceive themselves as stigmatized by the characteristics that would qualify them for group membership.

Family caregivers of persons in the initial stages of dementia often attempt to "cover up" and maintain an image of health and well-being for that relative for as long as possible (Blum, 1991; Perkinson, 1995). All too often, identification with dementia leads to avoidance by previous acquaintances (who "feel uncomfortable") and to eventual social isolation. Spousal caregivers admit to this cover-up even within retirement communities that house significant numbers of caregiving peers (Perkinson, 1995). By choosing to do so, these beginning caregivers cut themselves off from significant sources of information and support, since dementia caregivers often avoid talking about dementia and their caregiving experiences with noncaregivers, persons who might not understand what the caregiver was experiencing (Perkinson, 1995). Online discussion groups for dementia caregivers solve this dilemma by allowing persons to either "lurk," observing interactions and learning from other caregivers without disclosing themselves, or to participate in discussions without "going public" within their "real life" social environment. The importance of safety inherent in computer-mediated communications has been noted with other stigmatized groups (Correll, 1995).

Online communication also renders certain aspects of social interaction irrelevant. Social markers are absent (unless one consciously chooses to describe them). Physical appearance, age, sex, race, ethnicity, and other markers of status or position are invisible and individuals can interact unencumbered by such "baggage." The nature of the medium allows participants to ignore various external qualities that often categorize individuals and strongly influence the nature and quality of face-to-face interactions. Online participants by necessity focus more on the content of the message and the style in which it is conveyed.

This "refocusing" of social interactions may change the very nature of social bonds. Observers have commented on the deep level of involvement that often characterizes online exchanges (Cerulo, 1997; Walther, 1996). A "new brand" of relationship often develops in which intimacy occurs at the earliest stage of interaction and information about core characteristics of one's inner self is exchanged prior to disclosure of more mundane facts. Computer-mediated communication has been described as having the potential to "surpass normal interpersonal levels," resulting in "hyper-personal" communication (Walther, 1996). Others have noted the difficulty of conveying emotions online (Correll, 1995; Galinsky, Schopler, & Abell, 1997). Online groups have developed various conventions to show emotions or express moods, such as stating facial expressions (wink, smile); using capital letters to express yelling; using tails: Mary . . . sad; and using emoticons, such as :) or :(, for happy or sad, respectively (Correll, 1995; Jacobsen, 1996). The nature of computer-mediated communication requires the statement of feelings or emotions in an explicit manner, if they are to be expressed at all. This forces computer-mediated social interaction to be less subtle, more outright, and subject to less miscommunication. This may also account for the accelerated development of close bonds (or, conversely, conflict), since even initial interactions are by necessity less neutral and ambiguous.

One's sense of self or identity also can undergo radical change within the online social environment. Because of the enhanced ability to craft or control one's presentation of self, an individual can actively reconstruct his or her identity or self if he or she desires (Riva & Galimberti, 1997; Turkle, 1995).

Online communities are serving the needs of a growing number of people, as evidenced by the proliferation of web sites. Many of these sites are electronic support groups (Bliss, Allibone, Bontempo, Flynn, & Valvano, 1998; Klemm & Nolan, 1998; Miller & Gergen, 1998; Sharf, 1997; Winzelberg, 1997), and many of these support groups are specifically for older adults or their caregivers (Brennan, Moore, & Smyth, 1995; Mahoney, 1998; Smyth & Harris, 1993; Wright, Bennet, & Gramling, 1998). These support groups have therapeutic potential, offering validation, sympathy, acceptance, encouragement, and advice (Miller & Gergen, 1998). Participation in these groups has been shown to reduce caregiving stress (Bass, McClendon, Brennan, & McCarthy, 1998) and result in positive developmental outcomes (Wright et al., 1998). During their brief history, online groups have proven to be effective, low-cost tools for supporting family caregivers.

Because online groups are so new, social processes that lead to a sense of online community and to positive individual outcomes remain relatively unexplored. In an effort to understand the group dynamics of one virtual community, qualitative methods were used to analyze archival data from an online Alzheimer's discussion group. The group began in 1994 and is the oldest and largest of its kind. Analysis of the group's archives offered a unique opportunity to identify and document social processes as they changed over time within this computer-mediated group for persons dealing with dementia.

## Research Design and Methods

A grounded-theory approach was employed to analyze the archived data (Glaser & Strauss, 1967; Strauss, 1987). Rather than test specific hypotheses, this approach allows for the generation of hypotheses based on concepts and patterns that are "grounded" in the data. Nevertheless, this was not a totally inductive approach. The research interests stated above led to a variety of questions concerning group processes, emergent culture, online "careers," and shared strategies or norms for evaluating and managing dementia symptoms. Group processes investigated included: the negotiation of group values, norms, and goals; the development of conventions, especially those concerning communication, such as communicating emotions; the use of sanctions for inappropriate postings; mechanisms for establishing legitimacy and authority within the group; the development of various roles (e.g., jokester, medical authority, nurturing comforter, role models, leaders); and the communication process (e.g., the nature of discussions, disagreements, agreements, and norms concerning self-disclosure). Special attention was directed toward group processes that seemed to promote a sense of group cohesiveness and community.

In order to understand the processes that initiated community development within the group, analysis focused on the first year of archived postings. Even with this more focused approach, approximately 1,500 pages of text were available to be analyzed. The strategy for analysis was based on a two-step framework suggested by Miles and Huberman (1984), Lofland and Lofland (1984), and Strauss (1987). The first step entailed basic, categorical coding of the archived data. A code represents an abbreviation applied to a segment (e.g., a sentence or paragraph) of the archival data to classify or label that segment. A code is essentially a category (i.e., "a concept unifying a number of observations [or bits of data] having some characteristic in common") (Dey, 1993). For example, in coding the data for a category such as self-disclosure, an instance of a message revealing that the sender was 75 years old would be identified by the code SELF-DISCLOSURE-AGE. One of the goals in coding would be to identify all major types of self-disclosure.

One may create a "start list" of specific codes prior to fieldwork. However, this project began with a more general scheme for codes, a set of guiding questions (see above) that pointed to general domains in which codes would be inductively developed (Miles & Huberman, 1984). After an initial reading of the data set, a 6-page list of codes was generated, along with an accompanying 23-page codebook describing what each code meant. Once the codebook was developed and revised, each posting or segment of a posting was assigned its appropriate code or codes. These codes served as devices for organizing and retrieving data (Miles & Huberman, 1984). The computer program, The Ethnograph, was employed to assist in the mechanics of data management and retrieval by pulling out and assembling all segments in the data set that were assigned similar codes.

Coding is a first level of analysis, simply naming, classifying, or summarizing segments of data. As one reviews the assembled group of similarly coded segments, one searches for "repeatable regularities." In so doing, one identifies emergent themes or patterns, explanations that "pull a lot of material together into more meaningful and parsimonious units of analysis" (Miles & Huberman, 1984, pp. 67–68). "Pattern coding" groups codes into smaller numbers of overarching themes. For example, one theme associated with the earlier example of online self-disclosure indicated that caregivers engaged in self-disclosure under certain circumstances (e.g., they revealed professional credentials as a means of establishing authority or the legitimacy of their statements).

Patterns began to emerge, prompting the writing of "memos" (i.e., "the theorizing write-up of ideas about codes and their relationships") (Glaser, 1978). To elaborate, the major types of self-disclosure could be identified and the contexts in which each type occurred revealed, leading to a "theory of context for self-disclosure." In writing memos, one moves from the data to a more conceptual level, expanding codes, showing relationships among categories, and developing more integrated theory about events, processes, and outcomes (Miles & Huberman, 1984).

## The Process of Community Development: Negotiation of Group Norms

*Early Focus on Communication Style and Format.*   Early postings within the dementia list reflected an emerging articulation of group norms by both the list moderator and the group participants. These norms were guidelines or standards that indicated what did or did not represent an appropriate communication or posting. Some online behaviors were clearly taboo. For example, those attempting to advertise or sell products or reproduce published material in a posting (thus violating copyright laws) received unambiguous feedback from the list moderator and other list members, sanctioning such online transgressions. "Grassroots" decisions on what should not be posted were also reflected in various participants' concerns with "tying up the group," prompting some to opt for private communications through personal email when discussing topics that pertained to a small minority of group members. Others expressed concern over the "clutter" that had begun to accumulate on the site, and requested that members not fill up the list with what they perceived to be less essential items, such as confirmation notices. As they continued to define group norms regarding posting behavior, individual participants explicitly asked for feedback (e.g., wondering "out loud" whether a posting was too detailed or lengthy). The appropriate tone of a posting, as well as its content, was also subject to debate. One participant apologized for being "too blunt," and was promptly assured by another that it was good to "be upfront." While representing only a small proportion of the communications exchanged, these and other similar postings represented a negotiation of group norms, as various individuals commented on past online behaviors and how things should or should not be done. In the early months of the group, most of these normative statements and feedback pertained to style or format of communication.

*Expanding the Negotiation of Norms: What Is Appropriate Discourse?*   After an accumulated history of 8 months of online interactions, the process of negotiation of group norms underwent a significant change. A seemingly innocent request for information on medications prompted a "thread" of discussion that revealed significant subdivisions within the group and elicited explicit attempts to define the purpose of the list and the roles of its subgroups in contributing to those goals.

  It all started when a "newbie" introduced herself to the list and requested information from the group:

I have a mother in her early 70s who is in the middle stages (as I understand it) of Alzheimer's. I am interested in the newer generation of Alzheimer's medications that I read are coming into the market. Does anyone have information on what they are, what their status is, etc.

A physician promptly responded, describing his strategy and rationale for treating persons with Alzheimer's disease (AD). Although his posting was sent as a reply to the family caregiver's inquiry, it was worded in the manner of one medical professional addressing another. Using fairly technical jargon and concluding with his own request for additional information on drug interactions and side effects, the posting seemed directed toward medical experts in the audience:

> I have started treating most of my AD patients with tacrine plus deprenyl, theorizing that any benefit they get may be through different mechanisms and (perhaps) additive. There does not seem to be any undue toxicity associated with the combination, but I have seen no dramatic improvement, either. I am thinking of trying to add nicotine (gum or patch) or nimodipine. Any experience with this? Would side effects likely be less with nicotine, or might it exacerbate tacrine-related GI side effects? Is hypotension with nimodipine a major concern? Any other candidates for polypharmacy, like lecithin or vitamin E?

A member of a pharmacology department at a major university echoed the physician's questions concerning the therapeutic effects of the nicotine patch or gum on dementia. A second physician, the medical director of a memory program in a major U.S. university, promptly replied to both, describing in fairly technical terms the combination of drugs he used to treat patients. He concluded with a comment on the lack of rigorous, large-scale studies on the effects of using combinations of drugs, even though he felt polypharmacy for AD "makes sense." In the absence of large-scale clinical trials, he concluded that practitioners had little choice but to rely on case studies of combination therapies:

> Combination therapy makes sense since these drugs are believed to work by different mechanisms. Unfortunately, drug manufacturers won't support studies involving a "competitor's product". . . . I have added nimodipine (30 or 60 mg tid) to tacrine in an open-label pilot project with no untoward effects. Hypotension has not been a problem in these patients. Using lecithin with tacrine dates back to the early studies of THA [*Note:* A reference from a professional journal was provided to support this claim]. Some studies claimed increased benefit of the combination over THA alone, but (for unknown reasons) lecithin has not been used in any recent tacrine trials. In

general, the idea of polypharmacy in AD makes sense. However, the benefit of any of these agents is modest and it would take a very large patient population . . . to show a significant (cumulative) benefit from using them in combination. Until that happens, it is likely that combination therapies will remain case-report material.

In the middle of the technical debate among the physicians and pharmacist on combination drug therapy, two librarians posted information on a new caregiver publication that identified "emotional support resources" on the Internet for persons facing various chronic illnesses, including AD. A family caregiver's subsequent comment on this announcement implied her disappointment with the list in meeting emotional needs. Coming so quickly after the polypharmacy debate, and contrasting so dramatically in tone from that debate, the family caregiver's comments seemed to criticize the highly technical and somewhat impersonal discourse of the medical professionals:

> When seeing this posting this morning of the Guide to Emotional Support Resources I thought this ironic, since I thought that this list would itself be an emotional support resource when I subscribed.

This caregiver then introduced herself, spoke vividly of her personal suffering as a caregiver, and asked for help from the group:

> I am a primary caregiver for my aunt, who has advanced AD. She will soon be leaving my care to go and live in a board-and-care facility. . . . While I anticipate relief from daily caregiving, I am suffering from the knowledge that I am really losing her now . . . and her presence is my constant reminder of this suffering. I vacillate between looking beyond the present, to the future, and at the same time valuing these last days with her. This causes me to live on a kind of emotional seesaw. I would like to hear others' ideas on making it through this transition.

The list moderator promptly responded that emotional support was one function of the list, but reminded all that it was up to the subscribers to make the group what they wanted:

> (This list) *is* provided, in part, as an emotional support list. But there are many, many other places on the net that readers can also go to for information and support. (This list) is what its subscribers make it; more personal experience notes have to come from the readers, if that's what they want. . . .

A family caregiver commented on this debate and his perceptions of the purpose of the group. Testifying from personal experience, he spoke with gratitude about the powerful effect of the postings from group members who had shared both "technical" information and emotional support. Far from viewing these postings as impersonal exchanges, he referred to his online interactions as "talking to real people":

> "Talking" to the people on this list, both publicly and privately got me through a very difficult period over the last couple of months. All the self-help and support data can't take the place of talking to real people who can share technical information or provide a shoulder to lean on. Thanks, (list moderator), for making this list happen. And thanks to those who shared their thoughts and support to me over the last few months.

The next day, a third physician joined the earlier debate on polypharmacy in a lengthy, technical, and highly critical posting:

> Coming in late on this discussion, what's being proposed here seems naive at best. No series of anecdotes is going to establish whether a given therapy benefits your patients with AD. When pushed by behavior problems, we have to react empirically (though good studies are in process). To almost randomly throw meds, some of which are demonstrably ineffective and have no theoretical basis, at AD patients in hopes of transient cognitive benefits seems wholly irrational.

This physician continued and, in a discussion phrased in medical jargon, evaluated the available research on each of the individual drugs (nicotine, lecithin, etc.) mentioned in the earlier postings. Finding no compelling evidence at this point to prescribe these drugs, he concluded that physicians should consider other costs of polypharmacy:

> Finally, in addition to pharmacological and physiologic toxicities of these therapeutic adventures, one should consider the stress required by frequent monitoring visits and the VERY high cost for therapy that may not have any effect. As physicians, we often forget that one of the main side effects of our prescribing is poverty.

In an immediate reply, the physician who had initiated this debate responded to each point in this "scolding and condescending" post, in another lengthy and highly technical discussion (complete with bibliography). After discussing the merits of the available research, he concluded on a more philosophical note, pondering physicians' appropriate course of action given the incomplete data at hand:

> Ignoring Dr. _____'s scolding and condescending tone, I see this as an example of philosophical differences which often divides physicians. From a

scientific perspective, it is absolutely correct to say, we don't *know* something works until it is thoroughly studied. From a clinical perspective we often do what we think *might* work based on the incomplete data available. Alzheimer's is a terminal illness and patients and their families look to us to try to help them to the best of our abilities. When confronted with the question of whether there isn't *something* we can do, I am not comfortable sitting on my hands and saying nothing. (I also think it's *wrong*) Correct me if I'm wrong, but don't oncologists often embark on such therapeutic "adventures?" Like Dr. _____, I await the verdict of science. The question is what to do until the verdict comes in.

The next day, a family caregiver, while expressing appreciation for the diversity of the list participants, made highly critical comments of physicians as generally ignoring the psychosocial consequences of dementia. He voiced the "distance" he felt from the polypharmacy debate, and believed this discussion exemplified health professionals' disregard and lack of empathy for both patients and their caregivers:

I appreciate the diversity of this list: from practitioners and caregivers to clinicians and physicians. And I appreciate the empathy recently demonstrated by concerned list members to my dilemma as a caregiver. What I can offer is from my experience, and is for all.

He proceeded to describe a recent book that reinforced his stance on physicians. The book claimed that:

(Doctors) . . . treat the body as separate from the social being, and generally are unaware (or are prevented from being so) of the social consequences for the patient (or their families and concerned others) of their actions (and in general, those of the health care community). . . . What does this have to do with being an AD caregiver? I think we need to talk about it, and not feel that we are the only ones having a hard time (because we are just not strong enough, or clever or inventive enough). I bring this out because of the distance I personally feel from the physicians discussing pharmacological treatments for patients with AD. AD begins and ends with profound social consequences for those involved with an AD sufferer. (Yes, poverty is a side-effect of not just pharmacological treatment, but caregiving: depletion of mental and emotional resources). While I realize that physicians treat the diseased person, not their caregivers, I suggest that the caregiver becomes part of the AD patient as their 'alter-mind,' i.e., the caregiver makes meaning of the world for the AD patient, through interpretation, through empathy, through all of the many ways that the caregiver functions. Sometimes these functions are so subtle that we are not even overtly aware of them, only the feeling of being drained reminds us that we are really living for two minds, attempting to clarify the confusion, calm the anxiety, and provide comfort in the face of fear. It's hard work.

Shortly after this posting, the second physician in the AD drug debate expressed regret over the polypharmacological discussion. Although he believed such discussions among doctors were very important and should continue, he questioned whether the list was the appropriate setting for these debates. He feared list readers might misinterpret physicians' technical and sometimes speculative discussions and cautioned medical professionals to "be a bit more careful" about debating "in public":

> In looking over the postings from Dr. _____, Dr. _____, and myself on the subject of polypharmacy, I wonder if this is an appropriate setting for this type of exchange. This list seems to primarily be for, and composed of, caregivers. Those folks have to read our arguments. My first thought on reading Joe's response was that the shrill disapproving tone was intended for the caregivers who might see such a speculative discourse as a reason for renewed hope. That was certainly not the intention of this discussion. I do think that it is important for doctors to debate issues like these but we should be a bit more careful when doing so in public.

In this posting, he essentially called into question the identity and goals of the group. Should it focus primarily on addressing the emotional and information needs of the majority of its participants, the family caregivers, or should it also provide a forum for professional debates on dementia-related issues, including cutting-edge but currently unresolved topics? Should the "lay caregiver" be exposed to the often heated arguments and "speculative discourse" of medical professionals as these professionals attempt to make sense of the disease and piece together a reasonable plan of treatment?

The posting elicited a flood of comments in which participants, almost all of whom were family caregivers, expressed their appreciation and interest in medical debates and their desire for the list to remain "inclusive." In these postings, members explicitly stated their perceptions of (and hopes for) the purpose of the list. Most believed it should not be limited to either "a professional forum or a caregiver forum," but should be open to all, with the intent that both subgroups could benefit from exposure to the perspectives of the other (an exposure that did not often occur in the "real world"):

> I guess I am just a dumb caregiver. In reading all the stuff on polypharmacy, my conclusion is that there are still different opinions and still much research

to be done. At this point in my life, I feel that is all I need to know. I enjoy reading the messages from the researchers—even though in technical language. I feel I learn from them, but don't ask me to explain a message. I thought the original intent of the board was to provide a broad spectrum of information—from professionals to researchers to social workers and caregivers. My personal feeling is to see it continue that way it was last month. A little bit of stuff for all aspects of AD.

In spite of the misgivings expressed earlier by the physician, family caregivers in the group did not want to be sheltered from the "bad news" of ineffective treatments. Witnessing the online debates and musings of physicians and researchers as they grappled with various issues gave caregivers greater insight into "the mood, frustration, hope, and uncertainty" of the health care community in dealing with dementia. As one family caregiver wrote:

As the son of an AD victim, I am most interested in the type of discussions carried on by the health care professionals on the list. Aside from the knowledge gained from reading the messages, I find I am better able to understand the mood, frustration, hope, and uncertainty that the health care community deals with in trying to understand and treat the disease and to help the families cope with the problems related to the disease. . . . I think that those of us involved as primary and secondary caregivers have a thirst for knowledge on the subject. Dr. _____ may want to protect the non-professional from the frequently *bad news* about ineffective treatments and/or he may think that non-professionals will be confused or mistakenly encouraged by technical details of the issues discussed. However well intentioned his reasons for suggesting that technical discussions should not be held on the list, I would be disappointed if these discussions were curtailed.

Another family caregiver seconded the above posting: "An absolutely! to John's plea for 'hard' information." The list moderator also voiced her hopes for the list and how both groups could benefit from exposure to the experiences and perspectives of each other:

Many of us push for the practitioner to see the "client" (aka "patient") as a unit—i.e., the person with the disease plus significant others. From diagnosis to treatment, little can be done effectively without the caregiver(s)'s involvement. . . . And yes, the personal "burden" on the caregiver(s) can be quite significant and should not be underestimated. This is one of the reasons why I would prefer the list remain more inclusive—practitioners gain from hearing the experience and frustration of caregivers, and caregivers gain from hearing the knowledge (and frustration regarding inadequate information base) of practitioners.

A newcomer to the list from the United Kingdom reflected on the individual postings and the group's collective efforts to define the goals of the list. He observed that the difficulties of the two subgroups (i.e., health professionals and family caregivers) in communicating online and defining the nature of their appropriate roles on the list reflected similar problems between the two groups in the "real world," and suggested reasons for these difficulties:

> I have only been reading the comments for the last 10 days but have been fascinated by the discussion on the role of this list in regard to whether it is a professional forum or a caregiver support group. It mirrors exactly the ambivalent attitudes that prevail in the U.K. at present. . . . The problem as I see it centers around the often diametrically different attitudes of the professional and the carer. All medical students from the earliest days of training are taught that an attitude of professional detachment and rigorous clinical assessment of unproven therapies is essential for a career as a physician. It is not . . . possible to make the correct clinical judgements while one's mind is clouded by empathy or unwarranted enthusiasm. For this reason physicians are uncomfortable with empathy and unhappy with sharing thoughts with patients/clients. The family caregiver, on the other hand, has different priorities. They realize the essential part that empathy plays, especially in AD, and which is so clearly demonstrated by the messages from carers to this list over the past few days and they also have the *need* to be as fully informed as possible. Hence the difficulty of communication between the professional and carer evidenced in this list recently . . . professionals must be aware of the hunger that carers have for, firstly, understanding as far as that is possible and, secondly, for the emotional support that hope can bring. . . . On behalf of the families involved in this most cruel of diseases, I beg the professionals not to desert a multi-functional list such as this on the grounds that it is not a true professional forum. For the advancement in humane understanding of AD, if not its clinical resolution, they are an essential part of the dialogue that must co-exist between professional and family unit.

A spousal caregiver agreed that the list should be open to the postings and points of view of all concerned with AD. Although he did not always understand the technical debates of the health professionals, their discussions gave him a glimpse of the effort and dedication with which they approached their work. This was comforting and a source of hope for him:

> My choice is to have it opened to all who are concerned with AD and related dementias. When one professional questions another professional I do not see that as bickering—I see it as two people who are concerned about AD

and are really trying to do something positive. As a caregiver, it gives me great hope that some professionals are truly trying to help. I know it is too late for any help for my wife, but I pray that soon, nobody else will have to suffer the way she has, and the way I have. When I read here the messages of two or more different professionals who disagree with a medication, a potential cure, or a method of determining accurately who is high risk for AD, it gives me some relief of the worry I have for my children and grandchildren. Even though I may not fully understand what these professionals are talking about, I know they care and are trying. I see this forum as a great hope for all caregivers, and also for the professional members. . . . I still need additional help, and that is why I joined the board. It is a necessary part of my daily life to check and see if I have any email waiting for me. Even though I don't understand the message, it does help me as I know on a daily basis that others are concerned about my wife and me.

Other caregivers echoed these sentiments:

Over the past several months I have been reading both the caregiver and professional comments. Both are very important to me. I am a secondary caregiver for my mother who has AD. To be able to not only read how other caregivers are coping but also to read about the debates about possible research breakthroughs helps me to cope much better with my own situation.

In addressing his comments to the physician who had earlier questioned whether the list was an appropriate forum for professional debates, yet another family caregiver echoed earlier postings that the list should be open to all:

Joe: I appreciated your concern for the caregivers subscribed to this list. However, I'm concerned that the absence of such discourse would further contribute to the already existing separation between physician and patient or caregiver. . . . Personally, I am glad that physicians are willing to discuss their approach, methodology, visions, and concerns about the treatment of AD through this medium. Reading these discussions makes me feel that someone is trying very hard to "slay" the monster even if I could not follow all of it. I hope that this list serves to unite us all against this disease and at the same time provide the space for physicians, caregivers, and support givers to make their unique contributions and have their needs met.

## Conclusion

This dementia list began in 1994, when the Internet was relatively new to the general public. At that time, there were few existing online groups to serve as models. As one of the first online groups devoted to dementia and free to all interested parties, this foray into computer-mediated communication began as an attempt to efficiently disseminate the rapidly growing body of information on dementia and quickly evolved into a rather cohesive interactive community of professionals and lay caregivers.

An examination of the first year of the list archives revealed a change in the nature of communication from early postings of relatively impersonal questions and their replies to later disclosures of intensely personal encounters with dementia and a bonding among those who shared similar experiences. Through various comments (especially from newcomers to the list) asking for guidelines and through feedback from participants reflecting on what they thought was or was not appropriate for the list, the members of the group forged a generally shared sense of standards for online behavior.

Early comments focused on the basics of online communications—comments on the appropriate length and tone of a posting and what did or did not represent "clutter" or irrelevant communications. Well into the first year of its existence, reactions to a heated debate over the use of combinations of drugs for dementia revealed significant divisions within the list. This debate forced participants to consider basic questions regarding group membership, the appropriate content of postings and manner of online communications, and the essential goals or purpose of the group. Participants engaged in the negotiation of group norms as they discussed what they wanted from the list and openly testified to the benefits they had derived from it.

The medium—the fact that these debates and testimonials occurred online—had a major impact on the nature of group processes. Since all communication was written and participants had time to compose their thoughts and examine the communications of others, the negotiation of standards or norms for online communication was undoubtedly more explicit, self-conscious, and deliberate than typically occurs within face-to-face groups.

The online group offered obvious benefits in providing the opportunity for medical researchers and practitioners to exchange their latest findings and debate the pros and cons of various therapeutic practices. Dementia-family caregivers, many of whom admitted they were essentially housebound due to their caregiving duties, were given the opportunity to interact with a wide variety of caregivers who could readily empathize with their situation, offer concrete suggestions for dealing with particular problems, and provide sincere encouragement. The list also offered caregivers an opportunity to give support, as well as be supported. Several stated that this chance to "pay back" to others the support they had received earlier was part of "the healing process."

As important as these interactions were, they were not unique to the list. Health professionals can meet at professional conferences and seminars to exchange ideas and treatment strategies; family caregivers can do likewise in support groups. The list served to facilitate these interactions and enabled them to occur in a more convenient and extended manner.

The unique and seemingly unprecedented contribution of this new medium of online communication, as experienced through this particular list with its open-membership policy, was creation of a social arena in which categories of individuals who typically live very separate lives in the "real world" and whose face-to-face interactions were limited and highly circumscribed if they occurred at all, were exposed on an extended basis to the perspectives of each other. Family caregivers could observe current debates among physicians and researchers over medical treatments and thus better understand professionals' decision making—the lack of certainty, the diversity of opinion, the kinds of evidence on which they base their decisions, and the intensity and dedication with which many approach these issues.

Health professionals (researchers and clinicians), on the other hand, were exposed to intensely personal accounts of living with dementia and its vividly real and heart-breaking impact on everyday life and relationships. They undoubtedly gained insight into the needs, frustrations, and rewards of family caregiving.

In a world in which health professionals and lay caregivers are relatively isolated from each other's perspectives, online group interactions offered the opportunity to break down that separation and allowed members of each group much needed insight into the perspectives of the other. In the process of defining and negotiating the group's norms and articulating its goals, the participants in the list sensed the tremendous opportunity offered by the group. This was undoubtedly the reason that so many clamored for the continued presence of both groups, with unfettered debates open to all.

## Acknowledgments

[1]This research was funded as the study, "Group Dynamics of a Virtual Community of AD Caregivers," through the Washington University School of Medicine Alzheimer's Disease Research Center, National Insti-

tute on Aging grant P50-AG51681. The assistance of Joy Kiefer, PhD, throughout the course of this work is gratefully acknowledged.

# REFERENCES

Bass, D. M., McClendon, M. J., Brennan, P. F., & McCarthy, C. (1998). The buffering effect of a computer support network on caregiver strain. *Journal of Aging and Health, 10*(1), 20–43.

Bliss, J., Allibone, C., Bontempo, B., Flynn, T., & Valvano, N. E. (1998). Creating a web site for on-line social support melanocyte. *Computers in Nursing, 16*(4), 203–207.

Blum, N. (1991). The management of stigma by Alzheimer family caregivers. *Journal of Contemporary Ethnography, 20,* 539–543.

Brennan, P., Moore, S., & Smyth, K. (1995). Alzheimer's disease caregivers' use of a computer network. *Western Journal of Nursing Research, 14*(5), 662–673.

Cerulo, K. A. (1997). Reframing sociological concepts for a brave new (virtual?) world. *Sociological Inquiry, 67*(1), 48–58.

Correll, S. (1995). The ethnography of an electronic bar: The lesbian cafe. *Journal of Contemporary Ethnography, 24*(3), 270–298.

Dey, J. (1993). *Qualitative data analysis.* London: Routledge.

Downey, G., Dumit, J., & Williams, S. (1995). Cyborg anthropology. *Cultural Anthropology, 10*(2), 264–269.

Downey, G., Dumit, J., & Traweek, S. (in press). *Cyborgs and citadels: Anthropological interventions into technocultures.* Santa Fe, NM: School of American Research Press.

Escobar, A. (1994). Welcome to cyberia: Notes on the anthropology of cyberculture. *Current Anthropology, 35*(3), 211–231.

Galinsky, M. J., Schopler, J. H., & Abell, M. D. (1997). Connecting group members through telephone and computer groups. *Health & Social Work, 22*(3), 181–188.

Glaser, B. G. (1978). *Theoretical sensitivity.* Mill Valley, CA: The Sociology Press.

Glaser, B. G., & Strauss, A. (1967). *The discovery of grounded theory: Strategies for qualitative research.* Chicago: Aldine Publishing Company.

Goffman, E. (1959). *The presentation of self in everyday life.* Garden City, NY: Anchor Books.

Hakken, D. (1990). Has there been a computer revolution? *Journal of Computing and Society, 1*(1), 13–30.

Hakken, D. (1999). *Cyborgs @ cyberspace?: An ethnographer looks to the future.* New York: Routledge.

Haraway, D. (1991). *Simians, cyborgs, and women: The reinvention of nature.* New York: Routledge.

Harris, M. (1968). *The rise of anthropological theory.* New York: Thomas Y. Crowell Co.

Hess, D., & Layne, L. (Ed.). (1992). *Knowledge and society.* Greenwich, CT: JAI Press.

Ito, M. (1996). Theory, method, and design in anthropologies of the Internet. *Social Science Computer Review, 14*(1), 24–26.

Jacobsen, D. (1996). Contexts and cues in cyberspace: The pragmatics of naming in text-based virtual realities. *Journal of Anthropological Research, 52,* 461–479.

Klemm, P., & Nolan, M. (1998). Internet cancer support groups: Legal and ethical issues for nurse researchers. *Oncology Nursing Forum, 25*(4), 673–676.

Lea, M., & Spears, R. (1995). Love at first byte? Building personal relationships over computer networks. In J. T. Wood & S. Duck (Eds.), *Under-studied relationships: Off the beaten track.* Thousand Oaks, CA: Sage Publications, Inc.

Lofland, J., & Lofland, L. H. (1984). *Analyzing social settings: A guide to qualitative observation and analysis* (2nd ed.). Belmont, CA: Wadsworth Publishing Company, Inc.

Mahoney, D. M. (1998). Using a website for qualitative gerontological research: Issues and recommendations. Paper presented at the Gerontological Society of America, Philadelphia, PA.

Meyrowitz, J. (1997). Shifting worlds of strangers: Medium theory and changes in "them" versus "us." *Sociological Inquiry, 67*(1), 59–71.

Miles, M., & Huberman, A. M. (1984). *Qualitative data analysis.* Beverly Hills, CA: Sage Publications, Inc.

Miller, J. K., & Gergen, K. J. (1998). Life on the line: The therapeutic potentials of computer-mediated conversation. *Journal of Marital and Family Therapy, 24*(2), 189–202.

Parks, M. R., & Floyd, K. (1996). Making friends in cyberspace. *Journal of Computer-Mediated Communication, 1*(4), 1–15.

Perkinson, M. A. (1995). Socialization to the family caregiving role within a continuing care retirement community. *Medical Anthropology, 16,* 249–267.

Pfaffenberger, B. (1992). The social anthropology of technology. *Annual Review of Anthropology, 21,* 491–516.

Rheingold, H. (1993). *The virtual community: Homesteading on the electronic frontier.* Reading, MA: Addison-Wesley.

Rice-Lively, M. L. (1994). Wired warp and woof: An ethnographic study of a networking class. *Internet Research, 4*(4), 20–35.

Riva, G., & Galimberti, C. (1997). The psychology of cyberspace: A socio-cognitive framework to computer-mediated communication. *New Ideas in Psychology, 15*(2), 141–158.

Sharf, B. (1997). Communicating breast cancer on-line: Support and empowerment on the Internet. *Women and Health, 26,* 65–83.

Shedletsky, L. (1993). Minding computer mediated communication: CMC as experiential learning. *Educational Technology, 33*(12), 5–10.

Smyth, K. A., & Harris, P. B. (1993). Using telecomputing to provide information and support to caregivers of persons with dementia. *The Gerontologist, 33*(1), 123–127.

Strauss, S. G. (1987). *Qualitative analysis for social scientists.* Cambridge, MA: University Press.

Turkle, S. (1984). *The second self: Computers and the human spirit.* New York: Simon and Schuster.

Turkle, S. (1995). *Life on the screen: Identity in the age of the Internet.* New York: Simon & Schuster.

Walther, J. B. (1996). Computer-mediated communication: Impersonal, interpersonal, and hyperpersonal interaction. *Communication Research, 23*(1), 3–43.

Winzelberg, A. (1997). The analysis of an electronic support group for individuals with eating disorders. *Computers in Human Behavior, 13*(3), 393–407.

Wright, L. K., Bennet, G., & Gramling, L. (1998). Telecommunication interventions for caregivers of elders with dementia. *Advances in Nursing Science, 20*(3), 76–88.

Wixon, A., Furlong, M., Poole, T., & Rossman, L. (1998). A brave new world for elders: Building community on the Internet. Symposium presented at the 44th annual meeting of the American Society on Aging, San Francisco, CA.

# PART IV

# "Let's Talk"

# Introduction

## Nancy E. Schoenberg

In-depth interviews have a long-established place in qualitative research. Although the manifold ways of performing in-depth interviewing sometimes make this technique difficult to define and characterize, a common goal for most in-depth interviews is the collection of rich, person-centered, contextualized data through a collaborative participant-researcher effort based on good rapport. While some qualitative interviews consist of open-ended or semistructured questions appended onto larger structured interview schedules, more typically, in-depth interviews attempt to obtain a more profound level of understanding on a focused topic (Rubinstein, 1988). In addition, in order to represent accurately the analytic categories and perspectives of the research participant, in-depth interviewers often attempt to minimize, or at least make explicit, a priori assumptions. Put another way, in-depth interviewers often seek to understand the types and meaning of categories that people use to organize their lifeworlds (the *emic* approach) without preconceived notions from the researcher (the *etic* approach). Logically, such an orientation assumes the active agency of the participant in contrast with a more prestructured "empty vessel" approach to data collecting (see Gubrium & Holstein, chapter 8).

Another feature common to most in-depth interviews is the goal of capturing a rich and colorful mosaic of data, including extensive background on an individual's context and personal situation. Although it is possible to obtain insights about the topic of interest, as well as the environmental and personal characteristics of a research participant in one interview session, the in-depth interview process tends to be rather complex and often absorbs substantial amounts of time. As noted by Kaufman (1994, p. 128):

> Data emerge in the process of dialogue, negotiation, and understanding. Both co-producers will come to that dialogue with attitudes, values, personal

agendas, and conceptual frameworks that find their way into the context of the interview as it unfolds over time.

Consistent with a holistic and integrative approach, analyses often are conducted throughout data collection.

## The Nature of the Interviewer

Person-centered, meaning-oriented interviewing has been described as a concert performance and the qualified interviewer as a musician (Levy & Hollan, 1998). Prior to the actual performance of the piece, the interviewer must possess social, psychological, and interpersonal skills that facilitate optimal performance. Being able to read sheet music in no way assures a successful performance. Equally, familiarity with the mechanics of interviewing techniques does not insure a successful and illuminating in-depth interview.

Rather, skilled interviewers generally maintain a series of attributes—some acquired with experience and study and others seemingly inherent to the nature of the researcher—that generate a productive data-generating collaboration. These attributes include not only fundamental linguistic competence and the knack of showing up at the right time and place, but also the ability to engender trust, a true belief in the participant's expertise on the topics, and an understanding of and respect for local customs and norms.

While few would dispute the need for researchers to be conversant with the open-ended questions they will ask the participant or the need to wipe their feet at the door to someone's home, other unresolved and more controversial issues surround the interviewer. One of these issues is the insider/outsider debate, whether it is desirable for interviewer and interviewee to be matched according to significant personal characteristics (i.e., matching an Hispanic interviewer with an Hispanic elder, a female interviewer with an older woman, etc.). When a research participant is a member of a traditionally subordinated group, one could speculate that there might be a greater comfort level. Describing her return to her hometown of Eatonville, Florida, in 1929, anthropologist Zora Neale Hurston writes presciently about this debate, providing compelling testimony on why an outsider interviewer may obtain few insights from the group to which she is an insider.

And the Negro, in spite of his open-faced laughter, his seeming acquiescence, is particularly evasive. You see we are a polite people and we do not say to

our questioner, "Get out of here!" We smile and tell him or her something
that satisfies the white person because, knowing so little about us, he does
not know what he is missing. . . . The Negro offers a feather-bed resistance.
That is, we let the probe enter, but it never comes out. It gets smothered
under a lot of laughter and pleasantries" (1935, p. 4).

Others have warned against studying ones' own, owing to the potential for lack of objectivity and the inability to scrutinize perspectives and
circumstances if one assumes them to be "normal" (Myerhoff, 1978).
While far from resolved, few experienced interviewers contest that the
best way to generate meaningful data is to convey trustworthiness, reciprocity, and sincerity through active listening, respectful interaction,
and careful preparation.

## Sequencing and Approach

As in all study designs, the research question and desired outcome
shapes the research plan (with some flexibility due to logistical constraints, such as time and other resources). Interviewers sometimes
differ on the time input desirable for each research participant, although most would recommend as much time as possible. Some researchers claim that, since the degree to which rapport is established
directly relates to the quality of data elicited, extensive time needs to
be spent with each research participant. Other researchers propose
that excellent, pretested questions posed by a skilled interviewer can
streamline the number of sessions necessary to gather meaningful insights. Yet others maintain a relativistic stance—that the protocol depends on the study aims that, in turn, determine the number, breadth,
and depth of the interview sessions. These perspectives are not mutually exclusive.

Lack of preexisting guidelines and vague predictions, such as "When
you begin to make meaning, you will know . . . " can be frustrating
to those just getting started in the process of in-depth interviewing.
Moreover, a lack of prescribed number or expected time expenditure
may even foster the perception that in-depth interviews lack procedural
rigor. From the perspective that in-depth interviews seek to create meaning through collaborative discussion and trustful rapport, each session
represents an unfolding of meaning. To determine the exact number
of sessions requires taking into account the preparation and skill of the
interviewer, the nature of the topic, the bonds between the researcher-
participant, and the precision and validity of the questions.

Since the questions that comprise the in-depth interviews are designed to initiate and sustain discussion, the researcher often must invest a significant amount of time in order to create the interview protocol and must be an active and involved listener. A specific and well-crafted set of questions and a conversational exchange have the capacity to elicit the participant's sense of meaning.

> The multidimensional sense of identity proposed to be the intervening process in this research is not residing in an individual's memory bank, waiting to be printed out if we can discover the right command. Rather, this sense of self is more like an incomplete, fragmented, and usually simply understood theory of one's life. When confronted with a particular set of questions by the social scientist, this theory is articulated, more-or-less completely (Dressler, 1991, p. 291).

In summary, it is worthwhile to maximize the potential to elicit what, at first glance, appear to be extraneous comments or tangential stories, as these often provide telling insights into a participant's lifeworld. An engaging dialogue invites participants to construct their meaning in the presence of the researcher, rather than simply providing "just specific answers to specific questions" (Rubinstein, 1988, p. 131).

## Ethical Considerations and the Interview Relationship

As in all qualitative inquiry, researchers who engage in in-depth interviewing often encounter ethical situations that may, less often, confront researchers who remain more detached from their participants. During in-depth interviewing, gathering personal, intimate, and sometimes potentially harmful information about people's lives is often routine, since the researcher and participant often develop an interaction based on trust and driven by the desire to learn and to self-disclose. As a result, ethically sensitive situations often arise. Steps need to be taken:

> . . . on the part of the researcher to ensure that the research does not harm the participant and that the privileged position of access granted the researcher will not be used to the participant's detriment . . . (Sankar & Gubrium, 1994, xiv).

As Rubinstein cautions (see chapter 7), since inequalities between the status of the interviewer and participant often lay the groundwork for privileging of researcher assumptions, special care also should be taken to accurately represent the participant's perspective.

Seemingly more innocuous, but no less important, is reciprocity. Building trustful human interactions, whether interviewing or otherwise, is often predicated on reciprocity. While many interviewees feel honored to be included in a study, enjoy a "give and take" conversation, and do not object to their time being used to contribute to science, there may be more to reciprocity than simply paying attention to an elder. Other means of paying homage to participants by engaging in reciprocal behaviors include helping an elder with transportation to run an errand, explaining an obtuse clause on a legal document (assuming the interviewer understands them him or herself), or disclosing personal information.

Another essential component of a balanced and ethical relationship is the provision of information to the interviewee. While most research protocols require that informed consent procedures be administered to a participant, explaining the meaning of such protocols in plain terms facilitates trust and confidence. Similarly, most people appreciate being told what to expect in an interview (number of sessions, weeks or months, types of questions, etc.) and how their input will contribute to a "greater good" (Kaufman, 1994). Finally, there has been concern expressed by in-depth interviewers about how to ethically withdraw, how much the researcher "owes" the participants, and how to exit without abandoning people with whom rapport has been established.

One simple response to this dilemma is the explicit disclosure of intention from the outset. Specifying researcher expectations up front ("I'd like to ask you questions about your health. I'm thinking we might meet about 5 or 6 times, if that's OK with you. . . . ") and confirming those parameters at the time of each visit keeps the participant aware of the impending departure. Finally, as is increasingly common scholarly practice, many researchers are returning to their informants for verification of conclusions and to provide feedback on study findings. This type of closure helps to satisfy not only the intellectual curiosity of the participant, but also assures the participant that he or she assisted in the creation of knowledge (Morse & Field, 1995).

### In-Depth Interviewing in Gerontological Research

Concerns and responsibilities inherent to in-depth interviewing may be complicated by a gerontological focus. Such complications include issues related to memory and cognition impairments, problems with proxy or surrogate consent, and the researcher's own discomfort and potential for stress working on challenging topics like nursing home life (Higgins, 1998). While some of these concerns may be valid, it is possible to exaggerate the problematic nature of interviewing older people. Stereotypes such as the belief that a frail-looking elder will tire quickly, that older people need the interviewer to speak very loudly, or that nursing facility residents are utterly despondent and generally incoherent only dehumanize and marginalize people (Kaufman, 1994). Such dangerous generalizations obfuscate the enormous and meaningful variations within the lives of elders. Indeed, it is the richness of such lives, understood through sensitive, careful, and engaging collaborative dialogue that is revealed through in-depth interviewing.

## REFERENCES

Dressler, W. W. (1991). *Stress and adaptation in the context of culture: Depression in a southern black community.* New York: SUNY Press.

Higgins, I. (1998). Reflections on conducting qualitative research with elderly people. *Qualitative Health Research, 8*(65), 858–866.

Hurston, Z. N. (1935). *Of mules and men.* Bloomington, IN: Indiana University Press.

Kaufman, S. (1994). In-depth interviewing. In J. F. Gubrium & A. Sankar (Eds.), *Qualitative methods in aging research* (pp. 123–136). Thousand Oaks, CA: Sage Publications, Inc.

Levy, R. I., & Hollan, D. W. (1998). Person-centered interviewing and observation. In H. R. Bernard (Ed.), *Handbook of methods in cultural anthropology* (pp. 333–364). Thousand Oaks, CA: Sage Publications, Inc.

Morse, J. M., & Field, P. A. (1995). *Qualitative research methods for health professionals* (2nd ed.). Thousand Oaks, CA: Sage Publications, Inc.

Myerhoff, B. (1978). *Number our days.* New York: Touchstone.

Rubinstein, R. L. (1988). Stories told: In-depth interviewing and the structure of its insights. In S. Reinharz & G. D. Rowles (Eds.), *Qualitative gerontology* (pp. 128–146). New York: Springer Publishing Company.

Sankar, A., & Gubrium, J. F. (1994). Introduction. In J. F. Gubrium & A. Sankar (Eds.), *Qualitative methods in aging research* (pp. vii–xvii). Thousand Oaks, CA: Sage Publications, Inc.

# CHAPTER SEVEN

# The Qualitative Interview With Older Informants: Some Key Questions

## Robert L. Rubinstein

"We see ourselves from our own point of view; that is the
privilege of the weakest and humblest of us."
Henry James, *Portrait of a Lady*, Vol. 1, p. 167 ([1881] 1951)

While there are many distinctions between quantitative and qualitative research, there is no more telling difference than their
attitudes to "talk." For quantitative research, talk that takes
place in the research setting is an element of a stimulus-response paradigm. The underlying belief here is that a given verbal stimulus (a
question or "item") produces an acceptable range of responses (e.g.,
"a lot, a little, or not at all"). These stimuli are then subject to statistical
manipulation that examines correlates and underlying structures. Meaning is stripped away in the design of the instrument and then added
as privileged interpretation after the fact (Mischler, 1986).

Qualitative research, in contrast, sees talk as culturally meaningful
interaction. The process of research talk leads to revealing and establishing meaning through the narrative and conversational presentation of
experience. "Experience," then, is the object matter of interviewing.

As this book attests, qualitative gerontology is not a new discipline.
It has matured and grown in sophistication over the last few decades.
Yet it has retained its role as an approach to understanding human life
and, in particular, as an approach to understanding experience and
meaning. A central point of this chapter is that we must recognize the
complexity of the qualitative interview as a data-gathering tool. As part
of attending to this complexity, the chapter emphasizes a variety of

key questions, or unsolved puzzles, that need to be addressed when conducting and analyzing qualitative interviews. These include questions about the structure of qualitative interviewing; the complex nature of experience as elicited through interviewing; the tension between "constructed meaning" in contrast to "collaborating to create meaning"; variety in the length of interviews; the understanding of "themes" as opposed to what may be called "reflected subjectivities"; issues of narrative versus conversation in interview content; the nature of listening; and the limits of meaning.

While a focus on key questions or unsolved puzzles may, at first glance, be viewed as an admission of problems with qualitative interviewing, it is rather a statement of the strength and maturity of this approach. The human sciences are difficult, and no approach is perfect. Humans are meaning makers; meaning is identified through experience. Qualitative interviewing is one of the very best ways of coming to understand meaning through examining experience.

In this chapter, I draw on several research projects in which I have been involved over the last few years. Our metric will be both the qualitative interview—the single session conversation—as well as the interview series—the multiple verbal interactions that constitute a complex research interaction over time.

All the projects referred to in this chapter have used various interviewing techniques as a centerpiece of ethnographic inquiry. They range from interviewing over a single, rich sitting of 1 or 2 hours, often focused around a single topic, to interviewing of multiple sessions (e.g., three to five) over the period of a month, to interviewing that is broad and continuous over a longer period (up to 2 years) and is nested within the context of ongoing participant observation. While, as noted, I draw on several sources, I will, in particular, focus on a project designed to study death and dying in nursing homes. This project involves several separate researchers conducting both participant observation-based formal and informal interviews and interview-only formal qualitative interviews.

## The Structure of Qualitative Interviewing

Let us begin by focusing on the base structure of the interview: the interviewer or researcher and the informant, "collaborator," or subject. The interviewer is structurally one-up over the subject, empowered as the inquisitor. In this power imbalance, the interviewer is gazing upon, examining, leading, or interrogating the informant.

There may be a direct relationship between the type and duration of the interview and the structure of power in research. In this way, shorter, more formal interviews may grant more power to the interviewer in relationship to the informant, because there is a greater degree of rigidity and control, a more pressing agenda, and less chance for the informant to emerge and take charge.

The tension over power is expressed through the structure of research itself. Because of the lack of interview time and mutual knowledge, the categories and topics raised by the interviewer represent the greatest degree of "outsideness" to those of the informant (Keith, 1986). Outsideness has the greatest potential for misunderstanding the lived world of the informant. In contrast, in lengthier interviews in which the informant and researcher get to know one another as persons, there is a greater equality of power since the relationship between the players may become more balanced over time. Ultimately, however, it is hard to know if the essential relationship as giver and taker of knowledge can be broken.

Some have sought to diminish the power imbalance in the research relationship by more conscientiously involving informants as collaborators in research. In this way, research becomes more under the control of informants, thereby eliminating the researcher as data middle person, by redesignating him or her as merely a catalyst. When "the natives" design research, it may combine scientifically compelling topics with a greater sense of community problem solving and personal agency by informants than standard qualitative and quantitative interviewing.

An account of the discourse of objectivity applies here. This view renders the supposedly "objective stance" of the researcher as false, minimally because science fails to account for the social positioning of the researchers (Rosaldo, 1989; Wikan, 1990). From this point of view, some argue, interviews in a traditional format can only go so far, are clearly distorted, and produce data that have been achieved in circumstances of unequal power between interviewer and informant.

Possible inability to produce intact, truly accurate data is also problematized by other structural features that emerge in interviews. Beside the general issue of power in research relationships, issues of gender, age, race and ethnicity, and class, encompassing power as well as other issues, are significant and may make research understanding difficult and lead to false conclusions.

In qualitative research, depending on the format of the interview, the degree of research commitment, and the degree of reflexivity of both interviewer and informant, these issues can be addressed within the interview format (e.g., upon completion of an interview, the interviewer might be requested to submit a written response to a question like, "How do you think the fact that you are a woman affects this interview?"). These structural features become issues that can be called into consciousness, held up for scrutiny, and reflected upon during the interview process itself. The body of qualitative aging literature, in large part, makes no reference to the nuances of cross-age interviewing (although, see Rubinstein, 1995). In sum, the light shed by reflexive interviewing is essential to consider.

In a related way, issues of transference can affect interviews in qualitative aging research, in that the interviewer and informant may see each other as parent and child, respectively, or in some other relationship, in an unconscious manner. This may particularly be the case if the interviewer is middle-aged or young and the informant is elderly. In the deep, rich interview, transference and countertransference as parent and child may occur and may subtly affect feelings and, therefore, questions and answers. In shorter interviews, these structural issues may act as powerful impediments to deep, rich engagement. While important data may be forthcoming, structural barriers in interaction may set limits on the depth of interaction or may shape the types of narratives produced.

Another structural issue in qualitative aging interviewing concerns variety in the length of interviews. Lengths of planned interviews may vary for different purposes, although what actually happens in the interview setting is another story. I have planned research that has utilized five weekly 1- to 2-hour interviews with each informant; a series of three 1- to 2-hour interviews with informants; a single interview of 1 to 3 hours, with an occasional second session if warranted; weekly interviews for up to 2 years; and occasional interviews of various lengths in the larger context of participant observation. What can we say about the length of interviews in relationship to meaning?

There is often a direct relationship between the length of interview series and the depth of interview data. With many elders, 1 or 2 hours may be the limit for one interview session, given the need for awareness of the fatigue potential of older informants, as well as the interviewer. What is varied, in fact, is the length of the interview series: the number of sessions and the frequency with which they occur. In general, in my experience, the longer the interview series, the greater the meaning depth, until some pattern saturation is hit. Nevertheless, short-interview series (e.g., one or two sessions) can be extremely worthwhile, as long as they involve the collection of biographical and other necessary background information, are focused on a specific topic or area, and can expand in new or interesting directions if necessary.

The nature of the informant is also important. Informants vary in terms of who they are, what they want to say, and the narratives they bring to the table. Only a small percentage of informants can become "key informants," those to whom one can go repeatedly for questions and discussion. Most informants stay mildly or moderately loquacious. Many older informants are just too busy to host more than an occasional interview. The exceptional informant has much to say, reflects on what is happening in the interview, is creative and inventive, and uses the experience in some way for him or herself, for example, to sort things out.

Finally, the nature of the topic is also suggestive of the length of the interview. Some topics demand a great deal of time. Others are focused and may require much less. One key is that the interviewer should always recognize the need to expand the sessions over what had been initially planned.

## The Complex Nature of "Experience" as Elicited in Interviews

Qualitative interviews serve as vehicles to elicit narratives and discussion of experience. There is, of course, a distance between actual experiences and the way they are constructed by individuals. There are many cultural and individual formats or templates that render what may have been an amorphous chain of raw material into a culturally appropriate experience and, thereafter, a narrative. One critical cultural format is the propensity for stories to have beginnings, middles, and endings, and to be structured in other important ways as well. Getting closure on an experience is a key cultural and therapeutic motif.

Another cultural demand of experience is that it be largely coherent. Consider this passage from an interview with the daughter of an elderly woman who died in the nursing home. The daughter is in the process of constructing a more-or-less coherent narrative from an uncertain memory to the structural demands of the interviewer. It is likely that no one has ever asked her for this information before.

*Interviewer:*    How long did your mother live in the nursing home?

*Informant:*    How long did she live in the nursing home? She went in, I think she was there a year and a half. You know, I'm not sure because she was in a nursing home before that, and then she was in a home down the street from me . . . a regular home. So the dates are kind of vague. But, I would say at least a year and a half to two years.

*Interviewer:*   Now, the year and a half to two years she was in the nursing home the whole time?

*Informant:*   No, when she first moved in here, I moved her from Centerville, which was out in, outside of North Town. She was there for like, she was there for maybe five, six years. Then she had to go to assisted living. She was in an apartment, she had to go to assisted living. And then because the assisted living jumped from whatever it was to whatever it was, it doubled [in cost], and she didn't have enough money to afford to stay there.

*Interviewer:*   Where is the assisted living, in the same place?

*Informant:*   What did you say?

*Interviewer:*   Where was the assisted living?

*Informant:*   In Centerville, there was not assisted living . . . so that . . . they just, they had assisted living, but her money only lasted for I think, a few months there. And I had to transfer her out because she was getting worse. There was not a nursing area there at all, you know. So, she moved from apartments to assisted living, for maybe five or six months maybe, and then when I saw that her money was getting low, I thought I had to do something else, so when I moved her to, umm, when I moved her to the nursing home, she had uh, she had a little bit left, she had enough to. I don't know how long it lasted but she had enough to pay, to get in there, and then to start living in assisted living there (assisted living affiliated with the nursing home), because I wanted her some place where she could go from there to a nursing home. . . .

This final statement by the daughter represents a more complete restatement, in narrative form, of her responses to questions and conversation. To put it another way, the conversation has helped turn an amorphous set of ideas, at first unrecalled or poorly conceptualized, into a more-or-less coherent, brief narrative.

This excerpt is important because it points to the complexity of experiences to which an informant (and an interviewer) must attend. In the larger interview, the daughter is reconstructing the experiences of her mother, as well as her own experiences and her own experiences of her mother's experiences, for the interview. There are many other molds into which experience is poured, as it is transferred from an internal and subjective phenomenon to one which opens onto the world through narrative interaction.

When topics to be investigated have been initially developed by panels or communities of informants, such groups may accept, revise, or reject the researcher's initial interests. Thus these topics (the ones the researcher is interested in versus the ones the natives are interested in) might not correspond. The "scientific paradigm" privileges the researcher's interests, but regardless of their incorporation of researchers' topical interests, successful qualitative interviewing will always follow informants' leads and issues of interest, for they are at the heart of an informant's personal-meaning system.

When the interviewer's topics structure the initial interviewer-informant interactions, the interviewer may work from a set list of questions, from a list of topics, or from a general notion of what he or she wants to inquire about, making up questions as the interview progresses. Work taken from a set list of questions, a common practice in qualitative interviews with older people, facilitates reflexive interviewing in two ways. First, a basic set of questions will introduce responses that engender new topics that had previously been unconsidered by the investigator; second, each response will be turned back by the interviewer into a new line or lines of questioning as each topic is fully explored. In such reflexive interaction, a technique at the heart of qualitative interviewing, the investigator is free to follow each line or topic wherever it goes, to get at the core of experience. Following a line of responses and making up new questions allows the researcher to sketch out the meaning context of the topic at hand and to be sensitive to key statements of experience.

## The Relationship Between Experience and Meaning

A central question for qualitative interviewing concerns the relationship between experience and meaning. Do experiences intrinsically have implicit meanings? Does the process of constructing coherent and presentable experiences (for narrative) imply that these experiences have been given meaning? Even a "bare bones" construction of a life story (e.g., "I was born in 1908. I went to school until I was married in 1929") derives some meaning from broadly shared cultural conventions, but what does it say about personal meaning?

These are central questions and, to be sure, one of the conundrums of qualitative interviewing concerns what we mean by meaning. The idea of meaning has been used in many different ways in qualitative aging research. "Types of meaning" may include personal meaning, cultural meaning, environmental attachment, strategies for living, adaptation, emotions, the management of life-course events, daily activities, semantic meaning, thematic meaning, spiritual meaning, ultimate meaning, as well as additional meanings.

Qualitative-aging researchers choose from among this wide variety of meanings. As a discipline, we are still struggling with agreement on central forms of meaning. Certainly, the elicitation of "themes" (or thematic meaning) seems a central construct. In my own work, I have found it useful to think about two types of meaning (interpretation and personal meaning system) and one psychosocial process (cultural meaning). First, *interpretation* is a meaning-making process representing reflection on personal experience and cultural ideals. This is the act of masking meaning undertaken by individuals in placing an experience in semiotic space. Interpretation draws together meaning and experience, although many of the specifics are not yet clear to me. Second, a *personal meaning system* is an individualized grouping of personal experience: life-course events, constructed biography, activities, cultural formats, and individual actions. This is a significant entity for older adults who reinterpret new and old experiences in the context of the evolving matrix of personal meaning. Finally, *cultural meaning* involves normative or idealized notions of important, shared, cultural practices. Many people share notions of what these practices are and, although they may not follow them, they remain mental images of how things should be.

It should be noted that these are abstractions of particular ways in which older people construct and construe experience. Again, they are hardly the full range of meanings, although in my view they are central to qualitative research on elders. It is important to note that this process and two types of meaning are abstractions of folk usages (what people naturally do as part of everyday life). Additionally, interpretation undertaken in the qualitative interview on the part of the informant should not be confused with data analysis, which may be interpretation on the part of the interviewer. A researcher's interpretation should not be confused with interpretation on the part of the informant, which may be considered both "natural" (what the informant does on her own) and "interview-specific" (what the informant does within the context of the interview; see below).

In many years of qualitative research with elders, it has become clear to me that one can understand very little about personal meaning or experience without understanding the informant's biographical context. Personal meaning is linked to life experience and biography. The manner in which the life course is meaningfully constructed as a present-day story of the past life course combines acts of interpretation of individual experiences, in the context of the past life course, its thematic issues, and cultural rules or conventions.

As a consequence of the central place of the constructed biography in the personal meaning system of elders, nearly all the research projects that I have conducted have utilized the collection of a brief life history as prologue to the elicitation of data about a specific topic. The question that has been used goes something like this: "Now that we have met and talked for a few minutes, I'd like to know more about you and your life. Could you tell me the story of your life, whatever happened along the way? Start where you like and take as much time as you need."

In many projects, this question has generally elicited narratives from 5 to 45 minutes in length, with 15 or 20 minutes more typical. This provides the meaning-context for data collected about more specific topics. For example, in a study of the lives of older men and women who did not have children, the experience of childlessness and its meaning could not have been understood without detailed knowledge of the life course and its key players. Similarly, a study of older women who have been poor all their lives found the meaning of later-life poverty to be placed in the context of the set of biographical experiences.

## *The Individual and the Collective*

The importance of contextualizing an informant's life history makes sense given the tremendous cultural focus on the individual and individualism in most western cultures. Indeed, one might argue that as research goes, the interview itself represents the technical application of cultural individualism to social science research. This suggests another puzzle for data collection and analysis in qualitative interviewing. There is a tension between the irreducible essence of individual interviews (i.e., personal meaning and experience) and the fact that these interviews are often analyzed as a collectivity. One might argue that this tension mimics that in society between the individual and the collectivity, which is itself an important part of American culture. Researchers handle this in different ways. Qualitative-aging researchers often present data on single cases because they are so compelling and illustrative of an issue under discussion. In general, plans of data analysis also look to the aggregation of data. For aggregate qualitative interviews, key themes or underlying structures to meaning that seem to appear generically in interviews are salient.

Nevertheless, the qualitative interview is noteworthy in its role as an entry point to the subjectivity of individuals. Ultimately, the data collected from each informant are unitary and whole. At some deep and significant level, the person is indivisible, representing a patterned whole. This tells us something important about experience. Ultimately, while experiences can be compared, shared, and can be said to be similar, they are irreducible. While experience can certainly be analyzed, in certain ways, because of its irreducibility, experience is not "analyzable," but rather something to be retold, representing only itself.

In sum, individual subjectivity can shed light on experience as both lived individually and in common. While experience is irreducible, because of cultural conventions and common social life, experience takes conventional forms in many instances. One experience may be illustrative of others in structure, feeling, or tone. Qualitative researchers frequently use a single or a few accounts to illustrate, as best examples, the experiences of many.

## The Tension Between "Constructed Meaning" and "Collaboration to Make Meaning"

Social scientists have generated very few accounts of the research relationship, although there are some notable exceptions in qualitative research (Behar, 1993). Little is systematically known about how the interview process affects outcomes.

In qualitative interviews with older people, there is a difference between material that is presented "fully born," in contrast to material that is generated from the struggle that takes place within the interview session itself. An experience that is common for both qualitative and quantitative interviewers is this: when initially arriving at the home of an elderly informant and without any specific prompting, the interviewer is greeted by a deluge of facts or an already-constructed life story or an episode story. An older informant may say at the outset, "I'm the kind of person who . . . ," and then go on to state a series of likes or dislikes or some other character-based statement. This "identity statement" sets up a particular relationship between informant and interviewer, which presages the desire of the informant to participate in the interview and to tell his or her story. Yet, this material announces an already "worked-through" surface story. A puzzle or question then is whether the informant will expand on this story in the interview or use it as a shield from the unpleasant task of discussing parts of his or her life that are at odds with the surface story. In either case, the initial presentation of a story by an informant may prefigure a formalistic, though well-developed story.

Such a surface story is a social thing. It is presented as having veracity, validity, facticity, and truthfulness, and it is "out there" in intersubjective space. It begins as a seeming "working through" of subjective experience into a more objective or externalized form of the story, one that can be told and retold and which stands for the informant's biography. That certain facts may be at odds with this story or that it may have telling gaps does not matter. Now externalized, the facticity of this story is projected onto intersubjective space between informant and interviewer. It derives its significance at this point from two sources, both as a symbol of the self and as an external projection for other people to encounter. This projection can also work as a mirror for the self so that the informant can see him or herself as well. While not as tangible as a material thing, the initial story can create objectivity or facticity from subjectivity, pure and simple, through the use of narrative structure, emotional color, and often-elaborate emplotment. That this should do so is a kind of miracle. This transformation from subject to object in qualitative interviewing is not well understood and remains a puzzle in many ways.

The interviewer must also struggle with the question of whether to go beyond this first-presented story. Some important questions here include: What is the meaning of this initial story? Why go beyond it? Is the researcher second-guessing the informant by going beyond his or her presentation? Is the story given in this way to avoid further subjectivity? What are the moral and ethical issues in going beyond this object-surface and entering the realm of pain? Who is to gain here? Moreover, the researcher must judge whether going beyond is consonant with the technical demands of his or her research project. For example, an interview that goes beyond may be structurally too much for a research project based on a single interview session with each informant.

Finally, we return to the question of meaning. How can we know about the meaning of a phenomenon if it is to be interpreted in the context of this overarching but limited story? Interpretation can only be taken as far as the initial story and any other material gathered in the interview session can carry it. One answer may be found in whether there are any indicators of data at odds with this initial story. Statements that do not appear consistent with the elder's reality, body language that does not fit, long periods that are absent from the story, important characters (e.g., parents, spouse, children, friends) who are never mentioned in the story, and both excessive emotional expression or flatness may indicate additional areas that might be examined.

For the situation in which the informant presents (as above) an initial story, "I'm the kind of person who . . . ," that is, the kind of statement in which the meaning is implicit and extraordinarily clear: this is what I make of myself; there are other questions. Other pathways to meaning may be gleaned by the interviewer through attentiveness to the material. What is the semantic or conceptual chain to which the story belongs? What evidence supports or contradicts it? What is its thematic content?

In contrast to this sort of story giving is the sort of interview interaction in which the researcher and the informant collaborate to make meaning, as Frank and Vanderburgh (1986) have suggested. This collaboration is quite different from the simple presentation of an identity story. In collaborating to make meaning, the inherent meanings of life events, episodes, cognitions, and affects may not be known at the outset. With the help of the interviewer and with the opportunity provided by the interview sessions, the informant attempts to make sense of disparate information for him or herself. Simply, informants may never have discussed the topic at hand with anyone before or the topic may be delicate, inchoate, or unobjectified.

We had such a situation when we interviewed older women who were childless. Nobody had talked much about childlessness with these women. Few of them had previously engaged in deep discussions of its meaning and impact. If they had referred to the topic at all, it was generally in passing or within some specific context. The task of sitting back and looking at being childless for the interview session was one that was generally new (as well as welcome) for these women.

Similarly, in this study it was difficult to elicit information through direct questions. A very great deal of the information we gained about the meaning of childlessness came through a discussion of some other event. For example, we might inquire about the life an informant had within her community and find that a discussion of Mother's Day or of grandchildren might be problematic for some informants.

Such working around and working through a sensitive topic can only be undertaken in settings in which the interviewer acts as a collaborator of sorts, providing the opportunity and the level of comfort necessary for the informant to discuss things and in which the informant is open to new possibilities. In a sense, such interactions may become less narrative in nature and more conversational (see below), although narrative may continue to play a part as new areas are explored. The goal, often unstated, is to come to some overt or "objective" version of experiences that initially are covert or unformed.

The issues discussed immediately above also relate to questions of narrative versus conversation. Some products of interview interaction are largely narrative in nature, with the informant responding in lengthy, coherent, and well-figured accounts. Sometimes, however, the interview proceeds in a conversation style, with brief back-and-forth discussion. This is often the case when informants are recalcitrant or do not really understand what is being asked of them. Thus, an important puzzle is: how do narrative and conversation relate in the qualitative interview? Do differences matter analytically? We tend to speak of qualitative interviews as a form of "eliciting narratives" or good qualitative interviews as a form of story telling by informants. We have described contexts for the production of narratives in some instances as, for example, when a life-history interview or question elicits a more-or-less coherent life story or when a loquacious informant expounds upon a long narrative when first meeting the interviewer. But responses to specific questions or general topics ("what I'd like to talk about today") are often narrativized and contextualized in terms of information that has been previously shared ("the things I told you already"). Interviews turn to conversational back-and-forth for a number of reasons, including the interviewer's attempt to clarify information, to expand inquiry, or to comfort the informant after the telling of a difficult incident.

## Listening

I have suggested at the very beginning of this chapter that qualitative research is, in large part, about talk. But talk itself presumes a larger system of talk, listening, and response. Often, the issue of response drops out of qualitative research. This is because the first order of business in interviewing is not to respond naturally, like one involved in an equivalent relationship, but to respond with a question, either a new one or one amplifying what has already been said. For a researcher, appropriate response to a statement made by an informant is a contextualized, appropriate question that in some way requests the informant to expand his or her statements. Such is always based on careful and attentive listening. The question of whether an interviewer should make reference to her or his own personal experience often comes up in qualitative research, and the response to this question must be dictated by the individual research context.

Nevertheless, the second element of this response system, listening, is critical to the research enterprise. Perhaps the most difficult thing to learn in qualitative interviewing is the ability to listen well. This is not necessarily a natural ability, but for many interviewers is gained after hard work at developing a manner of listening that is both attentive to the details of the narrative and, at the same time, creates a schema or mental model of who this person is, who key others are, the outlines of his or her life, the events, the main themes, and issues. It may be the case that interviewers are much better listeners in interview situations than they are in the rest of their lives. Tape recording and transcribing are ways of insuring the quality of listening. How much analysis is done through a careful review of the tape or the listening performed through rereading the transcript is not precisely known, but constitutes a large part of core data analysis.

## Understanding "Themes" Versus "Reflected Subjectivities"

This is a more difficult area to talk about and brings out concern for data analysis and meaning. Kaufman defines themes as "cognitive areas of meaning" (Kaufman, 1981). These are topics or areas to which an informant, in discussing his or her life, turns again and again. They are clearly central and key in the presentation of self. Examples might be "my family is my life," "family is central," "the nature of work," "I have been a victim," and many others. There are many examples in Shenk's recent interview-based book on rural elders (1998). The reader will almost certainly recognize these types of themes from work with older informants. They are summary statements or an index for the life narrative.

A question then arises: are these themes the end product of data analysis? That is, having discovered themes that represent categories of meaning in and across individuals, do we need to go beyond this in understanding the informant or groups of informants? The answer depends on the type of analysis we want to do. Discovery of themes does not necessarily tell all about the informant. Many themes are so obvious in the interview setting that they can be fed back to the informant as questions ("You've mentioned your family quite a lot. Is that really the main thing in your life" or "Are there ways in which you are completely independent of your family?").

The status of themes in qualitative research is complex. They may be discovered as immediately apparent or "at hand." They also may be "dug out" after the fact through data analysis by the researcher. We do not necessarily know very much about how these different types of themes relate to meaning systems. For example, while themes that are immediately apparent relate to a meaningful presentation of self, do those dug out by analysis reflect this overt meaning system or something more covert or separate from the consciousness of the informant? Do they relate to the presented meaning system or to the interpreted meaning system of the informant?

"Reflected subjectivity" here refers to the subjectivity of the informant that is reflected upon in the interview process. Thus, it refers to another level of insight into the material, specifically when the informant calls into consciousness previously unconscious statements. This is not merely a thematic statement such as, "My family is central to me." Rather, it refers to reflection on the role of that theme in the meaning system of the informant, to something more about it, to an informant's metalevel of analysis.

A critical distinction is now made. This higher-level reflexivity leads to the development of a meaning system within the context of the interview. That is, the meaning becomes a hybrid object, blending interview-specific new meanings with programmatic meanings (surface meanings) from the previously extant personal meaning system. This is truly collaboration to make meaning as constructed within the interview setting.

There is a further possibility, namely that the informant is conducting "life review" work of his or her own that corresponds or exists contemporaneously with the interviewer's project (Rubinstein, 1995). The new, more inclusive or abstract level of meaning making may have commenced prior to the onset of the interview, continue through the interview where it is expressed in some way, and be resolved after the interview is over.

## The Limits of Meaning

The final question to be dealt with here is that of the limits of meaning: What are the limits to meaning? Anthropologists and other qualitative social scientists often talk about meaning as the gold standard of research. But understanding what meaning is and the various types of meaning are not always clear. We have talked in this chapter about a variety of types of meaning (e.g., cultural meaning, the personal meaning system, and life-course meaning). There are also a number of triggers for meaning making, for example, the interplay between social structure and temporal organization, the occurrence of the life review, and others. How are we to sort all these out?

Consider this additional excerpt from a portion of the interview presented above:

> *Informant:* . . . Well, she had a, she did have a strong desire to live. Although I can remember her . . . she didn't, she knew she had to live as long as she

was supposed to live. But when you'd go in to see her, she said to me, she'd say to me a couple of times, "You know, I'm not going to be here much longer." And I really sensed that people have a sense of that before they die. And I said, "Well, what do you mean?" And she said, "Well, I'm not just going to be here any longer." And she, and she used to sit at the windows. I'll never forget as I look back now, she used to look out. I'd try to take her outside. I used to bring her out, I'd take her out to see my daughter, who lives in Warwicktown, way, way out, one day and she really enjoyed that. But if I went in there and I tried to take her out, and she wouldn't go out, she at least [would] sit near a window. And she used to watch the tree blowing, you know, she would look at the trees all the time. And very honestly, in my heart, very honestly, I think she knew, this is only . . . my conception, when the leaves fell off the trees, I think she knew she wasn't going to be here. . . . "

This passage suggests that meaning in qualitative interviews is to be gleaned with careful attention to how an informant situates events in a larger context, that is, how the informant interprets events within the context of the personal meaning system; how objective events (the mother did not have long to live) are given subjective meaning; and how the interview, and the interviewer's skill and informants openness, work to create meaning in this intimate setting.

Qualitative interviewing is like the shining of light onto an irregular surface: there will always be parts in the dark. In the same way, there will always be fundamental questions about this important research procedure. While we need to emphasize what we do learn, in contrast to that which we do not, we must at all times be aware of key questions in qualitative interviewing, in general an accounting of what we do not know.

In sum, questions remain about the nature of interviews as we continue to shape qualitative-aging research. These questions derive from our basic understanding of the research interview as talk and from our basic concerns with meaning, experience, and interpretation. Questions or puzzles concern that structure of qualitative interviewing, including issues of power, social positioning, transference, and the length of interviews; the nature of experience and how this is conveyed; a tension between constructed meaning and collaboration in making meaning, including questions of narrative and conversation; issues relating to understanding themes versus reflected subjectivities; the nature of listening; and the limits to meaning. We must seek to address these systematically as our science proceeds.

## REFERENCES

Behar, R. (1993). *Translated woman: Crossing the border with Esperanza's story.* Boston: Beacon Press.

Frank, G., & Vanderburgh, R. M. (1986). Cross-cultural use of life history methods in gerontology. In C. L. Fry & J. Keith (Eds.), *New methods for old age research.* South Hadley, MA: Bergin & Garvey.

James, H. ([1881] 1951). *Portrait of a lady* (Vol. 1). New York: Modern Library.

Kaufman, S. (1981). Cultural components of identity in old age: A case study. *Ethos, 9,* 51–87.

Keith, J. (1986). Participant observation. In C. L. Fry & J. Keith (Eds.), *New methods for old age research* (pp. 8–26). South Hadley, MA: Bergin & Garvey.

Mischler, E. (1986). *Research interviewing: Context and narrative.* Cambridge, MA: Harvard University Press.

Rosaldo, R. (1989). *Culture and truth: The remaking of social analysis.* Boston: Beacon Press.

Rubinstein, R. L. (1995). The engagement of life history and the life review among the aged: A research case study. *Journal of Aging Studies, 9,* 187–203.

Shenk, D. (1998). *Someone to lend a helping hand: Women growing old in rural America.* Amsterdam: Gordon and Breach.

Wikan, U. (1990). *Managing turbulent hearts: A Balinese formula for living.* Chicago: University of Chicago Press.

# CHAPTER EIGHT

# The Active Subject in Qualitative Gerontology

## Jaber F. Gubrium and James A. Holstein

An image of the aging subject always stands behind the actual individuals and interactions studied in gerontology. The image affects the researcher's basic understanding of how the older person fits into the world. This image does not directly pertain to the individual respondent who actually answers questions in interviews, nor does it refer to the real behavior and interactions observed in field research. Instead, the image depicts what researchers imagine animates these respondents and social actors as research subjects. This may range from a subject who is passively animated by external or internal forces, to one who actively shapes the world in his or her own right.

This chapter is concerned with how researchers imagine the subject in qualitative gerontology. It is not directly about research procedure, although research design is necessarily implicated. By comparing two different images of the subject—one passive and the other active—we hope to show the advantage of qualitative gerontology's particularly active way of imagining the aging experience. In our view, how researchers conceptualize the research subject is as important for understanding the logic of research and the value of results as are the actual research methods. As we will see, this implicates the subjectivity of researchers in the sense that there is also a subject behind the researcher.

Researchers often ignore the assumptions they make about their subjects, as well as their own place in the scheme of things. They are rightfully concerned with justifying research methodologies in grant applications, presenting details of research design and methods of procedure in publications, and otherwise legitimizing the technical details of their work. But one cannot expect to comprehend why qualitative gerontologists, in particular, pose the research questions they do, why they might be more concerned with allegedly small samples instead of larger ones, or why they orient to data interpretively rather than causally, without understanding how qualitative researchers in general orient to their subjects and subject matter. Oddly enough, questions related to sample size, the reliability of instruments, or the ostensible representativeness of findings are not their leading concerns, simply because these often derive from an entirely different way of imagining subjectivity. Unfortunately, standards based on an inappropriate set of methodological relevancies are often applied, resulting in the unfair evaluation of qualitative research and its findings. While we do not address such technical matters here, we do offer a framework for approaching their relevance to qualitative inquiry.

## The Image of the Passive Subject

We begin with the image of the passive subject, which will provide a basis for comparison with the more active subject envisioned by qualitative researchers (Holstein & Gubrium, 1995). We will also consider the equal importance of the counterpart image of the subject standing behind the researcher or interviewer. At one time, the image of the passive subject dominated social and behavioral research. Researchers formulated arguments centered on the impact of conditions, such as class, generation, health, and morale, on the experience of aging. While this is no longer as pervasive, the image still informs quantitative researchers of how to think about their questions and observations, how to apply them, and how to evaluate the results. More than anything, this passive image makes it reasonable for quantitative researchers to orient methodologically to their projects in the way they do.

*Respondents as Vessels of Answers.* In quantitative approaches, those studied are conceived as passive vessels of answers for questions put to them in the role of respondents. The subjects behind these respondents are assumed to be repositories of experience. They hold the answers to demographic questions related to matters such as age, gender, race, occupation, and socioeconomic status. They contain information about social networks, including household composition, friendship groups, circles of care, and other relationships. These repositories also hold a great deal of experiential data, including attitudes, feelings, and activities. In principle, the vessel-like subject behind the respondent passively possesses all the information the quantitative researcher wants to know;

the respondent merely conveys, for better or worse, what the subject already owns.

The distinction between the subject on the one hand, and the respondent on the other, is tacitly acknowledged in quantitative studies. Survey researchers, for example, regularly differentiate the attitudes of their subjects and the corresponding opinions conveyed in respondents' answers. The goal of survey questions is to obtain valid and reliable data about these attitudes, which come in the form of opinions communicated by respondents in interviews. As a result, there is continuing concern over whether opinions provided by respondents actually correspond to their attitudes. This then leads to questions regarding the accuracy of measurement and related issues of reliability and validity.

Given a passive subject, all questions surrounding the relationship between the respondent and the subject are necessarily methodological. The passive subject is, after all, just there; information about his or her experience is simply waiting to be more or less precisely obtained for research purposes. At no time are these subjects viewed as contributing to this information in their own right. Ideally, they merely release information to researchers, information that has been held uncontaminated within their vessel of answers.

In quantitative research, the trick is to formulate questions and provide an atmosphere conducive to undistorted communication between researcher and respondent. Much, if not most, of the methodological literature on interviewing deals with the procedural nuances of these complicated matters. For example, the vessel-of-answers view cautions interviewers to be wary of how they ask questions, lest their mode of inquiry bias the respondent and contaminate what actually lies within the subject. There are myriad techniques for obtaining unadulterated facts, most of which rely on interviewer and question neutrality. It is assumed, for instance, that the interviewer who poses questions that acknowledge alternative sides of an issue is being more neutral than the interviewer who does not. Researchers are advised to take this into account in elaborating interview questions. Valid results are believed to flow from the successful application of such guidelines.

All of this applies as well in quantitatively oriented observational studies. The subject behind the actor or informant is similarly passive and not engaged in the production of knowledge in his or her own right. If observation "goes by the book," is unobtrusive, and unbiased, it can be assumed that actors will validly present what their subjectivity merely holds within them—the unadulterated details of their conduct or way of life. Contamination emanates from undue research intrusions in the social settings being observed or from the self-presentational distortions that arise when actors shape their conduct for the observer.

*The Passive Subject Behind the Researcher.* The subjectivity of the researcher also distinguishes quantitative and qualitative work. In quantitative work, a passive subject lurks behind researchers. Interviewers, for example, are expected to keep the respondent's vessel of answers in view and not unduly interfere in data collection. This is a matter of controlling oneself as an interviewer so as not to influence what the passive interview subject, who, except for perhaps the recalcitrant respondent, is only too willing to communicate. Interviewers must shake off serious self-consciousness; they must not take to heart the possibility that their presence in the interview may itself be constructing a distinctive subject behind the respondent. Most of all, interviewers must not seriously consider that their very own questions supply a particular frame of reference for the respondent's answers. To the extent such frameworks are considered to exist, they are viewed as embedded in the subjects' world behind the respondent, not behind the researcher. If the interviewer is to be at all self-conscious, it is limited to being alert to the possibility that the interviewer may be biasing or otherwise unduly influencing the research process.

Interviewers are expected to keep their personal opinions to themselves. While, of course, some minimal, neutral reaction to answers is necessary to acknowledge what respondents communicate, nothing further is normally deemed acceptable. For example, should the respondent discuss various sentiments surrounding caregiving, the quantitative interviewer might confirm this, but only as a way of inviting the respondent to elaborate on what already has been communicated. Ideally, the interviewer uses his or her interpersonal skills to merely encourage the expression of, but not to help construct, the attitudes, sentiments, and behaviors in question. In effect, the image of the passive subject behind the interviewer is one of a facilitator. As skilled as the interviewer might be in practice, all that he or she appropriately does is to promote the expression of the actual attitudes and behavior under consideration, information that lies in waiting behind or within the respondent.

The image of the passive subject behind this interviewer encourages the interviewer to control the interview situation so as to facilitate candid, uncontaminated communication. Ideally, the interview should be conducted in private. This assures that respondents will speak directly from their vessel of answers, not in response to the presence of others. Curiously enough, this assumes that the researcher merely facilitates the expression of what otherwise remains unaffected by his or her presence. The presence of a merely facilitating interviewer, in other words, is not viewed as itself infringing on interview privacy. As Jean Converse and Howard Schuman (1974) note in their book on the informal aspects of survey interviewing, the seasoned interviewer learns that the "pull" of conversation, which might have an interpretive dynamic of its own, must be managed so that the "push of inquiry" (p. 26) is kept in focus. The hope is that the communicative pressures of conducting inquiry will produce "good hard data," facilitated by means of the interviewers' "soft" (p. 22) but not empirically intrusive conversational skills.

The watchword here is "control." Control signifies a passive subject behind the researcher, suggesting an interviewer who limits his or her involvement in the interview to a specific role, one that is constant, in principle, from one interview to another. Should the interviewer go out of control, so to speak, and introduce anything but variations on specified questions into the interview, the passive subject behind the interviewer is methodologically compromised. It is not the passive subject who is the problem, but rather the interviewer who has not adequately regulated his or her conduct or the situation so as to facilitate the pure expression of the respondent's vessel of answers.

## The Image of the Active Subject

What happens to research procedure if we *activate* these images? What happens if we view all participants in the research process as actively making meaning? This is precisely what takes place in varying degree in qualitative research. While there are technical differences as well as similarities between quantitative and qualitative research, the heart of the distinction centers on differences in their respective images of subjectivity. It is a hallmark of qualitative research that the image of the subject behind all participants in the research process is active to some degree. Whether it is the image of the subject behind the respondent in interview-based studies, the image of the subject behind the informant in observational research, or the subjectivity of the researcher him- or herself, the leading idea is that asking questions, eliciting stories, conducting participant observation, and the like requires us to consider that both those who are studied and those who conduct research actively assemble their lives and worlds in the process.

*The Active Subject.*   Construed as active, the subject behind the respondent not only holds the details of a life history of experience but, in the very process of offering them up to the researcher, constructively shapes the information. The active respondent can hardly "spoil" what he or she is, in effect, subjectively creating in the interview process. Indeed, the activated subject pieces experiences together before, during, and after occupying the respondent role. This subject is always making meaning, regardless of whether he or she is actually being interviewed.

Because the respondent's experience is continually being assembled and modified, the truth value of interview responses cannot be judged simply in terms of whether they match what lies in an objective vessel of answers. From a quantitative standpoint, the truth of interview responses can be assessed in terms of reliability (the extent to which questioning yields the same answers under similar circumstances) and validity (the extent to which inquiry yields the correct answers) (Kirk & Miller, 1986). Different criteria apply when the interview is viewed as a dynamic, meaning-making occasion. They center as much on *how* meaning is constructed as on *what* those meanings are. These "how" and "what" matters necessarily go together in qualitative research because active subjects construct meaning as an integral part of its communication (Gubrium & Holstein, 1997). This is not the case in quantitative studies; there, researchers hope that the *hows* can be separated from the *whats* so that the *what* issues become the exclusive focus of attention. Ideally, the *how* questions are treated as technical issues; that is, they are limited to what the researcher does to obtain reliable and valid responses.

If qualitative researchers attend to the meaning-making process as much as to the meanings produced, it is because the image of the active subject requires it. This is not an aesthetic indulgence or a peculiar habit of procedure. Indeed, not attending to meaning production in qualitative research would be most invalid procedurally. Because research is viewed as a dynamic, meaning-making process, different methodological criteria apply, centered on how meaning is constructed, the circumstances that shape meaning, and the meaningful linkages that result. Of course, qualitative researchers do vary in the extent to which they emphasize the *hows* over the *whats*, but they all combine interest in them to some degree (Gubrium & Holstein, 1997). As such, the validity of their data does not derive exclusively from the data's correspondence to meanings held within the respondent, but from the data's capacity to convey experiential realities in terms that are circumstantially comprehensible and accountable.

*The Active Researcher.* The counterpart to the active subject behind those studied is the active subjectivity of the researcher. It is characteristic of qualitative researchers that they are not comfortable conceiving of their role as composed of passive theorizing, a priori hypothesis specification, and detached data collection. Rather, these are actively and simultaneously engaged in qualitative research. More important, they must be engaged if the subject behind the researcher is activated. Again, this is not just force of habit or a matter of research tradition; the active subjectivity of the qualitative researcher requires it.

The activated researcher can move in a number of directions, each of which will be illustrated empirically in the next section. One of these is "grounded theory" (Glaser & Strauss, 1967). The grounded theorist is active in the sense that she or he realizes from the start that the premature formulation of a theoretical perspective or the a priori specification of hypotheses can significantly color findings. Realizing this, the grounded theorist studiously avoids shaping the empirical material in advance of data collection and, instead, turns to the world of meaning of those studied for theoretical direction. Theory formation and hypothesis setting are viewed as matters best taken up in relation to the empirical material, not beforehand. In other words, these are to be figured from the ground up, thus the term, grounded theory. Theory develops hand-in-hand with data collection and, in the process, the researcher "constantly compares" empirical material in order to increase the generality of the emerging configuration of categories and types.

A second direction is represented by the growing interest in life stories in social research. Here, the researcher actively seeks to document the narrative formulations and/or the narrative activity of the storyteller (Gubrium, 1993; Kaufman, 1986; Kenyon & Randall, 1997). Narrative research focuses on the ways life stories or other narratives of experience are put together by the storyteller, how this is accomplished, and the conditions that shape the process. The researcher actively seeks the narrative qualities and contours of the experiences in question. To the extent that the *hows* of the narrative process are emphasized over the *whats*, the researcher attempts to document the ways in which the respondent's own narrative competence organizes the story communicated.

A third path toward activation of subjectivity directs the researcher to the active use of social forms and categories by those studied. This centers on the social rhetorics of age in everyday life. Rather than focusing on the way a life story is assembled by the respondent, research deals with how accounts of all kinds are used to persuade and to accomplish various ends in particular circumstances (Gubrium & Holstein, 1998). The focus here is on what is done with these accounts to create particular contexts for making age-related decisions, not on the analysis of story contents per se. The narrative process and its social influences are highlighted, not the internal organizations of stories themselves. Many of these studies feature the actor as directly involved in particular ongoing concerns—households, support groups, clinics, hospitals, nursing homes, friendship circles—whose participants put a premium on interpreting the meaning of age in particular ways (Gubrium & Holstein, 1997; Holstein & Gubrium, 2000a, 2000b).

## Forms of Active Subjectivity

To illustrate how qualitative researchers activate their own subjectivity as a way of activating the subjectivity of those studied, consider the following research projects, which exemplify the three directions noted.

*The Active Subject of "Grounded Theory."* Kathy Charmaz's (1991) study of people who suffer from chronic illness—many of whom are elderly—is described in her book, *Good Days, Bad Days*, and is a fine illustration of a grounded-theory orientation to qualitative research. Following in the footsteps of Barney Glaser and Anselm Strauss, who pioneered grounded theory, Charmaz asks how it is that those who suffer from serious chronic illnesses, such as cancer, lupus, multiple sclerosis, arthritis, and cardiovascular disease, construct their lives in relation to their illnesses. Rather than theorizing her respondents' lives and adaptations in advance, Charmaz works from the ground up, beginning directly with the experience of chronic illness itself.

From in-depth interviews conducted over a number of years with 110 individuals, Charmaz quickly learns that chronicity implicates the self in a way that acute illness does not. From the outset, her data begin to suggest that this is a difference in kind, not degree. Assuming that one recovers from an acute illness, the illness runs its course fairly quickly and those affected return to their lives, taking up where they left off. In contrast, those suffering from serious chronic illness live in relation to their illnesses for long periods of time. This shapes the very meaning of these lives. The result is a process of life reconstruction that shifts in relation to the pains and inconveniences posed by the illnesses.

Charmaz orients to those with chronic illness as actively responding to the effects of their illness, not as long-term passive sufferers. These activated respondents are not simply there to be interviewed. Charmaz's activation of their subjectivity leads her to focus on the ways they expressly assemble their experience, distinguishing the approach as an interpretive form of grounded theorizing. A passive subject would be merely there to respond to questions about the personal sentiments and daily rhythms of the chronic illness experience. Charmaz views her activated subjects as doing more: they actively construct and reconstruct the complex meanings of the chronic-illness experience as that develops from day to day. This naturally turns her to the questions of how this is accomplished and what the end results are, which respectively require detailed descriptions of the processes entailed and consequences for the meaning of everyday life.

Charmaz discovers that there are different ways that individuals construct their illnesses, which are affected by their place in the trajectory of the illness, as well as by the problems of daily living posed by specific symptoms. Her presentation centers on three types of response to chronicity—chronic illness as interruption, as intrusive illness, and as immersion in illness. As she takes us through her material and we hear the respondents describe their lives and related illnesses, we learn that these are *ways* of experiencing chronic illness; they are not characteristic of particular individuals. The same individual may at times construct his or her illness, as intrusive in his or her life and, at other times, construct life as immersed in the illness. On "bad days," one may become immersed in one's illness, with the resulting pathological implications for one's identity. On "good days," one's illness may be experienced as merely intrusive, the individual otherwise being mostly engaged in the normal rhythms of daily living. As a result, we are witnesses to subjects who not only actively construct the meaning of chronic illness, but who deftly do so in relation to their illnesses' shifting daily symptomatology. These activated subjects are not experiential "dopes," adjusting wholesale to their illness, but take account of the changing experiential contours of chronicity in discerning who and what they are as sufferers.

Chronicity implicates the self in the process. As Charmaz explains, "Each way of experiencing and defining illness has different implications for self and for meanings of time" (p. ix). Repeatedly, her respondents couple their statements about the daily travails of their illness with thoughts about who and what they have become, how their lives have changed, and what this means to them in the immediate scheme of things. Serious chronic illness and its daily vicissitudes are not just another series of passing events of daily living, as successful recovery from surgery or a bout of the flu might be, but make for complex and continuing changes in the sense of who one is as a person. Chronic illnesses are more than sicknesses; their fluctuations serve to continually redesign the selves individuals live by. In this regard, we are witnesses to identities that are wounded on bad days and, in the same individuals, identities that resiliently spring forth positively on good days.

All of this might easily have been missed had Charmaz oriented to her respondents' subjectivity as simply being that of sick people passively responding to their illnesses. The underlying lesson here is that we do great damage to our understanding of these experiences when we do not allow distinctly active respondents to communicate them to us. Equally instructive, especially for social gerontology, is the suggestion that the experience of being old, insofar as that is linked with chronic illness and dependency, may be constructively transitory and not be fixed by a particular stage of the life course (Holstein & Gubrium, 2000b). Charmaz is informing us that the active subject can tell us *when*, not just *how* or *what* they are as particular selves, something which the typical passive subjectivity imposed by quantitative researchers commonly freezes in time. Indeed, if the activated subject behind the chronically ill respondent may, on good days, construct one self and on bad days construct another, the overall duration of one's experience with serious chronic illness may even add its own layer of meaning to self-construction. Clearly, this is no simple picture of passive responses to disease.

*The Active Subjectivity of the Storyteller.* A second direction for activating the subject stems from the view that experience is not just lived, but comes to us in the form of stories (Gubrium & Holstein, 1998). The analysis of life stories has been growing in popularity and, in the case of qualitative gerontology, is making visible the complex narrative quality of the aging experience. Narratively oriented gerontological researchers have shown that the personal story and related forms of communication construct and reconstruct experiences as part of the ongoing representation of everyday life (Birren, Kenyon, Ruth, Schroots, & Svensson, 1996; Kenyon & Randall, 1997, 1999; Kenyon, Clark, & de Vries, in press). From diverse quarters, we are being informed empirically that the personal past has not simply gone by, but is continually lived out in new terms as its storytellers speak of life (Gubrium, 1993). The present and the future are implicated as well, as narrativity designs experience through time.

The activeness of the storyteller varies in narrative studies. At one end of the spectrum is the existential storyteller, a subject whose emotionality is even creatively formulated (Douglas, 1985). Introspective skills can be an abiding concern, even while the emphasis on the free play of narrative expression at times seems excessive (see Ellis & Bochner, 1992). At the other end of the spectrum are studies in which the narrator is viewed as embedded within, or guided by, larger forces of storytelling, such as the historical events that shape both how stories are told and what is conveyed (Bertaux, 1981). The link between story-telling and historical events may lead to the formulation of overly typi-fied historical accounts for the experiences in question. The difference in emphasis results in deeply personalized and inventive accounts on the one hand and detailed, subjective articulations of historical events on the other.

The debate surrounding this variation in narrative activeness is a point of contention in Sharon Kaufman's (1986) book on the sources of meaning in late life, *The Ageless Self.* Kaufman takes a distinctively active orientation to her respondents' narrative subjectivity. She refuses to treat their life stories as the narratives of older people or as the narrative by-product of this generation's historical experiences. It is clear in respondents' commentaries that age figures into what is said in a complex way; certainly these are not the straightforward stories of elderly persons, even while all are over the age of 70. Rather, if age is a topic at all in the narratives, it is represented as a particular image of the self, rather than being a framework for conveying who these respondents are tout court. As Kaufman reminds us, "The old Americans I studied do not perceive meaning in aging itself; rather they perceive meaning in being themselves in old age" (p. 6).

Nor does generation specify these life stories. While most of the respondents lived through the Great Depression and World War II, these events do not govern their life stories. Interestingly enough, they do not even figure as major themes. Instead, the stories Kaufman elicits from her respondents are actively constructed in relation to a variety of narrative resources, many of them centered on personal values, but not especially on the historical events they experienced earlier in life (see Ruth & Öberg, 1996, for contrasting results).

Kaufman asks two questions of her narrative material: What the-matizes the life stories of these older Americans and from where do they draw meaning to construct their accounts? Sixty people participated in open-ended interviews, important elements of which centered on their life story. In the book, Kaufman focuses on three respondents in order to highlight active subjectivity in detail. Their narratives show how inventive respondents can be in constructing their experience when given the opportunity. Millie, who is 80 years old and had been living in a nursing home before Kaufman met her, constructs her story around affective ties. Kaufman explains that most of the conversations she had with Millie over the course of the 8 months she was interviewed, focused on her interpersonal likes and dislikes, especially who she was attracted to, cared for, or loved. Millie uses the word "attach" repeatedly in her narrative: "I grew very attached to him and he to me," "I am so attached to her," "We developed an attachment to one another" (p. 33). "Love," too, is part of her vocabulary, continually inserted to embellish her affectivity.

Ben and Stella assemble their stories around different themes. Ben, who is 74 years old, presents a dichotomous self in his story. According to Ben, his life has been a battle between his sober, responsible side and his carefree, romantic side. The theme crops up repeatedly as he talks of his past, his present, and the years to come. At one point, he speaks of looking into the mirror and seeing his father, who, he notes, was "a very serious," "no-nonsense guy." Ben explains that this is the kind of image he conveys to the world, even though, he points out, "I don't feel that way. I feel carefree and happy . . . and I could easily slide or slip into a romantic adventure" (p. 48). Other themes are drawn from his need for financial security and his religion.

Stella was born in 1897 in the rural South. The central theme of her life story is her achievement orientation. According to Stella, "I don't look back at all. I only look forward to what I'm going to do next." Even her past is something she competes with, not something she longs for. A second theme relates to the first—her aesthetic sense and desire for perfection. Stella links both themes with a need for relationships that, she explains, prompts her to create new roles for herself.

Although there are various ways the lives in question are given meaning, they have two important things in common. One is that none of them is thematized in terms of old age. Of course, age does come up in the accounts or is brought up by the interviewer, but it is tied to more significant narrative anchors. Another important commonality, which works against the idea that subjectivity passively reflects larger social contexts, is the lack of emphasis on major historical events. As we noted earlier, the two world wars and the Depression were key events in the lives of all 60 respondents, but the respondents draw very selectively from history to assemble their narratives. We find that these lives narratively unfold in the meaning-making context of vastly inventive storytelling, the constructive skills of their narrators weaving experiences together in varied and sundry ways, far removed from what a late life story of "this" particular generation might be presumed to convey.

## Actively Using Age to Construct Context

If Kaufman shows us how older people select from contexts other than old age and history to thematize their stories, James Holstein's (1990) ethnomethodologically informed study of involuntary psychiatric hospitalization hearings illustrates how age is used rhetorically to create persuasive contexts for interpreting experience. Holstein's fieldwork centers on the judges, attorneys, psychiatric consultants, witnesses, and candidate patients involved in the commitment decision. The leading question here is how is age used to build a case for or against involuntary commitment. Rather than treating age as a background variable that affects the likelihood of involuntary commitment, which would consti- tute passive subjects, Holstein views it as a narrative resource selectively applied to make a case for or against commitment (Garfinkel, 1967). The standard background factor of age, which typically explains life events, is adopted by participants to influence commitment decision making.

Combining a focus on constructive activity and on the use of age to construct context, Holstein presents narrative material to show how participants in involuntary commitment hearings themselves theorize old age for various purposes. As Gubrium and Wallace (1990) have argued, gerontological theorizing is not exclusively a gerontologist's concern, but is part and parcel of popular explanations of aging. For example, Holstein (1990) illustrates how vernacular versions of disen- gagement and activity theories are used by judges in two different hearings to account for their decisions. As extracts from the hearings show, these "theories-in-use" can be seen as ways of constructing useful contexts for action, rather than just being researchers' explanations for the causes or consequences of aging. The subjects involved in commit- ment decisions are not passive vessels of answers for testing gerontologi- cal theories of aging, but are shown to be theoretically active in their own right.

The following extract from proceedings at Metropolitan Court, which is a pseudonym for one of the settings studied, shows a version of "disengagement theory" being applied by a judge to construct an age- related context warranting a decision against further hospitalization. Henry Brewer's hospitalization was initially ordered because his family believed that he was, in their words, "depressed" and "responding badly" to his recent retirement. A psychiatrist had testified that Brewer was indeed "withdrawn" and "suffered from acute depression." After being assured that medications would control these conditions, the judge nonetheless assimilated Brewer's behaviors to his own theory of aging, effectively normalizing Brewer's conduct by casting it as the inevitable withdrawal associated with aging. As a folk-disengagement theorist, the judge suggested that Brewer's increasing detachment from prior roles and activities was typical of those entering the later years and not a basis for commitment.

I'm going to release Mr. Brewer if he'll agree to move back in with his daughter. It's pretty clear that he's slowing down a bit, but that's to be expected from a man his age. I think we just have to leave him to his own small pleasures and not worry so much about what he doesn't do anymore. As long as he's not causing anyone any trouble, and he's happy spending his time by himself, I don't see any reason for further hospitalization. We really can't expect him to keep up with the old pace if he doesn't feel up to it (Holstein, 1990, p. 124)

Compare this with the gerontological theorizing implicit in an extract from hearings at Eastern Court. Here, Dwight Berry's involuntary commitment is under consideration, and the extract illustrates a different explanatory context being constructed by the judge for his decision, in this case to continue hospitalization. The account in this illustration is more reminiscent of "activity theory."

Mr. Berry hasn't been responding very well to his [mental] disability and I'm afraid he's not ready to leave [the psychiatric treatment center]. I think part of it is something we're all going to go through someday. Here's an older man who's not working, and now everyone wants to take care of him and he's been taking care of them all his life. He's having trouble figuring out what to do with himself. He might be okay in a retirement home, but I don't think he's ready for that yet. I like the idea of keeping him at Willowhaven [the psychiatric treatment center] because they've got all of those programs to try to get him involved. I'm hoping they can fit him into one of their vocational programs and get him on track, give him something to do that he can care about. Maybe then we can talk about a [retirement] home placement (p. 124).

Here the judge views Berry's problems in terms of the typical difficulties of adjusting to the changing and reduced opportunities and demands of old age, in the judge's words, "something we're all going to go through someday." Berry has lost his well-defined roles, due, in part, to his age, which in the judge's opinion can be addressed by "[giving] him something to do that he can care about." The ending phrase, "that he can care about," suggests activities that have a positive valence. In contrast to the Brewer case, the judge here assembles an account justifying further remedial intervention rather than benign inattention.

At times, participants disagreed about how to classify a candidate patient in terms of age, focusing proceedings on the construction of age itself, not on explanations of aging. Note how in the following extracts, the local meaning of 51-year-old Lois Kaplan's age emerges in her commitment hearing in Northern Court. Kaplan's public defender initially argued that

. . . a woman her age should do just fine in a board-and-care facility because she's gotten to the point where she's not likely to be too difficult to look after. She seems to have stabilized and at her age she's not likely to go looking for trouble. The best part about Crestview [the board-and-care facility] is she'll be able to live on her own but there'll be someone there to look after her. She's at a point in her life where that won't take much (p. 125).

But the judge was skeptical about the public defender's claims of Kaplan's manageability and presented his own gloss on the consequential meaning of Kaplan's age, instead emphasizing vulnerability.

[To the public defendant] I'm not sure that I agree with you, Mr. Lyle. The problem with getting older is you sometimes need a little more attention. Little things seem like major problems. They seem to get out of hand a lot quicker. I know I have to do a lot more for my own mother now than just a couple of years ago. As far as I know, Crestview is a fine facility, but their policy is for residents to be able to pretty much do it on their own. I'm not convinced that Lois won't need more help than they can give her (p. 125).

Clearly, there was no consensus here over what it meant to be Kaplan's age, even while it was agreed that she was "getting older."

There were several further exchanges about Kaplan's age, specifically concerning how getting older related to whether Crestview could handle Kaplan's problems. The two perspectives were repeated and larded with other arguments. Eventually, the judge took a different tack, this time linking vulnerability to gender, not just age.

You know what's bothering me? I think it's the fact that we're talking about letting an older women live alone, even if there is someone looking in on her. I can't help but worry that she's going to do something and nobody's going to notice until it's too late. It's so easy for someone like her—mental problems, getting a little older, not able to do everything she once did—to do something that might really be dangerous, something that could hurt her real bad (p. 126).

In this context, "getting a little older" means that, as an older woman, Kaplan is more susceptible to harm.

Across the hearings, it is evident that age has no fixed meaning. Indeed, the same age may be used in a variety of ways to build contrasting contexts for the matters under consideration. In turn, these contexts supply warrantable answers to questions of aging as this relates to the consequential decisions. From this perspective, active subjectivity extends to the very sense that is made of these candidate patients as "aging" individuals.

## Conclusion

What are the empirical advantages of taking an active orientation to
subjectivity? First, and perhaps foremost, is that ultimately the perspectives of the older people we have discussed would not become available
to us as researchers if we did not activate our own subjectivity. Passively
orienting to the empirical world as quantitative gerontologists typically
do—being concerned with collecting information from the vessels of
answers that subjects are taken to be—would merely reproduce preexisting conceptions of age and related variables. We would not be attuned
to how these matters become distinct variables in the worlds of those
we study, nor be attentive to where and how they are used by those
whose lives are in question. Instead, a passive orientation would simply
accept that these matters exist with sufficient existential constancy to
permit their measurement and analysis for research purposes. An active
orientation, in contrast, continually resonates the leading concerns of
qualitative gerontologists, centering on when and how matters of age
and aging enter into experience.

A second advantage of adopting an active orientation to subjectivity
is that the researcher's world is not viewed as categorically separate and
distinct from the world of those studied. As researchers, we are charged
with recognizing that our own subjectivity helps to distinctively constitute the subjectivity of those we study. The resulting qualities of our
respondents' or informants' lives, indeed, are in some sense the responsibility of *qualitative* research. In the final analysis, this is precisely what
distinguishes our work from that of our quantitative counterparts: an
abiding awareness that the way subjectivity is conceived—whether passive or active—will significantly affect the kinds of data obtained. The
awareness creates a moral, not just a scientific, environment for research
efforts, the form of data collected being as much a matter of how we
choose to view subjectivity as it is a matter of how technically adequate
our research procedures are.

A third advantage of an active orientation is the ability to recognize
the deep complexity of lived experience. Much of the intricacy of everyday life is glossed over in research models that conceive of the empirical
world in terms of fixed variables, and research subjects as vessels of
answers. We ignore how empirically and theoretically astute those studied are in their own rights. For example, we fail to take account of the
shifting meaning of self in the later years as that is organized in relation
to the sense of whether life is surrounded by good days or bad days.
We ignore the existentially important worlds that active subjects construct on their own—the ones they assemble as they narrate their lives, as

opposed to the "larger" worlds we habitually place them in for research purposes. In general, we miss the opportunity to appreciate how much active subjects are like researchers themselves as they frame their views of empirical matters, proffer theories for why these matters work as they do, and account for the relation between the two.

A fourth and final advantage of an active orientation relates to the public relevance of scientific knowledge. It is our obligation as social researchers to inform the public of what we know about individual lives and social experiences. Here, subjectivity is crucial. An orientation to a passive subject leads us to report and inform in quite a different way than an orientation to an active one. In studies of later life, both passive and active approaches describe and inform the public about the aging experience, but it is to the credit of qualitative gerontology that it communicates the varied constructive activities and abilities that individuals exhibit in relation to the aging experience. Often overlooked by other frameworks, these qualities open to public view the complex workings of aging and the myriad ways there are to be and to grow old.

## REFERENCES

Bertaux, D. (Ed.). (1981). *Biography and society: The life history approach in the social sciences.* Beverly Hills, CA: Sage Publications, Inc.

Birren, J. E., Kenyon, G. M., Ruth, J. E., Schroots, J. J. F., & Svensson, T. (Eds.). (1996). *Aging and biography.* New York: Springer Publishing Company.

Charmaz, K. (1991). *Good days, bad days.* New Brunswick, NJ: Rutgers University Press.

Converse, J. M., & Schuman, H. (1974). *Conversations at random: Survey research as interviewers see it.* New York: Wiley.

Douglas, J. D. (1985). *Creative interviewing.* Thousand Oaks, CA: Sage Publications, Inc.

Ellis, C., & Bochner, A. P. (1992). Telling and performing personal stories: The constraints of choice in abortion. In C. Ellis & M. G. Flaherty (Eds.), *Investigating subjectivity* (pp. 79–101). Thousand Oaks, CA: Sage Publications, Inc.

Garfinkel, H. (1967). *Studies in ethnomethodology.* Englewood Cliffs, NJ: Prentice-Hall.

Glaser, B., & Strauss, A. L. (1967). *The discovery of grounded theory.* Chicago: Aldine.

Gubrium, J. F. (1993). *Speaking of life: Horizons of meaning for nursing home residents.* Hawthorne, NY: Aldine de Gruyter.

Gubrium, J. F., & Holstein, J. A. (1997). *The new language of qualitative method.* New York: Oxford University Press.

Gubrium, J. F., & Holstein, J. A. (1998). Narrative practice and the coherence of personal stories, *Sociological Quarterly, 39,* 163–187.

Gubrium, J. F., & Wallace, J. B. (1990). Who theorizes age? *Ageing and Society, 10,* 131–149.

Holstein, J. A. (1990). The discourse of age in involuntary commitment proceedings. *Journal of Aging Studies, 4,* 111–130.

Holstein, J. A., & Gubrium, J. F. (1995). *The active interview.* Thousand Oaks, CA: Sage Publications, Inc.

Holstein, J. A., & Gubrium, J. F. (2000a). *Constructing the life course* (2nd ed.). Dix Hills, NY: General Hall.

Holstein, J. A., & Gubrium, J. F. (2000b). *The self we live by: Narrative identity in a postmodern world.* New York: Oxford University Press.

Kaufman, S. (1986). *The ageless self.* Madison, WI: University of Wisconsin Press.

Kenyon, G. R., Clark, P., & de Vries, B. (in press). *Narrative gerontology: Theory, research, and practice.* New York: Springer Publishing Company.

Kenyon, G. R., & Randall, W. (1997). *Restorying our lives: Personal growth through autobiographical reflection.* Westport, CT: Praeger.

Kenyon, G. R., & Randall, W. (1999). Narrative gerontology [Special issue]. *Journal of Aging Studies, 13*(1).

Kirk, J., & Miller, M. L. (1986). *Reliability and validity in qualitative research.* Thousand Oaks, CA: Sage Publications, Inc.

Ruth, J.-E., & Öberg, P. (1996). Ways of life: Old age in a life history perspective. In J. E. Birren, G. M. Kenyon, J.-E. Ruth, J. J. F. Schroots, & T. Svensson (Eds.), *Aging and biography: Explorations in adult development* (pp. 167–186). New York: Springer Publishing Company.

# PART V

# Hybrid Vigor

# Introduction

## Nancy E. Schoenberg

T heories of "hybrid vigor" have a long-standing and credible tradition in the world of genetics and evolution. Such theories suggest that an organism derives strength from culling the most advantageous features of its ancestry and "evolving out" of disadvantageous qualities. Fortifying the advantageous and reducing the disadvantageous seems desirable.

Hybrid vigor in social science methodology follows a similar logic. If one combines the advantages of qualitative and quantitative orientations, then combined strengths reduce, overcome, or compensate for the weaknesses inherent in either approach. Most researchers acknowledge strengths of quantitative methods to include the production of objective, reliable and generalizable data, while qualitative designs have the potential to elicit rich and valid data that "usually leave the participants' perspectives intact" (Steckler, McLeroy, Goodman, Bird, & McCormick, 1992, p. 1). Each approach also has its particular limitations. Quantitative approaches are criticized for questionable ecological validity, a lack of holism, and limited representation of nonmajority groups. Critics of qualitative approaches note that the small sample sizes typical in qualitative explorations limit the generalizability and reliability of findings.

Recognizing the potential advantages of complementing methods, or at least the potential to circumvent disadvantages commonly associated with a particular methodological orientation, researchers have begun to combine qualitative and quantitative approaches. Increasing interest in seeking hybrid vigor through complementary or combining methods has raised a number of important questions, which are explored briefly in this introduction and elaborated in subsequent chapters. Specifically, these questions include: (a) What are typical ways of combining qualitative and quantitative methods to elicit the strengths of each and diminish their weaknesses? (b) what are the advantages

*174*

of complementary methods? and (c) what are the disadvantages of complementary methods?

Groger and Straker (chapter 9) outline many of the approaches to combining qualitative and quantitative methods. Fairly standard in this repertoire are qualitative designs that precede and inform the creation of an instrument to be administered during a quantitative study; quantitative studies followed by qualitative studies to offer explanations for the quantitative findings; quantitative investigations that test hypotheses derived from qualitative designs; and equally contributing qualitative and quantitative designs (Steckler et al., 1992).

There are also special techniques that make use of both qualitative and quantitative approaches, but do not necessarily mix methods (Rowles & Reinharz, 1988). These include such ethnoscientific methods used in primarily qualitatively oriented research designs, such as pile sorting and multidimensional scaling. Focus group activities, while traditionally qualitative in their data collection, often are analyzed through more quantitative content analysis techniques (such as the co-occurrence of certain words or frequencies of themes). David Morgan's chapter in this section provides insights into this technique of combined methods.

## Beneficial Features of Complementary Methods

The increasing popularity of combined or complementing methods arises, in part, from recognition that one approach (qualitative or quantitative) may be insufficient to examine a phenomenon of interest. Instead, selecting the most appropriate method sometimes requires drawing from various traditions, a direction consistent with contemporary trends of multidisciplinary and interdisciplinary scholarship. The changing culture of research is such that scholars now feel more at liberty to choose the best protocol for a research study rather than remain constrained by a limited array of designs consistent with a narrow and inflexible methodological training.

Researchers also have become attracted to complementary methods for their potential to either confirm or document the validity of findings across methods or to supplement or round out findings from one method to another. As discussed by Groger and Straker, integrating qualitative and quantitative approaches through triangulation may increase the reliability and the validity of data. For example, qualitative approaches that seek to identify domains of importance in previously unexplored or underexplored topics can provide a baseline of understanding. Quantitative follow up may bolster generalizability and reliability. Opting for a particular technique that combines qualitative and quantitative orientations may prove cost effective and efficient. For example, while most survey formats tend to limit the depth of insight an investigator can achieve, adding open-ended questions may round out and add insider perspectives on a topic. Similarly, techniques such as focus groups often acquire an extensive array and quantity of information in a relatively brief period of primary data collection.

A final, overarching advantage of methodological mixing or complementarity is the possible benefits derived from cooperation among members of a research team. Because complementary methods often involve several investigators, it is likely that researchers will engage in a mutually creative and enriching process. Each researcher will also need to clearly explain and justify the particular component of the design for which he or she is responsible, lending increased clarity and focus to the project. Finally, increased dialogue across methodological divides can enhance appreciation for and understanding of both qualitative and quantitative approaches.

### Problematic Aspects of Complementary Methods

Many scholars maintain that complementary methods are difficult to implement and theoretically problematic. Critics claim that using techniques that bridge qualitative and quantitative designs often fails to achieve the benefits inherent in either approach.

Theoretical problems with combining methods include concern about violating the paradigmatic assumptions of both qualitative and quantitative approaches by intermingling the two. Those who support such a perspective argue that fundamental differences in the goals, approaches, and designs of qualitative- and quantitative research approaches make it inappropriate to blend the two perspectives (Gubrium, 1992). Such a view ignores the rich and diverse theoretical and methodological traditions within both qualitative and quantitative approaches (Groger & Straker, chapter 9).

There are also numerous concerns about practical problems in combining methods. Since most researchers tend not to have both qualitative and quantitative expertise, the employment of complementary designs often requires a team approach. Research teams frequently struggle with division of labor, the desirable and practical sequencing of alternative research designs, issues of privileging one orientation over the other, or simply engaging in different discourses. Other practical concerns include the tremendous resources that are generally necessary to conduct two or more parallel studies and a lack of existing exemplars of the successful modeling of complementary projects.

Finally, concerns have been expressed about the ability of techniques that bridge qualitative and quantitative approaches to obtain the benefits of either design. Specifically, researchers from qualitative traditions have questioned what they have perceived to be the "quantification of qualitative" approaches (Schoenberg & Rowles, chapter 1). Such critics claim that methodologies, such as focus groups, and analytical tools, such as computer programs for qualitative data, undermine the quality of emically derived data by privileging a numerical orientation toward the collection and analysis of even the most subjective information.

There is a need for continuing thought and dialogue on the advantages and drawbacks of using complementary methods in gerontological research. While qualitative researchers may be skeptical, the increasing popularity of complementarity and methodological holism in scholarship reveals greater acceptance, indeed, an embracing of a fusion of qualitative- and quantitative-research orientations. Wherever we fall on a hybrid vigor or methodological purity continuum, it behooves us to explore the rationale behind the employment of complementary methods.

## REFERENCES

Gubrium, J. F. (1992). Qualitative research comes of age in gerontology. *The Gerontologist, 32*, 581–582.

Rowles, G. D., & Reinharz, S. (1988). Qualitative gerontology: Themes and challenges. In S. Reinharz & G. D. Rowles (Eds.), *Qualitative gerontology* (pp. 3–33). New York: Springer Publishing Company.

Steckler, A., McLeroy, K. R., Goodman, R. M., Bird, S. T., & McCormick, L. (1992). Toward integrating qualitative and quantitative methods: An introduction. *Health Education Quarterly, 19*, 1–8.

# CHAPTER NINE

# Counting and Recounting: Approaches to Combining Quantitative and Qualitative Data and Methods

Lisa Groger and Jane K. Straker

## *Introduction*

A number of researchers have written on the problems and challenges of combining qualitative and quantitative methods (e.g., Denzin & Lincoln, 1994, 2000; Fielding & Fielding, 1986; Fraenkel, 1995; Morgan, 1998, Morse 1991; Steckler, McLeroy, Goodman, Bird, & McCormick, 1992). Combining qualitative and quantitative methods in the same study raises a number of questions, both at the production end and the consumption end of the research process. At the production end, issues include whether one researcher carries out each component of the research or whether there is a division of labor among differently trained researchers. How likely is it that one person is equally well versed in both approaches? If there is a division of labor, how will the products of this division be integrated during any or all phases of the research? At the consumption end, one of the most pertinent questions is how likely is it that a reader is equally well-versed in both approaches? Have more than cursory efforts been made to describe exactly what methods were employed and how they were combined? We suspect that qualitatively trained readers are at risk of glossing over the technical aspects of the quantitative part, making it unlikely that they will detect methodological flaws in that part of the design and will accept or reject the findings solely based on the qualitative piece. On the other hand, quantitatively trained researchers may hold expectations for representative samples or for identical conduct of interviews in qualitative studies and thus dismiss an entire study based on misconceptions about the nature of qualitative methods. Only thoroughly "bilingually trained" persons, of whom there are relatively few, can evaluate the methodological rigor of both approaches and appreciate their relative contribution to a given study.

With few exceptions (Hammersley, 1992), writers on the subject encourage the mixing of methods where appropriate, although they are not always in agreement on how to accomplish this goal. Fielding and Fielding (1986) lamented the fact that calls for combining methods are seldom accompanied by explicit instructions on how to achieve this in an integrated way, a complaint that is no longer valid since the publication of several volumes that provide clear instructions on how to combine multiple methods (Brewer & Hunter, 1989; Creswell, 1994; Tashakkori & Teddlie, 1998). It is, therefore, all the more surprising that both editions of *The Handbook of Qualitative Research* (Denzin & Lincoln, 1994, 2000) do not include a chapter specifically on combining qualitative and quantitative methods, although the topic is embedded in several contributions to the volumes. It is unclear whether this lack of explicit guidance is the cause or the result of an apparently inherent difficulty of combining qualitative and quantitative methods. Some scholars consider the issue to be basically a technical problem that methodologists should be able to solve. Others consider the issue to be a more basic epistemological problem attributable to irreconcilable conflict between two paradigms (Gubrium, 1992; Morgan, 1998).

With advances in computer technology generally, and the proliferation of software for text analysis in particular, technical difficulties are becoming increasingly surmountable (Bazely, 1999; Richards & Richards, 1994; Weitzman & Miles, 1995). On the other hand, the epistemological debate has not been resolved. There is, however, no reason why a strictly technical and pragmatic approach to combining methods must necessarily violate paradigmatic assumptions rather than take them into consideration as dictated by a given research question (Bazely, 1999). Combining methods is most often used to achieve completeness or complementarity, with each method asking different questions about varying aspects of the phenomenon under study. The objective is to obtain a broader picture, either by using quantitative research to provide a larger context for a qualitative study, or by using qualitative research either to inform the development of a quantitative instrument or to throw light on findings from a quantitative study.

## The Myth of Two Paradigms

The notion of combining methods implies that they exist as mutually exclusive and categorically separate entities rooted in traditions whose adherents differ with regard to how they view the world and how they address questions of voice, generalizability, validity, and reliability. For example, Steckler et al. (1992) characterize quantitative methods as producing population-oriented, "factual," [sic] reliable, and generalizable data presenting the outsider's or *etic* perspective, in contrast to qualitative methods they describe as producing case-oriented, "rich, detailed, valid process data" presenting the insider's or *emic* perspective (p. 10). This dichotomy also has been stated in terms of "pro-numbers" or "anti-numbers" (Patton, 1990, p. 479); dominant versus emergent paradigms (Schwartz & Ogilvy cited in Lincoln & Guba, 1985); or positivist versus naturalistic inquiry (Lincoln & Guba, 1985). Implicit in all such juxtapositions is the assumption that quantitative methods, if designed and carried out properly, are capable of tapping one measurable and generalizable reality that exists outside and independently of the objective observer, and that qualitative methods produce nongeneralizable—some would say "episodic"—and nonreplicable insights into multiple subjective perspectives of which the observer effect is an integral part.

Juxtaposition of qualitative and quantitative methods is often expressed in terms of different paradigms, when actually neither is a paradigm. Atkinson (1995) points out the dangers and the error of considering, advocating, and codifying research traditions as paradigms. Following Kuhn's (1962) original definition, Atkinson defines paradigms as

> . . . reconstructed logics. Seen from this perspective, they are frameworks for the justification of research activities, rather than systems of motivation that determine action. Paradigms are recognized retrospectively, when scholars find patterns and reasons for their work and that of others" (p. 119).

In contrast to paradigms defined in this manner, qualitative and quantitative approaches should be seen not as paradigms, but as approaches comprising multiple methods and world views. Furthermore, when we talk about qualitative methods in such a global manner, we are lumping together theoretical traditions (symbolic interactionism, phenomenology, ethnomethodology), general research approaches (ethnography), strategies for analysis (grounded theory), and general world views or filters through which we interpret what we see (positivism, constructionism, deconstructionism, feminism, critical theory). Likewise, when we talk about quantitative methods, we are including multiple methods for data gathering (telephone, self-completion, interview); multiple strategies for research design (experimental, quasi-experimental, descriptive); multiple operationalizations of the same concept (consider the number of scales for depression in elders); and divergent viewpoints ranging from positivist to postmodernist. Some quantitative researchers would say with great faith that anything can be measured, while others will admit to some skepticism about the validity and reliability of their undertakings.

A dichotomous view of two paradigms has been criticized as a myth that is being perpetuated by those who control funding and jobs (Rowles & Reinharz, 1988). Fielding and Fielding (1986) argue "data are never rich in and of themselves, but are 'enriched' only by their being grounded in a refined theoretical perspective" (p. 31), and that "ultimately all methods of data collection are analyzed 'qualitatively,' insofar as the act of analysis is an interpretation" (p. 12). The dichotomous juxtaposition of qualitative and quantitative methods ignores the realities of options faced by researchers. Instead of a clear-cut distinctiveness in type of data, setting, focus, view of natural science as a model, relation to theory, goals, and epistemological position between the two approaches, there is actually "a range of positions sometimes located on more than one dimension . . . [where] many combinations are quite reasonable" (Hammersley, 1992, p. 51). Hammersley (1992), who blames the distinction of methods for a kind of cold war between practitioners of one or the other approach, likens the growing interest in combining the two to a kind of détente that he considers to be worse than a cold war because it "still preserves the dichotomy" (p. 40).

"Purists," who contrast qualitative and quantitative methods as distinctly different, often decry as "method slurring" any attempt at combining them (Atkinson, 1995, p. 121). They maintain that combining the two amounts to mixing incompatible paradigms, each of which dictates the use of fundamentally different approaches to data collection and analysis. "Situationalists" concede that each method could make a contribution to the same project, but that there is no possibility for true integration. "Pragmatists" see a less fixed connection between paradigms and methods and are open to combining methods where appropriate (Carey, 1993).

## Why Combine Qualitative and Quantitative Approaches?

Advocates for combining methods do not necessarily recommend this approach as a methodological panacea for limitations inherent in qualitative or quantitative approaches, but agree that the research question and purpose should dictate whether and what kind of combination to use. There has to be a compelling reason for combining methods. To do it effectively, researchers must decide first what their questions are, what data to collect to answer the questions, what methods to employ for obtaining the data, and what time-ordered sequence to choose.

The two broad reasons for combining methods are either to confirm or to supplement findings from one method with those from another. *Confirmation or convergence of findings* are often referred to as triangulation, a much used term that actually refers to a number of different approaches. *Data triangulation* refers to the use of multiple data sources; *investigator triangulation* refers to the cooperation among multiple researchers; *theory triangulation* refers to the application of multiple perspectives for interpreting data; and *methodological triangulation* refers to the use of multiple methods (Denzin, 1970; Fielding & Fielding, 1986). Triangulation that refers to two studies aimed at coming up with the same findings is an expensive, and, therefore, infrequently used way of documenting the validity of findings (Morgan, 1998).

Qualitative/quantitative combinations have been used to compensate for the weaknesses of one method with the strengths of the other (Denzin, 1970); "to maximize the strengths and minimize the weaknesses of each" (Knafl, Pettergill, Bevis, & Kirchhoff, 1988, p. 30); to gain in-depth understanding of a phenomenon (Fielding & Fielding, 1986); to establish validity of findings (Hennessy & John, 1995); to serve as "an alternative to validation" (Denzin & Lincoln, 1994, p. 2); and to salvage quantitative research with qualitative data (Weinholtz, Kacer, & Rocklin, 1995). Under the euphoric voices extolling the virtues of combining methods, we can hear voices of warning and skepticism. Fielding and Fielding (1986, p. 35) remind us that the "accuracy of a method comes from its systematic application, but rarely does the inaccuracy of one approach to the data complement the accuracies of another." Indeed, whatever combination of methods one may use, if they are not appropriately administered, it can actually increase the chance of error because of biases and specific threats to validity inherent in each method. Simply combining methods will not guarantee validity. Because the respective approaches used for methodological triangulation are by nature different, they may not tap the same issues and, therefore, produce results that are not truly comparable, or they may produce divergent results that are not always dealt with in an unbiased manner (Bryman, 1992).

## Approaches to Combining Methods

*Models.*   Much of the literature on combining methods is in the area of health, which lends itself particularly well to combining qualitative and quantitative methods because it covers many disciplines and topics (Carey, 1993; Morgan, 1998). Like health, the aging experience is influenced by a multitude of complex factors, making it not only incumbent on gerontologists to read across disciplines, but also appropriate to combine qualitative and quantitative methods to capture this complexity. For example, to fully understand the role of the nursing home in American society, one must read across a number of disciplines that have examined nursing homes. Anthropologists tell us what it is like to live or work in one; historians suggest why nursing homes have become what they are; psychologists and social workers have studied individuals' well-being and adjustment to institutional living; and policy analysts look at nursing homes in the larger context of the politics and economics of social policy in the United States. Only by drawing upon the knowledge generated by these different disciplines can one begin to understand the complex issue of institutional care and the forces that shape it. The methods used by these disciplines similarly cover the full array of quantitative and qualitative approaches either singly or in combination.

Most conceptualizations of mixing methods incorporate temporal (time) and hierarchical (relative importance) dimensions. Drawing on Morse's (1991) model and focusing on the technical or "practical aspects of research design," Morgan (1998) proposes the "priority-sequence" model, or four practical strategies for combining qualitative or quantitative methods based on priority and sequencing decisions. Having defined the purpose and goal of a study, and having determined that a combination study is appropriate, either for confirming or complementing findings, the researcher has to make two decisions: first, which method should be the principal and which the complementary one (priority decision), and second, which method should be the preliminary and which the follow-up one (sequence decision). These two decisions about how to combine two approaches result in four alternative strategies, presented in Table 9.1 as numbers 1 to 4, with arrows representing sequencing and capital letters representing priority decisions. The model proposed by Morgan does not reflect a truly equal design. Morgan acknowledges that the omission of "middle options" or designs that give equal priority or importance to each method is a weakness of the priority-sequence model, and he suggests that research-

**TABLE 9.1  Summary of Ways of Combining Qualitative and Quantitative Methods and Data**

| Combination | Timing of Data Collection | Purpose |
|---|---|---|
| 1. qual → QUANT | Sequential | Qualitative piece informs construction of instrument for principally quantitative study |
| 2. quant → QUAL | Sequential | Quantitative piece identifies subsamples for more intensive principally qualitative piece |
| 3. QUANT → qual | Sequential | Qualitative follow-up sheds light on principally quantitative study |
| 4. QUAL → quant | Sequential | Quantitative piece tests hypotheses derived from a principally qualitative study |
| 5. QUANT + qual | Simultaneous | Qualitative questions embedded in principally quantitative instrument to probe respondents' answers and/or allow for elaboration |
| 6. Quant + Qual | Simultaneous or Sequential | Integrated approach with both pieces contributing equally and enhancing each other's power |
| 7. Ethnography | Intertwined | Multimethod approach par excellence, using multiple methods and data sources |

*Note:* Capital letters indicate relative importance of each method (Morse, 1991).

ers become more proficient in mixing methods equally and simultaneously.

The model proposed by Steckler et al. (1992) includes four types of combinations: a qualitative piece informing the construction of an instrument for a principally quantitative study; a qualitative follow up shedding light on a principally quantitative study; a quantitative piece testing hypotheses derived from a principally qualitative instrument; and an integrated approach with both pieces contributing equally and enhancing each other's power. These combinations correspond to those listed under numbers 1, 3, 4, and 6 in Table 9.1.

In a similar vein, Rowles and Reinharz (1988) distinguish between "separate but equal" and "integrated" combinations of methods, with the former used to answer different questions, and the latter used as triangulation. Bryman's (1992) 11 approaches to integrating qualitative and quantitative research is basically a list of reasons for mixing methods and of ways in which it has been done, whereas the multimethod, "bidirectional," 16-step model by Sells, Smith, and Sprenkle (1995) combines qualitative and quantitative approaches in an equal and integrated way, such that one method provides feedback for the other at multiple junctures.

Applying a mixed-methods approach to clinical encounters, Miller and Crabtree (1994) outline four types of designs. *Concurrent design*, or the simultaneous and independent conduct of qualitative-clinical and quantitative-interpretive studies where description of the context involved in a clinical trial illuminates the trial results; *nested design* of a single study that integrates qualitative and quantitative pieces, such that the qualitative piece helps "identify and operationalize key variables" (p. 344); *sequential design* where the results of one study inform another; and *combination design* consisting of different *qualitative methods* for certain questions seeking to "grasp the rich complexity of context" (p. 344), an approach most often used by ethnographers and evaluation researchers.

*Techniques.*   Examples of techniques for combining methods include the construction of Likert-type or Guttman scales based on qualitative exploration (Mueller, 1986); pile sorting (Weller & Romney, 1988); the quantitative analysis of qualitative data such as in content analysis (Weber, 1990); and consensus analysis (Garro, 1990). Writers on the subject do not always distinguish clearly between combining methods, that is, strategies for data collection and combining data from different sources, that is, information obtained from different types of actors or different accounts of the same events. It has been pointed out that combining qualitative and quantitative data is not the same as combining qualitative and quantitative methods (Fielding & Fielding, 1986). Bryman (1992) identifies two incongruent, and therefore not genuine, combinations of qualitative and quantitative methods. The first is the quantification of qualitative data. He rejects this combination for epistemological reasons, arguing that the collection of qualitative data is based on epistemological assumptions that are violated if such data are then subjected to quantitative analysis. The second incongruent, and therefore not genuine, combination of qualitative and quantitative approaches is the inclusion of open-ended questions in an otherwise quantitative instrument that he rejects for practical reasons, arguing that the insertion of one format violates the expectations of the participant, and demands of the interviewer a shifting of gears that may be difficult to achieve. Judging from the many quantitative studies that include some open-ended questions, not everyone would agree with this view. Researchers who have used this quantitative approach with open-ended questions may argue that inserting these questions gives respondents a chance to clarify and elaborate their answers, and that it breaks the monotony and formality of closed-ended questions and thus enhances the quality of the data and our understanding of the phenomenon under study (e.g., Wenger, 1999).

*Integration.* Most calls for combining methods fail to include explicit instructions on how to achieve this objective in an integrated way, and few studies achieve true integration. Particularly rare are longitudinal studies that achieve an interweaving of approaches by employing methods alternately over time. Rather, integration often occurs in an unplanned manner where data are collected with a particular purpose in mind, only to reveal themselves as more useful for another purpose (Bryman, 1992). Fraenkel (1995, p. 116) describes true integration as an "idiothetic" approach in terms of "an ever-enriching spiral of movement between methods germane to the study of general features of human life, to methods more suited to the richness" of individual experiences. Such a high level of integration is captured in the multimethod, "bidirectional," 16-step model proposed by Sells et al. (1995). Within this model, findings from a qualitative piece lead to the formulation and quantitative testing of hypotheses, followed by more qualitative probing to explore findings from the quantitative analyses. While this may be the optimal and, therefore, most desirable way of combining methods, it will, in many instances, be thwarted by the reality of resource constraints.

## The Practice of Combining Methods

Table 9.1 provides an overview of the most obvious logically possible ways of combining qualitative and quantitative methods. In actual practice, some approaches are used more frequently than others; however, the mixing of methods does not always occur in one of these "pure" forms, making it sometimes difficult and often arbitrary to classify studies into one or another category. Frequently, authors mention that they used qualitative and quantitative approaches, without specifying how exactly they did this, and the relative contribution of each approach to the findings.

Using qualitative strategies such as focus groups or pilot interviews to inform the development of a quantitative instrument (combination #1 in Table 9.1) is a very common approach to combined methods. Researchers may begin construction of an instrument by gathering questions from previously used quantitative instruments, considering their established reliability and validity; summarizing them into a few broad subject areas and conducting focus groups and interviews to explore the degree to which these topics have relevance to their participants; listening to the words used by participants to discuss the topics; and hearing about other related topics that may not have been included in the original instruments. This approach ensures that the instrument is valid and makes sense to those who will later be studied in a quantitative way.

A good example of such an approach is Bar-Tur, Levy-Shiff, and Burns's (1998) "study of the inner world and intrapsychic processes not previously investigated" (p. 5) of a sample of 60 community-dwelling, retired, middle-class men between the ages of 63 and 83 residing in Sydney, Australia. The authors are unusually explicit and detailed in their description of how they combined qualitative and quantitative research strategies, and their account of the contribution of each strategy to the findings. Focusing on mental and emotional engagement with others as a measure of adjustment to the losses of aging, the authors argue convincingly that their research called for a combination of qualitative and quantitative methods: they were interested in aspects of the aging experience about which little was known, and they were guided by the assumption that participants' subjective perceptions of their individual situations would explain their behavior better than would their objective situations. An exploratory approach helped the researchers discover and formulate significant questions on this topic, and understand the participants' ways of coping with work, health, and financial and social losses.

The researchers conducted "lengthy," audio-taped, qualitative, pre-test interviews exploring "activities, interests, reminiscences, relationships, and thoughts . . . revealing the interviewees' inner and external worlds" (p. 5). Through these qualitative interviews, participants actively helped shape and rephrase questions about perceived losses, the definition of and difference between mental and emotional engagements with significant others, life events, and categories of losses. The interviews were subjected to content analysis, and the resulting concepts and categories were used for construction of a final interview schedule. The final quantitatively oriented interview consisted of five sections: background information, present and past mental engagements, present and past emotional engagements with significant others, losses in aging, and subjective well-being. Each section began with open-ended, discursive, exploratory questions, and was followed by forced-choice questions designed to synthesize and summarize major points touched on in the preceding discussion.

The section on background information included demographics, as well as questions on family status, physical and mental health, past work experiences and current activities, and reaction to retirement. The objective of this first section was "in part to establish rapport and reduce anxieties, and mainly to help the respondent recollect and assess as precisely as possible the losses in aging and his mental and emotional world" (p. 6). Similarly, the exploration of mental engagements started with open-ended questions about a respondent's "typical week in his present life, including daily routine, activities, hobbies, and interests" (p. 6), and ended with a series of forced-choice questions for which the qualitative part had paved the way. The researchers then proceeded in the same fashion to explore the remaining three sections of the interview, covering emotional engagements with significant others, losses in aging, and subjective well-being. The authors then performed correlation and multiple regression analyses to explore the effects of each of the different types of engagement on well-being. They found that each type of engagement was positively related to well-being, "but that only mental engagement with the present buffered the negative impact of loss of work and loss of health on well-being" (p. 1).

The contribution of this research lies in its subjective assessment of respondents' outer and inner worlds, a focus not addressed in existing research. The authors' detailed descriptions of these measures and of the processes they used to develop them enhance the credibility of their findings and make replication possible. The use of a qualitative approach to establish the content validity of the quantitative part of their instrument served to incorporate within one integrated interview "both the qualitative strengths of the personal interview and the rigor of standardized measurements" (p. 5).

Combination #2 in Table 9.1 involves using an existing database from a quantitative study to select a sample for a principally qualitative study. This strategy may be part of a planned research design in which responses to quantitative surveys identify a subgroup with particular characteristics that the researchers then recontact for a study using qualitative methods. Alternatively, this strategy may be a coincidental by-product of the collaboration of researchers, with a quantitative researcher having access to previously collected data that could help the qualitative researcher identify participants for a totally unrelated study. This is one of the logical combinations identified by Morgan (1998) and Morse (1991). The limited number of examples of where a qualitative study was used for selecting a sample for a principally qualitative study may be due to researchers' failure to make explicit their sampling procedures.

Combination #3 in Table 9.1 is similar to #2 except for the emphasis given to each method. Here supplemental qualitative methods are used to illuminate findings from a principally quantitative study. Woodruff and Applebaum's study (1996), using structured telephone interviews with 270 home-care consumers to examine their satisfaction with services they were receiving from Older Americans Act-funded agencies, is an example of this approach. The researchers were puzzled by most elders' high satisfaction with the quality of their care, in spite of the fact that some respondents reported serious problems like abuse by a worker. This, together with other findings, prompted the researchers to supplement their quantitative interviews with case studies and participant observations to explore the reasons for the seemingly inconsistent and contradictory results. The qualitative follow-up shed light on these inconsistencies by revealing that consumers had mixed feelings that were not tapped by the quantitative survey. This approach also underlined the importance of asking specific rather than global questions and of probing in response to participants' answers.

Combination #4 in Table 9.1 is similar to combination #1 in that a qualitative approach informs a later quantitative study. However, rather than developing a quantitative instrument, the qualitative piece is intended primarily for hypothesis-generation. In other words, combination #1 tells us *how* to study our topic in a quantitative way, whereas combination #4 suggests *what* we should be examining. An additional difference between combinations #1 and #4 is the closer linkage between, and greater integration of, the qualitative and quantitative pieces in combination #4. Furthermore, in combination #4 the qualitative piece is the major one that creates a quantitative instrument to be used on a larger sample for testing hypotheses that emerged from the qualitative piece. The time-consuming and labor-intensive nature of a major qualitative study as a prelude to a relatively minor quantitative study—both to be completed in a usually unrealistic time frame dictated by a funding agency—may well explain the infrequent use of this combination.

Combination #5 embeds some qualitative questions into a principally quantitative questionnaire. Quantitative questions may be used to screen or identify specific respondents to whom may be posed exploratory qualitative questions. Straker and Atchley (1999) used this strategy when conducting interviews with long-term care providers regarding their frontline worker-recruitment and retention problems. Providers were asked to indicate the extent of their problems in the work environment on a scale of 1 to 10, with 10 indicating a very serious problem. Those who rated their problem as 5 or above, presumably those for whom problems have the greatest salience, were then asked why they thought they had recruitment or retention problems. The assumption here was that these providers would be most aware of a variety of reasons for their workplace problems and thus reveal hitherto unknown insights. This method is more economical and perhaps valid than employing a purely quantitative approach in which the researcher anticipates ahead of time all of the reasons for problems that someone might mention.

While researchers have used qualitative questions for selective elaboration and description, qualitative questions are most frequently embedded in principally quantitative instruments to probe all respondents' answers and to allow for elaboration. Together with combination #1, this is probably the most common strategy for combining methods. Sometimes this combination is used to ascertain that respondents had "interpreted the questions as intended" (Sorensen, 1998). At other times, it is used to provide insights into the rationale or motivation for certain behaviors reported in response to quantitative questions (Kuehne & Sears, 1993) or to assess whether gender, ethnicity, or other attributes such as childlessness are salient dimensions in how respondents answer certain questions in a principally quantitative study (Miller & Kaufman, 1996; Wallhagen & Strawbridge, 1995).

Wishing "to elicit caregivers' perception of role demands and supports linked to marital status," Litvin, Albert, Brody, and Hoffman (1995, p. 375) embedded two open-ended questions about the advantages and disadvantages of five marital statuses in an otherwise quantitative, longitudinal study on caregiving with a sample of 522 respondents. As a first step in the analysis, they sorted and categorized the responses. Responses were grouped into six codes summarizing the main advantages respondents had mentioned: emotional, instrumental, no advantage, financial, lack of competing demands, and role model for children. Nine codes summarizing the main disadvantages were: competing demands, no disadvantage, lack of freedom in lifestyle, family conflict, financial stress, lack of instrumental support, lack of emotional support, lack of privacy, and worry about future caregiving responsibilities. The authors then recoded "the presence of a theme . . . as a dichotomous variable" and performed ANOVAs to compare women's responses according to measures of strain and support. In their presentation of results, the authors included excerpts from the transcripts to document their rationale for assigning the codes and to let the women express their feelings. The researchers used a qualitative exploration of the advantages and disadvantages of caregiving and concluded "that competing roles have the potential to both disrupt and enhance one's life" (p. 286).

Combination #6 simultaneously takes a qualitative look at some phenomenon, while collecting quantitative information—or vice versa.
Wenger (1993, 1999) provides an excellent example of an integrated
combination of qualitative and quantitative data in which both sources
contribute equally and enhance each other's power. Wenger (1993)
used qualitative interviews with 30 individuals, age 80 and over, drawn
from a sample of 534 elders participating in an extensive, quantitative,
longitudinal study of aging. The purpose of the qualitative interviews was
two-fold: to identify patterns of self-help and mutual aid as manifested in
different types of networks and "to support the quantitative data from
the survey interviews" (p. 27). The author also used findings from the
earlier quantitative survey to assist in interpreting qualitative findings.

Wenger's 1999 article demonstrates constraints and contingencies
that influence the choice of a particular research strategy. Recognizing
policymakers' preferences for large-scale, quantitative, problem-ori-
ented studies, Wenger proposed a survey as the core of her study.
However, her qualitative training and predilection compelled her "to
include open-ended questions, to request interviewers to record verbatim comments in certain areas, and to complete interviewer's reports
that described the overall situation of the respondent and the interviewer's interpretation of the larger picture" (p. 370). The large body of
quantitative data obtained from more than 500 elders in 1979, and
from decreasing numbers of survivors in five subsequent waves was
immeasurably enriched by the qualitative, contextual elaboration, probing, and clarifying throughout the interviews. To satisfy the funding
agency's interest in identifying the characteristics and needs of vulnerable elders, the quantitative portion of the interviews tapped issues such
as frailty, needs, and deficiencies. On the whole, the picture that
emerged from the quantitative data was much less bleak than had been
expected: most elders were in relatively good health, had good morale,
and had adequate social contacts and support. The qualitative data
added to this basically positive picture by fleshing out "what people's
day-to-day lives were like. It was a very different picture from that presented in most of the literature on older people that existed at that
time. Much of the earlier work had been done on client or patient
samples that presented a much more gloomy picture" (p. 372).[1]

Encouraged by the mutually enhancing complementarity of the two
approaches, Wenger was funded to undertake an examination of the
dynamics of social networks using a broad range of open-ended questions. In addition, questions raised during the first phase of the study
were added to test hypotheses elicited during the qualitative segments
of the first phase. This escalation of mixed methods led to an ever-

richer body of data in successive waves of interviews, with qualitative findings helping to interpret quantitative data, and quantitative methods testing hypotheses that emerged from the qualitative data. The longitudinal nature of the study allowed for such an evolution where findings from one approach would feed into more exploration by the other. What started as a quantitative survey eventually took on features more akin to ethnography.

Ethnography (combination #7) might be considered the multimethod approach par excellence to combining qualitative and quantitative methods and data sources. Social scientists, usually anthropologists, who are trained in some of the various systematic approaches to ethnographic data collection and analysis, talk with and observe the people they study, in addition to counting people, sheep, pigs, acres of land, or numbers of trips to the market. Such inclusion of quantification does not necessarily represent a mixing of methods in the sense we used in this chapter, where quantitative methods usually refers not only to the collection of numeric data, but also to statistical assessment of associations within the numbers obtained in surveys.

Garro's (1990) work in an Ojibway Indian community in Manitoba, Canada, provides an excellent illustrative example of mixing methods and achieving a high degree of integration through a technique called consensus analysis. Consensus analysis is a quantitative technique that provides a mathematical model of the knowledge a group has of a specific cultural topic. Garro used this approach to describe the "cognitive domain" of high blood pressure. She first conducted qualitative interviews with 26 individuals to discover the folk model for high blood pressure. Specifically, she asked informants "what caused the illness, why it started when it did, the history of the illness, the kinds of effects it has, what possible and appropriate treatments are, along with other related questions and additional questions that arose from the informants' responses" (p. 101). This explanatory interview allowed her to collect a wide variety of individual beliefs about blood pressure. She then presented her informants with 67 statements derived from earlier interviews with informants and asked them to identify these as either true or false. According to Garro, these two sets of interviews provided "somewhat different, yet complementary, information about illness. The explanatory model interview allows the informant to describe the illness and its consequences in terms of personal meaning and experience . . . [whereas] responses to the true-false questions draw upon general understandings about the illness" (p. 102). In addition, the true-false questions allow the researcher to examine agreement among informants. Garro found that, "on average 78 percent of the answers given reflected shared cultural knowledge for the domain of high blood pressure" (p. 106). The findings from these two steps of data collection informed more focused ethnographic interviews and allowed the researcher to arrive at a better understanding of the folk model. Such a sequential methodological triangulation generally is more powerful than a simple description of informants' beliefs about blood pressure would be.

## Challenges and Solutions to Combining Quantitative and Qualitative Methods

Debate about the relative value of qualitative and quantitative methods may undermine efforts at combining the two. As long as each school claims its method to be superior, adherents of one or the other are unlikely to talk across the ideological chasm, much less to bridge it by combining methods (Morgan, 1998). Disciplinary boundaries across which it is difficult to establish effective communication are also an obstacle to multimethod approaches (Carey, 1993). Simple questions of semantics pose problems as well: when we publish our results, do we call those we studied subjects, respondents, participants, or informants? Training in one method or the other necessarily creates differing definitions of concepts such as "model," "sample," and "interview schedule," to name only a few. All these issues are particularly pertinent to gerontology because of its multidisciplinary nature, making it a fertile testing ground for efforts at combining methods. As we move further along in our efforts to find appropriate combinations of methods to address salient questions, we also discover the potential pitfalls of and obstacles to this new endeavor.

The first of these is essentially an issue of practical constraints. In-depth interviews, participant observation, and focus groups generally consume a great deal of research time, and generally use small samples. Qualitative results are not intended to be generalized to a larger population; instead, they illuminate and describe with the goal of providing insights into the phenomenon of interest. On the other hand, quantitative research generally uses large samples to ensure generalizability to the population from which the sample is drawn. Because of time and money constraints, a choice is usually made between the need for generalizability and the need for in-depth explanatory information on the research question. Rarely do researchers have the luxury of collecting enough in-depth qualitative information to generalize to the larger population. Decisions about whether and how to combine methods are driven by budgetary and time constraints, as well as the ultimate purpose of the research. For example, national public opinion polls that rely on quantitative methods give us a snapshot of what people are thinking right now, but they fail to explain why they are thinking that way. Consider this finding: "Despite the fact that most adults anticipate that life will improve for older Americans and that there will be cures for life-threatening diseases during the next 50 years, only 27% say they would like to be 100 years old" (Takeuchi, 1999, p. 1). The public opinion poll reported here tells us *what* people are thinking, but obviously fails to explain *why* they are thinking it. Finding an answer to the *why* question would require probing into a number of contextual and situational aspects.

A second obstacle to combining methods involves the capabilities of researchers. Academic disciplines traditionally come with biases within their own methods. As mentioned previously, researchers are often trained in either quantitative or qualitative methods, but rarely in both. Accepted standards for sampling and questionnaire design in quantitative studies are seemingly violated by the purposive sampling and evolving interview schedules that can be used in qualitative research. Researchers trained in different methods must work hard to understand each other, to accept the legitimacy and assumptions of different methods, and to understand the benefits and limitations of an approach outside of their own expertise. When a team of researchers begins the project with shared assumptions, the collaborative effort will be greatly enhanced. However, when they share few assumptions, the task of collaboration is made even more difficult. Both qualitative and quantitative research have their own constraints, and attempts to combine the two may multiply the constraints and challenges.

Despite these philosophical and practical difficulties, research in gerontology is moving away from rigid, disciplinary-bound approaches, and toward increased emphasis on choosing the method that is most appropriate for the questions to be studied. This often requires mixing methods. Our examples show that combined approaches can shed light on complex issues that would remain unclear using a single method.

There are several solutions to the problem of a lack of convergent findings: combine methods with the aim of achieving convergence; conclude either that the findings from one method are invalid or that the whole study was conducted improperly; or give priority to findings from one piece or use divergent findings to achieve a higher level synthesis (Chesla, 1992). If multiple methods contributed unequal amounts of evidence, the results of the method that contributed more should take priority (Morse, 1991). Thoughtful researchers have learned to recognize the limitations of their preferred methods, and are learning new methods, new ways of collaborating, and new research approaches capable of integrating multiple methods into cohesive research designs. There are indications that students from all disciplines are increasingly cross-trained in a variety of research methods that make them both better producers and consumers of mixed-methods research.

## Discussion

Theorizing about models and principles of combining qualitative and quantitative methods seems easier and is probably intellectually more stimulating than actually doing it. Researchers who embark on such an enterprise may know the requirements for data versus theory triangulation. They may recognize the consequences of their priority and sequencing decisions, and they may appreciate the relative advantages of a concurrent versus a nested design. And for certain projects, they probably dream about Sells and colleagues' (1995) truly integrated 16-step model where each method feeds on, and provides more food for, the other. In the real world of contingencies and constraints, the combinations that emerge are less pure, more pragmatic, sometimes accidental, sometimes an afterthought, and probably sometimes aborted or botched and, therefore, not publicized.

In many cases, they are not adequately described, making it impossible for the reader to classify these studies into the neat categories dictated by theory. More important, such lack of explicit description of how exactly a study was carried out or why the methods were mixed makes it difficult to judge both the value of mixing and the relative contribution of each method. Given the space limitations imposed by most journals, many articles drawing on studies that used mixed methods report only on the results of one of the methods. Often, there is only a vague reference to the current article being part "of a larger study," which may or may not be referenced so that the reader keen on discovering the alchemy of the mix is in no position to track it down.

But we also learned from our excursion into this topic that diehard quantitative researchers are becoming less timorous about including open-ended questions into their protocols. Qualitative research has not only come out of the closet, but it has legitimated itself in some bastions of positivist rectitude. There seems to be a growing recognition that while quantitative methods involve counting, they also require of respondents that they translate their largely subjective experiences into empirical data. In addition, without understanding domains relevant to the respondent, quantitative instruments and consequent findings risk being devoid of meaning and irrelevant. In some ways, combining qualitative and quantitative questions in the same protocol can be seen as an effort at joint translation by the respondent and the researcher. This is definitely indicated and increasingly practiced where the researcher knows too little about a topic to formulate valid forced-choice questions or when an explication of the findings is needed.

There is, however, still the latent assumption that numbers are more objective and, therefore, more scientific than stories. How else does one explain the preference of gerontologists for a clinical diagnosis of depression based on scores on the Geriatric Depression Scale rather than individuals' stories of their symptoms and feelings? Social scientists' attachment to quantitative methods grew out of their desire to be accepted as scientific and supposedly value-free, an aspiration that was shared by early gerontologists. The increasing practice of mixing methods in gerontology in all sorts of combinations and constellations attests to the fact that we have been able to let go of an obsession with "science" and "fact" in favor of the quest for utility and meaning. As a result, more gerontologists are ready to acknowledge that they can—and sometimes must—merge their scientific perspective with the voices of their informants.

## Note

[1]The fact that Wenger (1999) "was criticized by advocacy groups and elected representatives for painting an unrealistically positive picture" (p. 372) provides an illustration of the extent to which qualitative research can be politically subversive.

## REFERENCES

Atkinson, P. (1995). Some perils of paradigms. *Qualitative Health Research, 5,* 117–124.

Bar-Tur, L., Levy-Shiff, R., & Burns, A. (1998). Well-being in aging: Mental engagements in elderly men as moderator of losses. *Journal of Aging Studies, 12,* 1–17.

Bazely, P. (1999). The *bricoleur* with a computer: Piecing together qualitative and quantitative data. *Qualitative Health Research, 9,* 279–287.

Brewer, J., & Hunter, A. (1989). *Multimethod research. A synthesis of styles.* Newbury Park, CA: Sage Publications, Inc.

Bryman, A. (1992). Quantitative and qualitative research: Further reflections on their integration. In J. Brannen (Ed.), *Mixing methods: Qualitative and quantitative research* (pp. 57–78). Aldershot, UK: Avebury.

Carey, J. W. (1993). Linking qualitative and quantitative methods: Integrating cultural factors into public health. *Qualitative Health Research, 3,* 298–318.

Chesla, C. A. (1992). When qualitative and quantitative findings do not converge. *Western Journal of Nursing Research, 14,* 681–685.

Creswell, J. W. (1994). *Research design. Qualitative & quantitative approaches.* Thousand Oaks, CA: Sage Publications, Inc.

Denzin, N. K. (1970). *The Research Act in Sociology: A Theoretical Introduction to Sociological Methods.* London: Butterworths.

Denzin, N. K., & Lincoln, Y. S. (1994). Introduction: Entering the field of qualitative research. In N. K. Denzin & Y. S. Lincoln (Eds.), *Handbook of qualitative research* (pp. 1–17). Thousand Oaks, CA: Sage Publications, Inc.

Denzin, N. K., & Lincoln, Y. S. (2000). *Handbook of qualitative research* (2nd ed.). Thousand Oaks, CA: Sage Publications, Inc.

Fielding, N. G., & Fielding, J. L. (1986). *Linking data.* Beverly Hills, CA: Sage Publications, Inc.

Fraenkel, P. (1995). The nomothetic-idiographic debate in family therapy. *Family Process, 34,* 113–121.

Garro, L. (1990). Explaining high blood pressure: variation in knowledge about illness. *American Ethnologist, 15,* 98–119.

Gubrium, J. F. (1992). Qualitative research comes of age in gerontology. *The Gerontologist, 32,* 581–582.

Hammersley, M. (1992). Deconstructing the qualitative-quantitative divide. In J. Brannen (Ed.), *Mixing methods: Qualitative and quantitative research* (pp. 39–55). Aldershot, UK: Avebury.

Hennessy, C. H., & John, R. (1995). The interpretation of burden among Pueblo Indian caregivers. *Journal of Aging Studies, 9,* 215–229.

Knafl, K. A., Pettengill, M. M., Bevis, M. E., & Kirchhoff, K. T. (1988). Blending qualitative and quantitative approaches to instrument development and data collection. *Journal of Professional Nursing, 4,* 30–37.

Kuehne, V. S., & Sears, H. S. (1993). Beyond the call of duty: Older volunteers committed to children and families. *Journal of Applied Gerontology, 12,* 425–438.

Kuhn, T. S. (1962). *The structure of scientific revolutions.* Chicago: University of Chicago Press.

Lincoln, Y. S., & Guba, E. G. (1985). *Naturalistic inquiry.* Newbury Park, CA: Sage Publications, Inc.

Litvin, S. J., Albert, S. M., Brody, E. M., & Hoffman, C. (1995). Marital status, competing demands, and role priorities of parent-caring daughters. *Journal of Applied Gerontology, 14,* 372–390.

Miller, B., & Kaufman, J. E. (1996). Beyond gender stereotypes: Spouse caregivers of persons with dementia. *Journal of Aging Studies, 10,* 189–204.

Miller, W. L., & Crabtree, B. F. (1994). Clinical research. In N. K. Denzin & Y. S. Lincoln (Eds.), *Handbook of qualitative research* (pp. 340–352). Thousand Oaks, CA: Sage Publications, Inc.

Morgan, D. L. (1998). Practical strategies for combining qualitative and quantitative methods: Applications to health research. *Qualitative Health Research, 8,* 362–376.

Morse, J. M. (1991). Approaches to qualitative-quantitative methodological triangulation. *Nursing Research, 40,* 120–123.

Mueller, D. J. (1986). *Measuring social attitudes: A handbook for researchers and practitioners.* New York: Teachers College Press, Columbia University.

Patton, M. Q. (1990). *Qualitative evaluation and research methods.* Newbury Park, CA: Sage Publications, Inc.

Richards, T. J., & Richards, L. (1994). Using computers in qualitative research. In N. K. Denzin & Y. S. Lincoln (Eds.), *Handbook of qualitative research* (pp. 445–462). Thousand Oaks, CA: Sage Publications, Inc.

Rowles, G. D., & Reinharz, S. (1988). Qualitative gerontology: Themes and challenges. In S. Reinharz & G. D. Rowles (Eds.), *Qualitative gerontology* (pp. 3–33). New York: Springer Publishing Company.

Sells, S. P., Smith, T. E., & Sprenkle, D. H. (1995). Integrating qualitative and quantitative research methods: A research model. *Family Process, 34,* 199–218.

Sorensen, S. (1998). Predictors of anticipating caregiving in multigeneration families: An exploratory study. *Journal of Applied Gerontology, 17,* 499–520.

Steckler, A., McLeroy, K. R., Goodman, R. M., Bird, S. T., & McCormick, L. (1992). Toward integrating qualitative and quantitative methods: An introduction. *Health Education Quarterly, 19,* 1–8.

Straker, J. K., & Atchley, R. C. (1999). *Recruiting and retaining frontline workers in long-term care: Usual organizational practices in Ohio.* Oxford, OH: Scripps Gerontology Center.

Takeuchi, J. (1999). *PBS Special: "Stealing time" study: A summary of findings.* Washington, DC: AARP.

Tashakkori, A., & Teddlie, C. (1998). *Mixed methodology: Combining qualitative and quantitative approaches.* Thousand Oaks, CA: Sage Publications, Inc.

Wallhagen, M. I., & Strawbridge, W. J. (1995). My parent—not myself. *Journal of Aging and Health, 7,* 552–572.

Weber, R. P. (1990). *Basic content analysis* (2nd ed.). Newbury Park, CA: Sage Publications, Inc.

Weinholtz, D., Kacer, B., & Rocklin, T. (1995). Salvaging quantitative research with qualitative data. *Qualitative Health Research, 5,* 388–397.

Weitzman, E. A., & Miles, M. B. (1995). *Computer programs for qualitative data analysis.* Thousand Oaks, CA: Sage Publications, Inc.

Weller, S. C., & Romney, A. K. (1988). *Systematic data collection.* Newbury Park, CA: Sage Publications, Inc.

Wenger, G. C. (1999). Advantages gained by combining qualitative and quantitative data in a longitudinal study. *Journal of Aging Studies, 4,* 369–376.

Wenger, G. C. (1993). The formation of social networks: Self-help, mutual aid, and old people in contemporary Britain. *Journal of Aging Studies, 7,* 25–40.

Woodruff, L., & Applebaum, R. (1996). Assuring the quality of in-home supportive services: A consumer perspective. *Journal of Aging Studies, 10,* 157–169.

# CHAPTER TEN

# Maximizing Methods: Interviewers as Informants

## J. Kevin Eckert and Sheryl I. Zimmerman[1]

The term "key informant" has a long history in anthropological and sociological research, especially in ethnography. Traditionally, the key informant was the ethnographer's primary link to and source of information on the group he or she studied. Such individuals often developed a special relationship with the researcher, serving as teacher, translator, and friend. By definition, key informants are insiders, or members of the group being studied, who are willing to act as a guide and interpreter of cultural mores, individual and group behaviors, jargon and language. By virtue of their position and stature, they provide the ethnographer with access to the group, guidance on how to avoid mistakes, and insight on interpretations. For example, without the help of Doc in William Foote Whyte's *Street Corner Society* (1943), it is doubtful that Whyte would have been able to penetrate the depths of urban society to conduct his classic study.

Ideal key informants are often seen as people with special characteristics. A hallmark of a good informant is total familiarity with the culture drawn from either being a member or long-term exposure. Other frequently mentioned characteristics include being currently involved in the culture, having available time to spend with the researcher, and having a nonanalytic or common sense understanding of the group or setting. In addition to these characteristics, researchers are often advised to interview several key informants so that multiple and varying perspectives might be represented (Fontana & Frey, 1994).

In a chapter discussing key informants in primary care research, Valerie Gilchrist (1992) offered a broader conceptualization of key informants. She writes, "Rather than thinking of key informants as distinctly different from any other individual or informant, I think it is more helpful to view key informants as individuals who can teach the researcher" (p. 74). In her view, key informants are not defined by rigid criteria, but by their ability to teach or mentor. They may be individuals who possess special knowledge, status, or communication skills, but above all they have access to perspectives and observations denied the researcher and are willing to share them (Goetz & LeCompte, 1984). Gilchrist's perspective, combined with the observation that the knowledge and experience of survey interviewers is underutilized in quantitatively oriented studies, led the authors to experiment with the use of interviewers or evaluators as key informants.

## The Collaborative Studies of Long-Term Care

The Collaborative Studies of Long-Term Care (CS-LTC) is a program of study of 233 residential long-term care/assisted-living facilities and nursing homes across four states: Florida, Maryland, New Jersey, and North Carolina. These states have well-developed residential-care/assisted-living industries, yet exhibit sufficient variability to provide a broad perspective on issues related to quality of care, resources of facilities, and staff-client activities and exchanges. In each state, residential-care/assisted-living facilities were randomly sampled in three strata to further capture existing variation. First, were facilities with fewer than 16 beds ($n = 113$). A second stratum comprised facilities with 16 or more beds that reflect components of purpose-built, new-model assisted living designed to promote aging-in-place ($n = 40$). The third residential-care category consisted of facilities with 16 or more beds that are more "traditional" and do not meet the new-model definition ($n = 40$). Nursing homes ($n = 40$) constituted a fourth stratum. Baseline data for the CS-LTC were collected from October 1997 through November 1998 on facilities and residents over the age of 65 ($N = 2,839$). All residents from the small facilities and approximately 20 residents from each of the larger facility types were recruited. A team of highly trained interviewers made site visits and conducted interviews with residents, staff, and administrators. They assessed participating residents' mental and physical functioning, interviewed care providers about residents' status and administrators about facility policies, and completed observational measures of structural characteristics of the facilities. A complete description of the methods and measures is available in Zimmerman, Sloane, and Eckert (in press).

The conceptual model behind the CS-LTC was the structure/process/outcomes approach to quality that was developed for health-care settings (Donabedian, 1966). Within this model, structure (traits and resources of the physical and organizational setting) and process (activities taking place between those providing and receiving care) were evaluated using quantitative measures deemed relevant to medical and functional outcomes for residents. A qualitative component, focusing on CS-LTC evaluators as informants, was added to the study when, during the course of data collection, it became apparent that the evaluators could provide valuable insights on residential care that could not otherwise be captured.

As is the case in most studies employing structured interviewers, extensive training was conducted on how to administer interview protocols so as to reduce interviewer bias and minimize errors. Use of a stimulus-response interview format assumes that properly phrased questions will be answered truthfully, interviewer differences minimized, and the effects of context neutralized. However, early informal comments of CS-LTC evaluators made it clear to the investigators that the interview process was revealing more than required in the closed-ended questionnaires. The interviewers, as perceptive individuals, were observing, experiencing, and reacting to the contexts in which they conducted their work.

## Evaluators as Key Informants

The same interviewers/evaluators collected data in more than one state and across a range of residential-care/assisted-living facilities and nursing homes. In the course of conducting formal interviews, they were exposed to multiple dimensions of everyday life within each facility. The observations and experiences of evaluators were systematically gathered to provide a qualitative perspective on the phenomenon under study. To accomplish this goal, evaluators were asked to maintain a journal of experiences, observations, and stories associated with what was going on around them as they performed formal interviews and structured observations. Although not key informants in the traditional sense (i.e., they were not members of the group or culture under study, although they were immersed in the cultures of the long-term care facilities), they possessed important information on life within facilities that could not be captured by standard quantitative methods.

Qualities of good informants include knowledge of the subject, an understanding of the nature of the information required by the investigator, and the willingness and ability to communicate. As noted by Bernard (1994), if an investigator is willing to become a "student," a good informant is an educational source. Collaborative Studies of Long-Term Care evaluators met these and other important criteria: they were trained, observant, articulate, knew how to tell a good story, and interested; they conducted interviews across the range of actors in residential-care/assisted-living facilities and nursing homes, including residents, caregivers, administrators, and families; they were in facilities on multiple days and at different times of day; they were sensitized to carefully observing the physical and social environment; and they were eager to tell a story about what they saw and to elaborate on their experiences while in the field. As multiple observers with systematic exposure to a wide range of facilities within a concentrated time frame, evaluators were able to corroborate observations and subjective interpretations, thereby increasing the trustworthiness of their observations.

The 14 evaluators for the CS-LTC had diverse and manifold experiences visiting residential-care/assisted-living facilities and nursing homes. By the conclusion of the study, all evaluators had visited at least 50 long-term care facilities in conducting this and related studies of long-term care; nine evaluators had visited more than 100 facilities. This level of immersion into the long-term care environments enhanced the veracity of the evaluator's observations. In addition, the diverse backgrounds of the evaluators fostered diverse vantage points—12 of 14 evaluators were female, 13 were Caucasian, and 1 was African American. All had at least some college education and seven were trained as nurses. The contrasting backgrounds of the evaluators provided variations in perspective that contributed to the comparative value of their observations.

## Data Quality and Sources

Questions of validity are often difficult to address in qualitative research because of its nonlinear design and dependence on the investigator(s) as the central instrument of data gathering. In this study, validity—the trustworthiness of the data—was enhanced through various forms of triangulation of observers and methods (Crabtree & Miller, 1992). First, in many instances, more than one evaluator made multiple visits to the same facility. Second, in most cases, evaluators spent multiple days within the same facility. Third, multiple methods were used to gather observations and experiences of the evaluators. Three types of qualitative data were collected from the evaluators: field journals, information from personal interviews, and material gathered from structured debriefing sessions.

*Field Journals.* Evaluators maintained field journals to gather and record impressions, reactions, events, and incidents observed in the field.
To structure observations and note-taking, each evaluator was asked to
comment on six broad features of the long-term care context they were
assessing: the physical environment, staff, residents, social interactions,
care-giving philosophy, and community setting. For convenience, pre-
formatted journal pages were placed in three-ring binders. In addition
to the six characteristic codes mentioned above, each page provided
space for the interviewer identification, facility identification, facility
type, state, and date/time of observation.

*Individual Interviews With Evaluators.* Face-to-face interviews approximately 1 hour in length were conducted with all 14 evaluators. Interviews
were tape recorded and transcribed. Each interview was conducted by
the first author (JKE) and began with the evaluator responding to the
general question: "What were your most memorable experiences while
conducting interviews for this study?" Interviews were reflexive, allowing
evaluators to elaborate on their responses, tell stories, and reflect on
themes inherent to the overall study, such as the quality of care, social
interactions, community setting, and physical characteristics of the
facilities.

*Group Debriefing Sessions.* Two debriefing sessions were conducted with
the evaluators. After completing baseline data collection in North Carolina and Florida, a 4-hour debriefing session was conducted with seven
evaluators, principal investigators, project staff, and a consultant. A
second 2-hour debriefing session with eight evaluators (six of whom
had participated in the first debriefing session) was conducted at the
completion of baseline-data collection in the remaining two states. In
each session, evaluators were encouraged to share experiences, impressions, and stories about what they observed while in the field. Both
sessions were tape recorded and transcribed.

## Analysis of Qualitative Data

The three sources of data were entered into an analytic database for
qualitative analysis using Qualitative Solutions and Research's NUD*IST
(Non-numerical Unstructured Data Indexing Searching and Theorizing) software (Qualitative Solutions and Research, 1997). The software
facilitates coding data in an index system, searching text or searching
patterns of coding, and theorizing about the data. The coding scheme

was developed through an iterative process that incorporated a priori coding categories reflecting the interest of the investigators, as well as categories emerging from the text.

The process began by reading the text of the first debriefing session and applying codes reflecting components of the process and structure of care paradigm. This process resulted in 26 indexing (or content) codes. The investigators then reread the coded texts, collapsing and combining related and overlapping categories and creating new ones to reflect the content. The final indexing system comprised the following content codes: philosophy of care (subcodes: small residential care, large residential care, nursing home); dementia care; staff-resident interactions; resident-resident interactions; facility-community integration; resident recruitment; selecting a home; dislocation from family and friends; family concerns-involvement; resident-facility congruence; caregiver ethnicity; religion; quality (subcodes: positive dimensions, negative dimensions); aging-in-place; and research in residential-care/ assisted-living. The three sources of data were then recoded using the emergent indexing system.

## Uses of Qualitative Data

Qualitative data from the indexing and coding system were used in several different ways: to complement and add breadth to largely quantitative analyses, as stand-alone analyses of emergent themes, and to inform the process of research itself.

*Adding Breadth.* Qualitative interviewer narratives were identified and isolated for selected substantive topics (e.g., aging-in-place, Alzheimer's and dementia care) and made available to the authors to inform the interpretation of quantitative data. For example, analyses related to residential-care/assisted-living and dementia illustrated the lived experience within facilities. The following interviewer narrative provides insight and understanding by placing residents in context.

> There was a place in Florida with thirty-five residents suffering from psychiatric problems and dementia. It was an unusual place. The administrator had over twenty years experience in running psychiatric facilities and was knowledgeable about dementia, drugs, and psychiatric diagnoses. He worked closely with physicians in teasing out the best medications for each resident. He expected families to participate in the care of their loved ones. Families reported that they had seen remarkable changes in their relatives since enter-

ing the home. Some reported that previously bedridden relatives were now up and walking. The administrator's philosophy was that residents should be as ambulatory as possible. He said, "They might fall, but we will pick them up and put their Band-Aids back on." He believed that it was better for them to have freedom. He had a computer that was connected to arm bands that they wore. Residents could wander a certain distance from the facility before the computer would alert staff to their location. They would go find and return them. The staff seemed very happy; they wanted to work in this open and seemingly chaotic environment. All sorts of people were coming to visit from the community. It was a highly stimulating environment.

Although the evaluators' impressions were kept distinct from the quantitative data that were being collected (data collection forms were completed before impressions were provided), such impressions made invaluable contributions to interpretation of the data, especially in those cases where objective assessment failed to capture the lived experience of life within a facility or class of facilities.

*Stand-Alone Analysis.*   A second important use of qualitative data from the evaluators is as stand-alone analyses that identify or discover new themes or support existing themes. For example, as the panel of investigators read and discussed the coded texts derived from the evaluators' journals, transcripts of interviews, and transcripts of debriefing sessions, the strength and quantity of evaluators' comments on residents' interactions with people and place emerged as a central theme. We refer to this central theme as "connectedness." Content codes associated with the theme of connectedness included: staff-resident interaction, resident-resident interaction, facility-community integration, dislocation from family and friends, family involvement/concerns, resident-facility congruence, selecting a home, and resident recruitment. The eight coding categories associated with connectedness accounted for more than one quarter of the coded texts and ran through each of the three types of qualitative data.

While connectedness is not a new concept, the quantitative measures tended to capture only select dimensions within this theme. Typically, staff-resident interactions are assessed by recording behaviors such as eating together, meeting residents' needs for assistance with functional activities or social/recreational activities. The importance of staff, however, extends beyond tending to residents' physical needs to psychological and emotional needs as well. The ability of staff to show empathy, kindness, and affection (personal attributes not easily quantified) toward residents was illustrated in evaluators' descriptions of quality.

For good quality the staff should be attentive both to the physical and emotional needs of residents. Staffs need to make time for them. To sit down and talk to them. To sit down and have tea with them. To know when their family hasn't been in to see them and they are upset. This makes it seem like family too. The human part of it is by far most important.

The main ingredient [of quality] is being concerned about mother as a person. Knowing what she likes and what is good for her and knowing her correct name. I've been in facilities where I've called a family member and referred to Helen and the family member says, 'it's Ellen.' The family says, 'I got this form from the nursing home about your study and they spelled her name wrong. I've told them several times over the past several months that this is my mother's name and they still have it wrong.' Personalization is very important.

Across the three types of data (field journals, personal interviews, and debriefing sessions), the evaluators' narratives were more likely to make references to the benefits of small homes than larger homes. Smaller sized homes have been characterized as unique in their potential to provide an environment more conducive to the development of close, personal relationships, individualized care, and a family-like atmosphere (Sherman & Newman, 1988; Morgan, Eckert, & Lyon, 1995). Moreover, Silverstone (1978) suggests that smaller environments can offer relatively permanent primary-group relations, where needs for individualized attention, including the need for affection, can be realized. The following two narratives are examples of how evaluators came to subjectively understand the contribution of facility size to generating a family or homelike atmosphere and allowing caregivers to have more personal relationships with residents.

In smaller homes, the people always looked like they were in a family. The large homes were institutions. No matter how nice the nurses were, which they were, it was more like 'I have a patient, and these are my nurses.' The small homes were homier, more like a family.

My impression is that small facilities have staff who really know the residents. A larger facility with a lot of privacy does not allow for as much staff-resident contact. For example, when interviewing a nurse for the study, she said, "No one reads." I had just interviewed a resident who put down his Eric Segal novel to talk to me.

Evaluators' subjective assessment of small facilities as homelike or like a family, in contrast to larger homes as like an institution or impersonal, in spite of their beauty or "upscale" look, was a powerful theme throughout the qualitative data.

The theme of shared characteristics and background had no parallel in the quantitative data and serves to illustrate the value of evaluators as sources of qualitative insight. Similarly, evaluators observed the powerful influences of shared religious beliefs and ethnicity in amplifying resident connections and interaction. They also noted that the ethnic background of staff sometimes facilitated interaction, especially among non-European heritage care providers with a "cultural bias" toward elders. The first two examples illustrate how sharing religious beliefs and experiences transcends the potentially alienating effects of large size and the different physical capabilities of residents.

> One of the most memorable places was a large church home. They really made you feel welcome. They were admitted there because they worked as missionaries for years out in the field. That was one of the requirements for them to be admitted. It was a particular religious group. It was Protestant. You could have worked as a janitor all your life if you were part of the religion. They all had this in common. They were quite friendly with one another. They talked about their experiences all the time. You could go from room to room and hear them conversing about what had happened in the past. I was impressed. They had a lot in common even though they were from different economic brackets. They went from janitor, cook, up to professors. There were more men in this home, which was highly unusual. Some were more able to do things for themselves than were others. Most were pretty able to move around and take care of themselves. They all had private rooms. Three or four of us were there for three or four days. This was a different place.
>
> There were a few homes that were religiously oriented that even brought the people closer together because they all had a common bond. I found that this was the case in both smaller and larger places. In the Jewish homes I visited the people seemed very close.

Ethnicity not only connects people through shared background and history, but also serves to increase sensitivity to elders through cultural beliefs that value old age.

> In Florida, it was the Filipinos, in Maryland there was a Nepalese run home. In these homes everyone was interacting with everyone else. This applies to the Black run homes too. They were culturally oriented toward older folks. If this wasn't the case, you could walk into a home and everyone would be like robots; meaning the residents didn't really talk to each other. They would roll in and have their breakfast, not talk, then go sit and watch TV, then eat lunch, then take a nap.

These and other observations, captured from systematically engaging the CS-LTC evaluators as key informants, suggest the importance of religious and ethnic affiliations as distinctive organizational and structural features of residential-care/assisted-living facilities. Such features may take on added significance as increasing numbers of people from diverse backgrounds grow old in these settings.

*Informing the Dominant Approach.*   A third way in which the qualitative component of the CS-LTC informed the dominant quantitative approach was through evaluators' comments on the conduct of the research itself. For example, the evaluators noted that observational data were not being collected at the time of day that was most relevant for the study aims. Specifically, they reported that resident activity levels, which were being observed in the afternoon, were not a valid indication of true resident involvement in day-to-day activities. To address this concern, a pilot study was conducted during which quantitative observations were made in both the morning and afternoon. While the findings indicated similarity of activity regardless of the time of day, the evaluators' perceptions resulted in documented validity and reliability of quantifiable observational data that will be used in multiple analyses.

In another instance, several evaluators questioned whether the measures of quality used in the study were sensitive to human interaction dimensions of quality of care. As one evaluator stated:

> There is a humanness in some facilities that the instruments really don't pick up on. . . . The questions seem kind of sterile. You are getting more of that from our journals and these interviews with us. The interviews are probably better than the journals since most folks can express themselves better in words than in writing.

The subjective and difficult-to-measure side of quality appraisal presented dilemmas for evaluators when they attempted to assign seemingly objective rankings to various aspects of facilities.

> I don't think the instruments are getting at the emotional side of quality. Sometimes when I walk through a home I really like, I find that I can't give them credit for what I feel, but instead have to downgrade them because of something I see or don't see. I feel bad about it. I try to be objective. I try to weigh it according to what the instruments want me to do, but inside my head I'm saying that I hate to give them a six when I really feel they should be an eight. It happens frequently enough that I am aware of it; and so are the other evaluators. How can we give them a higher rating when we've already shown on paper in numbers something else?

The preceding narrative illustrates the tensions as well as insights that arise when multiple methods are employed simultaneously in a

study. The defining characteristics of the positivist/postpositivist paradigm (e.g., objectivity, reliability) are challenged by the personally informed and subjective understandings of the sophisticated observer. In
this instance, each view can inform the other by challenging reduc-
tionism and loss of context when numbers are aggregated.

Aggregate, quantitative measures of the process of care in CS-LTC
facilities included measures in three domains: requirements for residents, individual freedom and institutional order, and provision of
services and activities. When compared with larger "new model" and
traditional residential-care/assisted-living facilities, small facilities
scored less favorably in most areas. For example, in the domain of
individual freedom and institutional order (includes measures of policy
choice, resident control, policy clarity, and the provision of privacy),
small facilities scored less favorably than either larger new-model or
traditional board-and-care facilities. The greatest disparity was in policy
clarity and privacy. A low score in the measure of policy clarity suggests
that small residential-care facilities have fewer institutional mechanisms
for defining resident behavior and communicating ideas, while a lower
privacy score indicates less privacy given to residents. In each case, lower
scores can be interpreted as deficiencies rather than normative features
of informal, primary relations associated with small groups.

Qualitatively derived stories and descriptions of facilities highlight
the complexity and cautions required in interpreting these data. The
following two vignettes contrast evaluators' experiences in a larger,
upscale home, and a small home serving the poor.

> I did a large private facility which was terrible. Upscale, private, no Medicaid,
> no nothing. If you don't have the money, you don't go there. Staffing was
> terrible. It was short-staffed; they were pressed, they wouldn't give you the
> time of day. Some of them wouldn't even look at me because they were afraid
> I would ask them something. The place was beautiful and the landscaping
> was gorgeous, but the residents weren't happy. You know that saying, "Money
> can't buy happiness."

In sharp contrast, one evaluator, describing her experience in a small
facility, noted:

> I was upset when I first went there and wanted to get out as soon as possible.
> It was a small facility in a rural area. Physically the place looked bad, but they
> were doing for these people what they needed. There were both men and
> women residents and these were very poor people; the state was the guardian
> for many of them. I could tell the people were very happy by the interactions
> they were having with each other. The staff was very attentive; their philosophy

was to allow them to be who they wanted to be. The atmosphere was happy, the staff were helpful and extremely open.

The subjective observations of evaluators offer differing perspectives on how residents might experience formality of communications and staff behaviors, and how these factors might relate to such outcomes as resident satisfaction and happiness.

## Summary

Combining qualitative and quantitative approaches in a single study has become an accepted design in social and behavioral research (e.g., Campbell & Fiske, 1959; Denzin, 1978; Steckler, McLeroy, Goodman, Bird, & McCormick, 1992). Triangulation of data sources, investigators, and methods serve to neutralize bias while enhancing validity. Grant and Fine (1992) provide rich illustrations of such combinations, ranging from free-form observations supplemented with structured, quantitative observations, through the mixing of ethnographic and experimental research designs, to combining surveys with qualitative procedures. Evaluators or survey interviewers often are overlooked as important sources of information and insight in quantitative studies. The richness of their collective knowledge and impressions, gained in the process of conducting structured observations and interviews, are lost or "neutralized" by too rigidly adhering to the cannons of quantitative survey research. In the CS-LTC research, viewing evaluators as informants who possess special knowledge gained from exposure to the field of study, provided an efficient and enriching qualitative component to an otherwise quantitative study.

## Acknowledgments

[1]The research presented in this chapter was supported by grants from the National Institute on Aging (R01 AG13871 and R01 AG13863). The authors wish to acknowledge Dr. Phillip D. Sloane, P.I., project associates, evaluators, facilities, residents, and families participating in the Collaborative Studies of Long-Term Care.

## REFERENCES

Bernard, H. R. (1994). *Research methods in anthropology: Qualitative and quantitative approaches* (2nd ed.). Thousand Oaks, CA: Sage Publications, Inc.

Campbell, D. T., & Fiske, D. (1959). Convergent and discriminate validation by the multitrait-multimethod matrix. *Psychological Bulletin, 56,* 81–105.

Crabtree, B. F., & Miller, W. L. (1992). *Doing qualitative research: Research methods* (Vol. 3). Newbury Park, CA: Sage Publications, Inc.

Denzin, N. K. (1978). *The research act: A theoretical introduction to sociological methods* (2nd ed.). New York: McGraw Hill.

Donabedian, A. (1966). Evaluating the quality of medical care. *Milbank Memorial Fund Quarterly, 44,* 166–196.

Fontana, F., & Frey, J. H. (1994). Interviewing: The art and science. In N. K. Denzin & Y. S. Lincoln (Eds.), *Handbook of qualitative research* (pp. 361–376). Thousand Oaks, CA: Sage Publications, Inc.

Gilcrist, V. J. (1992). Key informant interviews. In B. F. Crabtree & W. L. Miller (Eds.), *Doing qualitative research: Research methods* (Vol. 3, pp. 70–89). Newbury Park, CA: Sage Publications, Inc.

Goetz, J. P., & LeCompte, M. D. (1984). *Ethnography and qualitative design in educational research.* Orlando, FL: Academic Press.

Grant, L., & Fine, G. A. (1992). Sociology unleashed: Creative directions in classical ethnography. In M. D. LeCompte, W. L. Milroy, & J. Preissle (Eds.), *The handbook of qualitative research in education* (pp. 405–446). New York: Academic Press.

Morgan, L. A., Eckert, J. K., & Lyon, S. M. (1995). *Small board and care homes: Residential care in transition.* Baltimore, MD: Johns Hopkins University Press.

Qualitative Solutions and Research, QSR NUD*IST. (1997). Scolari, Sage Publications Software. Thousand Oaks, CA: Sage Publications, Inc.

Sherman, S. R., & Newman, E. S. (1988). *Foster families for adults: A community alternative to long-term care.* New York: Columbia University Press.

Silverstone, B. (1978). The social, physical and legal implications for adult foster care: A contrast with other models. In H. K. Haygood & R. E. Dunkle (Eds.), *Perspectives on adult foster care.* Cleveland, OH: Case Western Reserve University Press.

Steckler, A., McLeroy, K. R., Goodman, R. M., Bird, S. T., & McCormick, L. (1992). Toward integrating qualitative and quantitative methods: An introduction. *Health Education Quarterly, 19,* 1–8.

Whyte, W. F. (1943). *Street corner society.* Chicago: University of Chicago Press.

Zimmerman, S. I., Sloane, P., & Eckert, J. K. (in press). *Assisted living: Residential care in transition.* Baltimore, MD: Johns Hopkins University Press.

# CHAPTER ELEVEN

# Seeking Diagnosis for a Cognitively Impaired Family Member: Evidence from Focus Groups

## David L. Morgan

This study had its origins in an earlier project on social support for families who were caring for a cognitively impaired older person, either in the community or in a nursing home (Morgan, 1992; Morgan & Zhao, 1993). Since that study purposely dealt with the later stages of dementia caregiving, I was curious to examine some of the issues that occurred nearer to the beginning of caregiving. In addition, the earlier study was quite exploratory, so I wanted to pursue some of the issues it had raised concerning how families made decisions about caregiving.

That earlier research experience thus led to this study of the factors that influenced family caregivers' decisions to seek diagnosis for problems related to increasing cognitive impairment (i.e., Alzheimer's disease (AD) and other progressive forms of dementia). Although there was already a considerable literature on the kinds of symptoms that medical experts used to detect Alzheimer's disease or other progressive dementias, there was much less research on how families made this determination. This is an important topic, since research indicates that family requests are the source that typically lead doctors to examine older patients for possible dementia (Boise, Camicioli, Morgan, Rose, & Congleton, 1999).

One of the most common products of a clinical diagnosis of dementia is a score indicating the patient's level of cognitive impairment—most typically measured through the Mini-Mental State Examination or MMSE (Folstein, Folstein, & McHugh, 1975). The MMSE measures several aspects of cognitive functioning, including orientation, memory, attention, calculation, language, and cognitive imagery. As a clinically assessed measure of cognitive functioning, the MMSE provides a valuable indicator of a person's degree of impairment at the time of diagnosis.

It would be surprising if most families sought diagnosis when their family member was only slightly below a perfect MMSE score of 30, since such small declines in cognitive functioning are difficult to detect without a rigorous assessment. Diagnosis is also rare with scores that fall below 10 points on the MMSE, since this corresponds to a level of impairment where the patient can barely maintain a conversation. In the range between 10 and 29, one likely pattern for the distribution of MMSE scores at initial diagnosis would be the familiar bell-shaped normal curve. The center of the curve would correspond to the typical level at which cognitive impairment became obvious to family members, while the spread around this central tendency would correspond to families who sought diagnosis at levels of impairment that were either milder or more severe. Within this context, a secondary intention of this study was to examine the meaning of MMSE scores for family members who make judgements about the needs of elders.

The first order of business was to investigate the MMSE scores for the clinics involved in this project. Examination of medical records for 100 consecutive patients who had been diagnosed as having probable AD or a related dementia showed a uniformly flat, rectangular distribution of MMSE scores, rather than the anticipated normal curve where diagnosis was more common in the middle range and less common at either extreme. From a statistical point of view, this indicated that the decision to seek diagnosis had no correlation with clinically assessed symptom severity. Thus, a first specific research goal that emerged in this study was a desire to understand this apparent disconnection between symptom severity and diagnosis seeking.

One source of the widespread differences in the level of cognitive impairment at which families sought diagnosis could have been special problems that arise in detecting and interpreting symptoms of dementia. In particular, the patient's loss of short-term memory typically means that family caregivers have the primary responsibility for seeking diagnosis. This task is complicated by the nature of AD and other age-related dementias, where the first symptoms typically involve memory failures that may not have distinctive, recognizable, or visible impacts on immediately observable behavior. As the disease develops, more extensive cognitive impairment leads to disorientation and limitations in independent functioning. Beyond this general pattern, however, the progression of specific symptoms is highly idiosyncratic for each person, and the essentially unpredictable nature of AD produces considerable frustration for caregiving families (Gubrium, 1986; Cohen & Eisdorfer, 1986).

At this point, a literature review located a promising line of previous research on how people made decisions about whether symptoms merit diagnosis. This was the distinction between *recognizing* health problems and *responding* to them (Leventhal, Leventhal, Schaefer, & Easterling, 1993). This approach emphasizes a two-part process that begins with the recognition that some change in health or behavior might be interpreted as a symptom. Once potential symptoms have been detected, the next concern is the appropriate response. A diagnosis of probable AD may occur at milder levels of cognitive impairment when caregivers *both*: a) recognized relatively small changes in their family member as potential symptoms, and b) responded to these changes as a medical concern that required a diagnostic work-up. Alternatively, the diagnosis may not occur until further into the progression of cognitive impairment if there were either a failure to recognize mild symptoms or problems in deciding that diagnosis was an appropriate response.

Recognizing and responding to symptoms were treated as sensitizing concepts. As such, they did not generate specific questions in the interviews that would "test" correctness. Instead, the goal was to understand the relevant issues or domains of recognizing and responding to symptoms that underlie a caregiver's decision making.

The most basic question in this study is whether symptoms of dementia, in and of themselves, played a major role in decisions about seeking diagnosis. This issue is especially complicated by the nature of diseases that involve cognitive impairment, since the patients' memory problems limit their ability to detect, interpret, and describe symptoms. This gives family members the responsibility for making decisions about a set of symptoms that are ambiguous at best. Under these difficult circumstances, how do caregivers decide when to seek diagnosis for a family member who may have AD?

## Collecting the Data

A concern with how caregivers explained their help-seeking decisions led to the choice of focus groups as the core method (Krueger, 1994; Morgan, 1997; Morgan & Krueger, 1998). The strengths of focus groups were particularly well matched to this goal because group conversations gave the participants an opportunity to share accounts of their decision making. Through a process of "sharing and comparing" in group discussion, caregivers provided not only detailed statements about how they made their decisions, but also offered explanations for why they acted as they did.

Although it certainly would have been possible to collect data on this topic using individual, qualitative interviews, focus groups had at least two distinct advantages. The first was largely logistical: this design used only six group interviews to solicit information from 38 caregivers. It is impossible to know how many individual interviews it might have taken to generate an equivalent amount of data, but judging by the two interviews that were collected as preliminary data, that approach would certainly have involved the analysis of far more than the nine hours of tapes produced by the focus groups.

The second advantage that focus groups provided was the production of a large amount of very rich data, because each caregiver could use what the others said as a "context" for presenting their own experiences and beliefs. This process of sharing and comparing is one of the key elements of focus groups (Morgan, in press). In these groups, the participants were keenly interested in learning how others had dealt with the same problems that they themselves had faced. They became quite involved in sharing and comparing their experiences in seeking diagnosis, as well as the reasons why they had made the choices they did. The result was a tightly focused set of discussions in which the participants were interested in understanding precisely the portions of each others' lives that were central to this project.

In addition to the focus groups, the participants completed a brief survey questionnaire that provided complementary, quantitative data. The project thus followed a design for combining multiple methods (Morgan, 1998), where the core, qualitative method was supplemented by a smaller quantitative data collection.

*Selecting the Research Participants.*   The caregivers who participated in this study were located through the medical records of a large, private, nonprofit hospital in an urban area. This hospital was well known for its work in geriatrics and dementia. Members of the research team reviewed records from relevant clinics to generate the names of caregivers whose family members had been recently diagnosed as having probable AD, along with a few cases of other progressive, age-associated dementias that the clinics treated as outwardly indistinguishable from AD. Although the staff members in these clinics were careful to describe their diagnoses as "probable AD," the participants in this study consistently talked about the person they were caring for as having AD. These families used the specific label "Alzheimer's disease" for cases that a clinician might have characterized more generally as progressive, age-related dementia.

The source for the sample consisted of all cases diagnosed during an 8-month interval, although actual recruitment was done in two separate 4-month intervals to ensure that the diagnosis would still be recent at the time of the interview. Cases were excluded when records indicated that the family was seeking a second opinion for an earlier diagnosis; when there was no listing for next of kin; or when listed family members lived more than 100 miles away. The clinics' nursing staff reviewed this pool and recommended exclusion of a small number of cases due to known problems in the family situation (e.g., two cases involved caregivers with substance abuse problems, while another involved a lawsuit).

Cases were divided into higher and lower levels of impairment according to their scores on the MMSE (Folstein et al., 1975) at the time of diagnosis. The median MMSE score for patients in these clinics was the basis for recruiting families. When patients scored in the 19 to 29 range, their caregivers participated in focus groups of families who all had sought diagnosis at a lower level of impairment; when patients scored in the 10 to 18 range, their caregivers participated in groups of families who had sought diagnosis at a higher level of impairment.

The goal in the recruitment was to find participants for three focus groups of families who had responded to lower levels of impairment, as well as a similar number who had responded to higher levels of impairment. The screening of medical records produced a pool of 137 caregivers who received a brief explanatory letter from the hospital. This was followed by a telephone call from a recruiter on the project staff who gave more information about the nature and purpose of the research. If the person reached was unable or unwilling to come to the session, the recruiter asked if there was another similarly knowledgeable and involved family member who could participate in a focus group. The recruiters were able to find the desired number of participants through telephone calls to 78 families, of whom 38 (49%) participated in the research, representing 21 cases with higher levels of impairment at diagnosis and 17 cases with lower levels of impairment. Among those who did not participate, the primary reason given was constraints imposed by their caregiving (no funds were available to provide respite care for patients while their family members participated in the focus groups).

In their discussion of sampling in qualitative research, Luborsky and Rubinstein emphasize the importance of "sampling for meaning" (1995, pp. 101–102). This study used two of the principles they recommend. First, using the point of diagnosis as an opportunity to explore the experiences of families allowed the data collection to occur within the context of what Luborsky and Rubinstein term a "defined social process" that had meaning to participants. Second, the sampling strategy emphasized a comparison of families as "representatives of different experiential types," through the comparison between participants who had sought diagnosis at different levels of impairment. All participants were selected because they had recently experienced a meaningful event. They were divided into two distinct subgroups to search for differences between families who sought diagnosis in the presence of higher or lower levels of cognitive impairment.

*The Focus Group Sessions.*   The focus groups were held in conference rooms at the hospital where the diagnosis had been made. Since the hospital's staff routinely used these conference rooms to meet with families, this was a familiar environment for the caregivers. There were three groups for both levels of impairment, yielding a total of six groups. The focus groups ranged in size from four to eight, with a total of 38 families participating. All group interviews lasted 1.5 hours and were moderated by the author.

Upon arrival, each caregiver spent approximately 15 minutes completing a brief questionnaire that covered items on background characteristics and demographics, questions on the severity of a list of possible symptoms that paralleled the MMSE, and questions about limitations in both basic and instrumental activities of daily living (Fillenbaum, 1988).

One unanticipated aspect of the data collection was that several families brought more than one person to the focus groups. This created a disparity in comparing those families where the person we had spoken to on the telephone was the only one who attended. When families did bring more than one person, a member of the research team explained the need to ensure that every family would be equally represented in the discussion; consequently, we asked families to designate one person as their primary spokesperson. We then arranged the group so that this spokesperson would sit directly at the table, with the other family members seated behind him or her, away from the table and out of his or her view. This not only allowed us to direct all questions to the family's spokesperson, but also reduced the influence of the other family members on their spokesperson. We did, however, encourage the spokesperson to ask other family members for help in answering questions, and we allowed the other family members to raise their hands to volunteer additional information when they believed it was important to do so. In addition, families who brought more than one caregiver to the group worked together to complete a single questionnaire. Fortunately, this spontaneous adaptation of our original procedures worked quite well, and subsequent comparisons of both the questionnaires and the focus-group transcripts showed no discernible differences due to how many family members were in attendance.

Turning to the interviews themselves, focus groups can use either a more or less structured approach (Morgan, 1997; in press). These group discussions used a relatively structured format, with the moderator following a similar sequence of questions in each of the six groups. The advantage of this approach in the present study was the ability to collect a large amount of information from each participant, due to the small size of the groups, while creating a high degree of comparability across groups, due to the structured questioning strategy.

The moderator's interview guide consisted of three sets of questions organized around the theme of taking a "history" of how each family decided to get a diagnosis. The first set of questions in the focus groups asked about the caregivers' perceptions of the earliest symptoms, changes in symptoms over time, and how people in their family shared this information among themselves; these questions generated data on the links between symptoms and decision making. The second set asked about the decision to contact a doctor or other health professional, as well as how the family chose this particular hospital for the diagnosis; these questions generated data on access issues. The final set of questions asked the participants to think about factors that had led them to act sooner or had kept them from acting more quickly, and concluded with a question about the advice they would give to other families facing similar decisions; these questions explored other "barriers" and "facilitators" that influenced the decision to seek diagnosis.

It is important to note that the interview questions all emphasized the participants' own experiences and beliefs, rather than asking directly about researcher-generated topics, such as recognizing and responding symptoms, as well as access issues. The strategy was first to hear from participants in their own words and then to analyze whether their accounts corresponded to concepts from previous research.

*Analysis Strategy.*    Analysis proceeded in two phases. The first involved statistical analyses of the preliminary quantitative data designed to identify factors that distinguished the families who had sought diagnosis at higher and lower levels of symptom severity. Because the data consisted of a small, nonrandom sample, the quantitative analyses were descriptive and sought to identify patterns in the quantitative data that could be explored in more depth through the qualitative data (Morgan, 1993). The combined analysis strategy thus moved from establishing differences between the two categories of caregivers, to generating explanations that accounted for those differences.

The core of the qualitative analysis consisted of comparisons between the three groups where the families sought diagnosis at lower levels of assessed impairment and the three groups where the families sought diagnosis at higher levels of cognitive impairment. This process emphasized systematic group-to-group comparisons, searching for themes that were common in one category of caregivers, but either absent or notably modified in the other category of caregivers. To assure that these themes applied as broadly as possible, the qualitative analysis included the construction of a case history for each of the 38 participating families.

## Decision Making and Diagnosis

*Descriptive Results From Quantitative Data.* Data from the questionnaires that participants completed prior to the focus groups showed that families who acted in response to milder or more severe levels of cognitive impairment were indistinguishable on all background characteristics, their relationship to the patient, the patient's age, and the patient's place of residence. This effectively eliminated any differences in the caregivers' demographic characteristics as an explanation for differences between families who sought diagnosis in the presence of low or high symptom severity.

The questionnaire also asked about symptoms related to memory, speaking, behavior, and personality, as well as functional limitations in both instrumental and basic activities of daily living. Among these problem areas, instrumental activities of daily living (IADLs) stood out. Specifically, families who sought diagnosis at lower levels of clinically assessed cognitive impairment reported few IADL problems, while higher levels of cognitive impairment at diagnosis were accompanied by more problems with independent living. Regression analyses showed that once differences in IADLs were taken into account, none of the others symptoms (including problems with memory, communication, behavior, and personality) were related to the patients' levels of cognitive impairment at diagnosis. In other words, functional limitations showed the strongest relationship with clinically assessed levels of cognitive impairment at diagnosis, and none of the symptoms that were more closely related to cognitive functioning had any additional impact.

The remaining quantitative analyses examined variables that had been coded from the focus-group transcripts. These content analytic codes were generated using The Ethnograph software package (Seidel,

Kjolseth, & Seymour, 1995). One set of codes matched the same sets of symptoms that were measured in the survey questionnaire, another set coded access issues, another captured barriers and facilitators, and a final set of codes captured social support through positive or negative mentions of other people. A further set of regression analyses showed that only one of these variables had an effect, above and beyond the impacts of IADLs: negative mention of other family members. Thus, the quantitative analyses showed that seeking diagnosis at higher or lower levels of assessed impairment was primarily associated with reports of more problems in instrumental activities of daily living, with family conflict having a smaller but significant effect.

These quantitative results proved especially useful in the analysis of the qualitative data on the issues that families faced in recognizing and responding to symptoms. Hence, the next four sections summarize the qualitative analyses with regard to, first, the effects of IADLs and family conflict on the recognition of symptoms, and then, their effects on the response to symptoms.

*Instrumental Activities of Daily Living and the Recognition of Symptoms.* Since the recognition of symptoms must precede a response to them, and since IADLs had a much stronger relationship to the timing of diagnosis than did family conflict, the qualitative analysis began by examining whether and how IADLs affected the recognition of symptoms.

The IADL scale contained items about the independent ability to use the telephone, get around by car or bus, go shopping for groceries or clothes, prepare meals, do housework, take medications, and handle money. One obvious reason why problems in these areas triggered caregivers' identification of increasing cognitive impairment was their recognizability in comparison to memory problems. Although symptoms related to short-term memory typically are the earliest manifestations of AD, caregivers consistently reported that memory problems were hard to distinguish from common "forgetfulness" or occasional "confusion." In contrast, families who reacted at higher levels of cognitive impairment told how they could not dismiss more tangible problems, such as getting lost while driving in a familiar area, failing to file income taxes, or not eating while food was rotting in the refrigerator.

For families that reacted to lower levels of assessed impairment— before IADL limitations were apparent—relatively small departures from a prior pattern of behavior triggered the recognition of symptoms. Although these caregivers seldom reacted to the first appearance of memory problems per se, they did note related things that they believed marked a distinctive change in the patient. In some cases, this involved ceasing some characteristic activity, such as reading, shopping, cross-word puzzles, sewing, and so forth—or just generally "losing interest in things." In other cases, the recognition of symptoms that were directly related to cognitive impairment involved repeating oneself (e.g., telling the same story twice within a single occasion) or becoming disoriented in relatively familiar environments (e.g., at a daughter's house or while driving in a nearby city).

Those who recognized relatively low levels of impairment were especially likely to note changes in fundamental aspects of personality, as illustrated by a spouse in one of the higher impairment groups in her reply to the moderator's opening question about what were the first symptoms she noticed and how long ago they started.

*Participant:* Oh, I'd say about a year and half ago. He was a bit agitated and so I had my daughter take him to the family doctor, and he more or less diagnosed him at that time.

*Moderator:* Now when you say "agitated" [pause].

*Participant:* Oh, he'd get angry at things.

*Moderator:* Like what, can you tell me a story?

*Participant:* He is a very even-tempered person—he was. But little things would make him angry, and then he'd say, "You guys make me mad." . . . [In the family business,] he'd do what he wanted to do, which may not always be the things that needed to be done, but he'd go ahead and do them anyway. So, they'd say, "Dad, that's not what we want to do right now." Well, he'd do it anyway. That's what I mean when I say he'd get angry then because he thought he was always right.

By comparison, the families who sought diagnosis at higher levels of impairment differed in two major ways: either they did not detect the things that previous families did, or, if they did notice such things, they interpreted them as nothing out of the ordinary. Starting with the failure to detect milder symptoms, long-distance caregiving was one factor that made a major difference. Because caregivers who lived in other cities would have less contact with their family members, they were less likely to notice the more subtle symptoms that accompanied memory loss. Counting mentions of long-distance caregiving from the transcripts showed that it was mentioned in 43% of the higher impairment cases, compared with 18% of the lower impairment cases.

Several families who were living farther away had low levels of contact with the family member until they had to deal with problems with independent living. After the family became involved due to an IADL problem, they often became aware of a wider and graver range of symptoms, as reflected in this account by a son in one of the higher impairment groups who was moving his mother from another state to live with them.

> I had spoken to her over the phone several times to say I'm coming at this particular time, and have you contacted the movers, and how are you coming with organizing all of your belongings, and so forth. And I arrived, and she couldn't find the airport, and so it was about four hours later [before] we eventually got back together. So that was a reinforcement of a previous incident. Then when I finally, we got to her apartment, I looked at it and she was not ready to move. She kind of thought that she was. And it just became clear to me that her ability to think abstractly and to organize was just not there. . . . So anyway, we drove back and moved, but at that point I knew. I had learned a lot of things. . . .

A second barrier to the recognition of symptoms occurred when caregivers detected problems, but came to the initial conclusion that this did not depart from their family member's ordinary behavior. Caregivers in those families often normalized whatever changes they noticed by interpreting them as falling within the patient's predictable range of behaviors. Normalization is a well-known problem in the recognition of mental health problems, going back to the classic work of Clausen and Yarrow (1955). In particular, Perrucci and Targ (1982) cite normalization as one of the key "alternative interpretations" that families use prior to concluding that they are dealing with a case of mental illness.

As the next section shows, there was more than one way that these caregivers used normalization as an alternative interpretation for potentially problematic behavior. What made the present form of normalization distinctive was the fact that caregivers interpreted their family member's potential symptoms of AD as falling within a range of behaviors that had already been observed repeatedly. For example, the caregivers might say that their family member had always been forgetful, or "flighty," or "difficult." The following quotation from a daughter whose mother had a high level of impairment shows that dealing with such family members often involved a mixture of sadness and humor.

> Our family calls her the squirrel because we figure she's nuts. And we say that lovingly, but we always called her Grandma Squirrel. . . . I was so used to the way that she was.

It was especially difficult to recognize symptoms when the person in question had a long-standing pattern of erratic or antisocial behavior. When the mental stability of family members was already open to question, caregivers found it quite challenging to separate the early manifestations of AD from what they had long since accepted as "normal" for this person. Physical health problems could also mask the recognition of new symptoms, as in two cases where hearing loss provided an alternate interpretation for the source of inappropriate remarks and behavior. Only in retrospect did any of these families interpret the changes that they observed as symptoms of probable AD.

Once the family member could no longer function independently, lack of competence was clearly viewed as a departure from the past. Instrumental Activities of Daily Living problems thus broke down attempts at normalization, because families were no longer able to use continuity with previous behavior as an "alternative interpretation" for the troubles they were observing. Even a caregiver who lacked a clear baseline of normal behavior could recognize functional limitations as a change that threatened their family member's ability to live independently without assistance.

In contrast, families who sought diagnosis in the presence of lower levels of cognitive impairment typically detected mild symptoms in the form of fairly minor changes in behavior. These symptoms were easier to detect when family members had relatively frequent contact with the potential dementia patient. It was also easier to recognize symptoms when family members considered the potential dementia patient's behavior to be predictable and consistent, rather than flighty or erratic.

Seeking diagnosis in the presence of lower levels of cognitive impairment was thus most common in families who had the opportunity to observe changes in a stable pattern of baseline behavior. In families who lacked these opportunities, symptom recognition often did not occur until their family member's cognitive impairment progressed to a level that generated functional limitations.

*Family Conflict and the Recognition of Symptoms.* To this point, there has been little attention to the fact that multiple family members were often engaged in the process of recognizing symptoms; however, the ambiguity of cognitive symptoms in early AD meant that there could easily be different opinions about what was happening. Those who thought they were detecting symptoms often sought a consensus or validation. When others in the family denied the existence of any "real" problems, this produced doubts for those who thought they were perceiving symptoms. For example, in reply to a general question about

the first time anyone could remember discussing symptoms with someone else, one adult daughter in a high impairment group began by
recounting her attempts to convince her father that her mother was
having problems; she then described her further efforts to get others
in the family to recognize symptoms that included her mother's inability
to cook or drive.

> I went to my siblings and I said, This is what I see. Is it just me or are you
> seeing things also? And there was denial. We don't want to hear it, and that
> sort of thing. . . . I needed them to know that there was something, and I
> also needed the reaffirmation that they were seeing the same thing.

Family conflict was relatively rare, but when it did occur, it could
disrupt the recognition of symptoms by raising disputes about whether
symptoms existed at all. When family members disagreed about whether
there were recognizable symptoms, this often delayed action until IADL
issues created difficulties in maintaining independence. This change
in functioning shifted the balance in favor of those who claimed there
were problems. By comparison, the relative absence of conflict in families who sought diagnosis in the presence of milder symptoms meant
that caregivers who noticed smaller problems were taken seriously by
other family members.

*Instrumental Activities of Daily Living and the Response to Symptoms.*
Even if caregivers did recognize problems and took them seriously, this
did not necessarily result in action, since there might be delays between
recognizing symptoms and responding to them. The families in this
study had all sought diagnosis, so the real issue was how IADLs were
related to this symptom response.

Recognizing symptoms of cognitive impairment without responding
to them was most likely when families nullified the threat from the
disease by perceiving these problems as part of normal aging. In essence,
this was a second form of normalization, which eliminated the need to
pursue the diagnosis-treatment process that underlies Western medicine. In contrast to the previous form of normalization, these caregivers
did recognize a meaningful change in the family member, but they
attributed this change to a taken-for-granted aspect of life, rather than
to an abnormal disease process. Comments such as, "She's 87, for gosh
sakes," denied any need to visit the doctor. Indeed, several caregivers
explicitly stated that one of the reasons for not visiting the doctor was
that their family member was so healthy, by which they meant an absence
of physical problems.

For families who saw normal aging as the source of problems, this was an alternate interpretation that once again interfered with the translation of symptom severity into a medical response. Ironically, diagnosis seeking was most powerfully blocked when members of the medical community pronounced normal aging as the source of whatever problems the family had recognized. The effort required from the caregiver to challenge a physician is illustrated by one participant in a lower impairment group, who began by reassuring another who had to leave her regular doctor and find a specialist in order to get a diagnosis.

> I really agree with that, because even as good as my family doctor is, without my asking specific questions, he would not have told me anything, and there were times when I would have this great big question mark. . . . I can just see my doctor [ignoring the problem] if I had not pressed him into a corner and said, "What's going to happen?" They just don't want to deal with it, I don't know, maybe they do, maybe they don't, I don't know.

When caregivers interpreted symptoms of cognitive impairment as due to normal aging, this did not lead to "inaction" so much as a lack of medical action. In essence, these caregivers selected self-care as the appropriate response because they believed their knowledge and resources were sufficient to deal with the problem. If the problems were due to normal aging, the implication was that family caregiving was the only appropriate response, at least until the aging process was so advanced that nursing-home care was more appropriate.

When families initially responded to symptoms of cognitive impairment as normal aging, it was relatively easy for them to provide care as long as the cognitive impairment was mild. In contrast, when IADL problems increased the demands on these families, it was often the emerging reality of AD caregiving that drove their decisions to seek diagnosis. As one caregiver put it, "I was looking for guidance, how to more realistically cope with my father." Indeed, several of the conversations in the high impairment groups clearly showed that some of these caregivers were seeking diagnosis to legitimate their decisions about IADL issues, such as driving, living arrangements, or managing financial and legal matters. As another caregiver explained, she and her husband sought the diagnosis "to professionalize the decision" they had already made about relocating her father-in-law.

Overall, families who used a normal-aging interpretation of symptoms were less likely than those not normalizing symptoms to respond to the symptoms of dementia that they did detect, since they saw these problems as routine and even inevitable. Those families who responded to lower levels of cognitive impairment were more likely than those who sought a diagnosis at higher levels of cognitive impairment to interpret the symptoms that they detected as problems that needed to be solved.

The key impact of a normal-aging interpretation of cognitive impairment was thus to inhibit an active response to the earlier stages of dementia because these problems were normal. Ultimately, the progressive course of the patients' cognitive impairment did lead the families to seek diagnosis. Ironically, it was usually their own caregiving needs, rather than the patients' actual symptoms, that led these families to seek help.

*Family Conflict and Response to Symptoms.* When conflict did occur, one of the primary sources was disagreement about whether caregiving itself was really an appropriate response to the problems the family had detected. For example, when the caregiver quoted in the previous discussion of family conflict described why she consulted her brothers and sisters about the need for a diagnosis, it was because, "I did not want to make a choice by myself—I needed their blessing."

Resolving conflicts about caregiving through an outside expert's judgment was a major reason why families sought diagnosis. This use of the diagnostic assessment to address conflicts over the need for caregiving was reinforced by two policies used by the clinics from which these participants were drawn. First, whenever possible, the clinicians gave their diagnostic conclusions at a full-scale "family conference." This provided an opportunity for the family to ratify one of their members as the primary caregiver. Second, these conferences were not limited to diagnostic information, but also included the clinicians' opinions about changes that needed to occur in the immediate future, such as restricting the patient's driving or relocating the patient to an assisted-living environment. Both of these policies could have a decisive effect in an ongoing family conflict by throwing the weight of expert judgment behind one of the parties.

Overall, there was a fundamental similarity between disputes that produced family conflict over the response to symptoms and disputes about the recognition of symptoms. In the present case, family members who disagreed about how they should respond to symptoms of cognitive impairment were unlikely to act until functional limitations from IADL problems shifted the balance in favor of those who wished to seek help. When family conflict was absent, it was easier to produce consensus on an appropriate response.

## Conclusions

Conclusions from this research must be tempered by limitations of this study. One set of limitations comes from the sample. Compared with general population surveys of caregivers (e.g., Stone et al., 1987), these caregivers had notably higher levels of income and education. This fits with the fact that using geriatric clinics, such as the one that provided this sample, requires a degree of sophistication in accessing services. Consequently, these results are most likely to apply to other users of expert diagnostic units. Whether they would apply to caregivers in general remains to be seen.

Another limitation is that the sample consisted only of diagnosed cases. These data provide no information about the decision-making processes of those who do not seek expert diagnosis. This points to the need for prospective studies that locate both diagnosed and undiagnosed cases in representative, community-based samples.

Despite these limitations, the current results make it clear why IADLs and family conflict were the key predictors of seeking diagnosis at higher levels of impairment. Although it was the quantitative data that initially pointed to the importance of IADLs in caregivers' decision making, it was the qualitative analyses that clarified why IADLs were so important. When families did not recognize or respond to relatively subtle symptoms associated with lower levels of cognitive impairment, the development of IADL problems eventually required action as these caregivers confronted their family members' inability to function independently.

The quantitative finding that family conflict was associated with seeking diagnosis at higher levels of cognitive impairment also fits well with the qualitative analysis. Because of the uncertainty surrounding both the recognition and response to symptoms of cognitive impairment, conflict within the family on these issues greatly increased the difficulty of making decisions. Family conflict was a further obstacle in making a decision that was already difficult.

Taken together, these results show how the severity of cognitive impairment influenced families' decisions to seek diagnoses for dementia. For some families, relatively mild symptoms of cognitive impairment were enough to produce both recognition and a response. For other families, a variety of factors blocked either the detection of symptoms or action on those symptoms until the affected family member could no long function independently.

For all of these families, a diagnosis of dementia was not only a statement about the patient but also about the caregiving responsibilities of the other family members. Consequently, the point at which a family sought a diagnosis was as much a demonstration of their capacity to take on caregiving as an indication of the severity of their relative's cognitive impairment. Seen in this light, the decision to seek a diagnosis for dementia often depended on the implications that such a decision would have for the family as a whole.

As with many other chronic illnesses (Charmaz, 1991), progressive dementia redefines the needs of both the person who is ill and the obligations of significant others. When an illness requires caregiving, the diagnosis generates a series of realignments in relationships between the patient and his or her significant others. In Zola's (1973) terms, it creates a disruption in the ongoing "accommodations" that the family members have worked out with each other. Then, as family members attempt to sort out caregiving responsibilities, this can have further impacts on the accommodations that underlie their relationships. Dementia caregivers must consider how their decisions will have impacts that go beyond the patient into their own lives, and the lives of other family members as well.

Realizing the importance of caregiving also helps in understanding why IADLs were an important marker for when families sought diagnosis. Because IADL problems signaled a limited ability to live independently, they raised questions about the need for caregiving. While expert clinicians in geriatric-assessment clinics may routinely detect less intrusive symptoms, many of these families detected and responded to cognitive impairments only when those problems threatened to disrupt their lives. In essence, it was the need to provide assistance in the form of caregiving that triggered the actions of families who sought diagnosis at more severe levels of cognitive impairment.

Although the Health Belief Model (Strecher, Champion, & Rosenstock, 1997) includes the concept of "triggering events" as a factor in seeking help, there has been very little research in this area. One likely reason for this lack of attention is the fact that triggering events tend to be quite specific. Examples of the actual events that led to diagnosis among the families in this study included: a man who left a gym locker full of rotting food; a formerly fashionable woman who wore the same soiled dress for days on end; and a woman who became lost in a supermarket where she had shopped for years. At one level, each of these events was so specific that it might not have happened in another family—or it might have had a different meaning if it did occur. At another level, however, all of these events raised broader concerns about whether the older family member could maintain an independent life. As a result, the survey measure of IADLs captured a whole class of triggering events because it was the best available indicator of the patient's ability to live independently.

Another important finding of this study is that rather than a single primary caregiver, networks of family relationships often are involved in complex and conflict-ridden, decision-making processes. Despite all of the discussions about "family caregiving" in social gerontology, we have somehow managed to pay too little attention to the concept of "caregiving families"—a lesson that first became apparent in this study when families, rather than individual caregivers, showed up for the focus groups. We need to consider the extent to which concentrating on the "primary caregiver" reflects the research needs of social gerontologists, rather than the experiences of families. In particular, future studies of caregiving should treat family members as bound up in a web of mutual obligations, where anything that changes one person's ability to meet her or his responsibilities can have reverberating effects on each of the others.

## REFERENCES

Boise, L., Camicioli, R., Morgan, D. L., Rose, J., & Congleton, L. (1999). Diagnosing dementia: Perspectives of primary care physicians. *The Gerontologist, 39,* 457–464.

Charmaz, K. (1991). *Good days, bad days: The self in chronic illness and time.* New Brunswick, NJ: Rutgers University Press.

Clausen, J. A., & Yarrow, M. R. (1955). The impact of mental illness on the family. *Journal of Social Issues, 11,* 3–66.

Cohen, D., & Eisdorfer, C. (1986). *The loss of self: A family resource for the care of Alzheimer's disease and related disorders.* New York: Norton.

Fillenbaum, G. G. (1988). *Multidimensional functional assessment of older adults: The Duke older Americans resources and services procedures.* Hillsdale, NJ: Lawrence Erlbaum Associates.

Folstein, M. D., Folstein, S. E., & McHugh, P. R. (1975). Mini-mental state: A practical method for grading the cognitive competence state of patients for the clinician. *Journal of Psychiatric Research, 12,* 189–198.

Gubrium, J. F. (1986). *Oldtimers and Alzheimer's: The descriptive organization of senility.* Greenwich, CT: JAI Press.

Krueger, R. A. (1994). *Focus groups: A practical guide for applied research* (2nd ed.). Thousand Oaks, CA: Sage Publications, Inc.

Leventhal, E. A., Leventhal, H., Schaefer, P., & Easterling, D. (1993). Conservation of energy, uncertainty reduction, and swift utilization of medical care among the elderly. *Journals of Gerontology: Psychological Sciences, 48,* P78–P86.

Luborsky, M. R., & Rubinstein, R. L. (1995). Sampling in qualitative research: Rationale, issues, and methods. *Research on Aging, 17,* 89–113.

Morgan, D. L. (1992). Designing focus group research: Applications to primary care. In M. Stewart, F. Tudiver, M. J. Bass, E. V. Dunn, & P. G. Norton (Eds.), *Tools for primary care research* (pp. 177–193). Thousand Oaks, CA: Sage Publications, Inc.

Morgan, D. L. (1993). Qualitative content analysis: A guide to paths not taken. *Qualitative Health Research, 2,* 112–121.

Morgan, D. L. (1997). *Focus groups as qualitative research* (2nd ed.). Thousand Oaks, CA: Sage Publications, Inc.

Morgan, D. L. (1998). Practical strategies for combining qualitative and quantitative methods: Applications to health research. *Qualitative Health Research, 8,* 362–376.

Morgan, D. L. (in press). Focus group interviewing. In J. F. Gubrium & J. Holstein (Eds.), *The handbook of interviewing.* Thousand Oaks, CA: Sage Publications, Inc.

Morgan, D. L., & Krueger, R. A. (1998). *Focus group kit* (6 vols.). Thousand Oaks, CA: Sage Publications, Inc.

Morgan, D. L., & Zhao, P. Z. (1993). The doctor-caregiver relationship: Managing the care of family members with Alzheimer's disease. *Qualitative Health Research, 2,* 133–164.

Perrucci, R., & Targ, D. B. (1982). *Mental patients and social behaviors.* Boston: Auburn House.

Seidel, J. V., Kjolseth, R., & Seymour, E. (1995). THE ETHNOGRAPH: A user's guide (Version 4.0) [Computer software]. Amherst, MA: Qualis Research Associates.

Strecher, V. J., Champion, V. L., & Rosenstock, I. M. (1997). The health belief model and health behavior. In D. S. Gochman et al. (Eds.), *Handbook of health behavior research, Vol. 1: Personal and social determinants* (pp. 71–91). New York: Plenum Press.

Zola, I. K. (1973). Pathways to the doctor: From person to patient. *Social Science and Medicine, 7,* 677–689.

# PART VI

# Looking and Seeing

# Introduction

## Graham D. Rowles

In 1966, Eugene J. Webb, Donald T. Campbell, Richard D. Schwartz, and Lee Sechrest published, *Unobtrusive Measures: Nonreactive Research in the Social Sciences*. Despite the authors' reputation as well-respected methodologists, the book did not quite fit within the prevalent epistemological ethos of the time. With its emphasis on novel and, in some cases, seemingly quirky sources of scientific data, the volume provided a testament to the ingenuity of creative researchers. A chapter on the inferential use of physical traces cited techniques, including the measurement of tile wear in the area surrounding museum exhibits as an indicator of their popularity, the use of devices to monitor the frequency of drivers tuning to particular radio stations as an indicator of cultural preference, and analysis of people's garbage as a measure of their material lifestyle. There were chapters on the innovative use of archival material, on the critical analysis of personal documents, and on the use of observational technologies, such as one-way mirrors and electromagnetic movement meters for unobtrusive observation. By the authors' own admission, the "occasionally bizarre content of the material" (p. v) resulted in a liberating, groundbreaking contribution that not only became immensely popular, but also began to erode entrenched and restrictive methodological conventions. Emphasizing ingenuity, innovation, and imagination both in content and presentation (chapter 8 comprises a single paragraph and the concluding chapter 9 the single line, "From symbols and shadows to the truth."), through its advocacy of *multiple operationism* and the use of unusual sources of information, this volume legitimized a critical broadening of vision in an era of methodological orthodoxy.

Just as *Unobtrusive Measures* emerged in tandem with intellectual currents that transformed American society, so too does the promise of a new "age of aging" offer immense potential for imagination in qualitative gerontology. In the final segment of this volume, we provide two exemplars of the manner in which artifacts of a liberated, postmodern information and communication age—literature, poetry, journalism, photography, and even art—become vibrant and revealing sources of insight as we progress "from symbols and shadows" toward a "truth" of the aging experience.

## Auditory and Visual Media

As the way we come to understand ourselves and others becomes ever-more shaped by the often unidimensional images broadcast on radio and television and in other media, there arise a profusion of opportunities for critical interpretation of attitudes toward and understanding of the aging experience. As we listen to our car radios on lengthy cross-country trips, we are suffused with auditory messages, ranging from the crude stereotyping inherent in ageist humor to the more subtle and gentle inculcation of images of growing old in the upper Midwest as Garrison Keiller whimsically pervades our consciousness with monologues on the citizens of the fictional Lake Wobegon. Although radio broadcasts seem to reflect societal preconceptions of growing old, there are few content analyses that have employed this untapped reservoir of material to reveal how our culture creates and views its elders and the experience of aging.

There is even richer potential for powerful, poignant, and theoretically instructive perspectives on the process of aging and societal attitudes toward elders from a large and ever-growing genre of films, both full-length feature films and made-for-TV movies, that incorporate both auditory and visual representations of the aging experience. The subtle insights on reminiscence and feeling for place encapsulated in Ingmar Bergman's *Wild Strawberries* (1957) and Geraldine Page's anguished rendering of Mrs. Watts in *The Trip to Bountiful* (1985) can be contrasted with more direct social commentary on the issues and meaning of aging provided by popular films spanning several decades, such as *I Never Sang for My Father* (1970), *Harry and Tonto* (1974), *Cocoon* (1985), *The Whales of August* (1987), *Strangers in Good Company* (1991), *Waking Ned Devine* (1998), and *Tea with Mussolini* (1999). There are a few examples of critical interpretation of film in gerontology, and *The Gerontologist* now features an audiovisual review section that critiques contemporary films (Yahnke, 1999). However, the potential for penetrating content analyses of this medium remains largely untapped.

Some gerontologists and social commentators have begun to explore the potential of the creation and interpretation of still photographs as a window on the aging experience (Clark, 1995; Leonard, 1993; Magilvy, Congdon, Nelson, & Craig, 1992). Clark's photographs of aging athletes confront stereotypes of decrepitude. Leonard's creation of photographic collages reveals the creativity with which photography can be used to poignantly express relationships among generations. In the chapter that follows this introduction, Dena Shenk, an anthropologist, and Ron Schmid, a professional photographer, explore this approach to qualitative gerontology as they reflect on their work photographing rural elders in a variety of environmental contexts. They raise a series of compelling questions regarding both the potential for bias (through unwarranted inference and the deliberate framing of photographs) and the opportunity for revelation (through the interpretation of poses and backdrops) that cannot be derived from any other approach.

Finally, in recognizing the instructive power of empathy, gerontology must begin to acknowledge and harness the potential of sculpture and painting to convey essential features of the aging experience that may be unavailable through other means (McLerran, 1993). For example, in 1997, an exhibition of the paintings of older artists was held at the National Gallery in conjunction with the national meeting of the Gerontological Society of America. Through careful perusal and contemplation of the exhibit's portrayal of the diverse works of older artists, we can learn much from the way in which these artists represent themselves and capture, in the evolution of their work on canvas or in clay, what it means to be old (Ravin & Kenyon, 1998). Even without personal expression of identity, artistic representation of aging experiences has merit. For example, Pope (1999) commissioned artist Margrith Fritschi to visually represent the essence of her terminal subjects' lives as encapsulated within self-defining abstract "portraits" that integrated the nature and meaning of their "being" as an elder, as they reflected on their lives during their final hours.

## Literary Gerontology

Some of the most telling insights into the aging experience are provided by creative writers and poets who are able to capture subtle nuances of the aging experience through the skill with which they evoke image and emotion in writing about the later years of life (Achenbaum, 1989; Berman, 1994; Waxman, 1999). Such contributions include sensitive, perceptive, and largely autobiographical reflective works of writers, such as Florida Scott-Maxwell (1968) and Doris Grumbach (1991, 1993), as well as the sometimes phenomenally perceptive writings of "extra"-

ordinary people such as Mel Kimble (1993), who writes, "At a certain point one's perceptions of aging become intertwined with perceptions of oneself" (p. 27). Literary gerontology also has an emerging tradition that involves diverse representations of age and aging developed by critical readers of literary works (Yahnke, 1993). Finally, there is a fledgling genre of interpretations of the aging process that use literary sources as basic data in the creation of literate original insight into the aging experience. The essay by Maria Vesperi (chapter 13) that concludes this section provides an example of this genre. As Anne M. Wyatt-Brown (1993) writes, "Literary gerontologists seek to challenge the preconceptions about aging that influence our thinking about later life."

From appreciation of the value of the insights of novelists and essayists, it is but a short step to acknowledgement of the power of poetry as a medium for conveying the starkness, vibrance, ambiguity, clarity, complexity, angst, simplicity, contradiction, warmth, fear, satisfaction, desolation, pleasure, and pain that form the many conflicting facets of aging (Maclay, 1977; Schutz, 1974). For poets such as William Butler Yeats, aging and death provided an underlying motif of a portion of their work: "Did all old men and women, rich and poor, who trod upon these rocks or passed this door, Whether in public or in secret rage as I do now against old age?" For others, such as Robert Browning ("Grow old with me! The best is yet to be. . . . ") and Henry Wadsworth Longfellow ("It is too late! Ah, nothing is too late Til the tired heart shall cease to palpitate. . . . "), aging was viewed more positively, or the theme was only touched on tangentially (Browning, 1864; Longfellow, 1890). Finally, playwrights often have important insights for us in their creation of performance ethnography (Denzin, 2000), as they capture situational aspects of aging with both clarity and poignancy (Kastenbaum, 1994; Luke, 1987). In sum, it behooves gerontologists to embrace and seek to understand the powerful insights of those who are sometimes able to express aspects of the aging experience that transcend everyday discourse. As Barbara Frey Waxman (1999, p. 523) concludes: "This writing humanizes individual elders, complicates readers' notions of later life, and is evidence of the intellectual and spiritual contributions people can make to society, well beyond midlife."

## Some Limitations

While it is helpful to embrace alternative modes of knowing with enthusiasm, cautions are in order as we seek to reconcile the abacus and the rose, and move toward a blending of science with art in gerontology. It is important to grapple with the issue of "truth." Each literary and artistic perspective is just that—a perspective. It is an interpretation colored by the filtering and generally distorting lens of the observer, participant, or commentator who seeks to represent the complexity of the aging experience through an expressive medium. While phenomenologists would argue that the medium may capture the "essence" of the aging experience, others would contend that it can only represent "a" truth rather than "the" truth. As such, its value lies in its usefulness in helping us obtain a more sophisticated, refined, and, perhaps, more authentic perspective that is more closely aligned with "lived experience" than alternative approaches to insight.

A second caution is the need to avoid the unwarranted elevation of literary and artistic expression to a status beyond its potential. It is important to avoid undue romanticism and "preciousness" in interpretations of aging that may arise from blind reverence for alternative ways of knowing. While a perceptive autobiographical novel or highly emotive sculpture may capture the essence of the experience of a disadvantaged elder eking out an existence in an inner city slum and may have significant political impact, the raised consciousness arising from such a portrayal does not necessarily put food on this individual's table. It is necessary to view such work in concert with, and as a stimulus for, more traditional forms of inquiry that seek to reveal both the quantitative dimensions of the problem and its structural context.

Finally, it is important to acknowledge that both moral and ethical issues are raised as we employ literary and artistic forms to probe into and express intimate, and sometimes highly personal, dimensions of the aging experience. Paradoxically, and somewhat ironically, we commenced this introduction with reference to the essentially quantitative treatise of Webb and his colleagues. In their volume, these authors note: "In presenting these novel methods, we have purposely avoided consideration of the ethical issues which they raise. We have done so because we feel that this is a matter for separate consideration" (Webb et al., 1966, p. v). Qualitative gerontology cannot adopt this stance. Rather, the very essence of contemporary qualitative scholarship entails an acceptance of responsibility and an obligation to consider the implications of the approach. As we develop relationships with participants and photograph them in their daily lives, as we view a set of paintings and make inferences about the artist's view of aging, and as we selectively synthesize the writings of commentators, poets, and playwrights in the process of creating *our images* from theirs, ethical integrity demands that we explicitly consider the potential distortions and misrepresentations that are inherent in our images. We must accept responsibility for and ponder the consequences of the images we create.

## *Looking and Seeing: A Gerontological Gaze?*

Novelists, poets, photographers, and even journalists are in the business of representation. Their skill lies in an ability not only to look at and report on the human condition, but also to see beyond the surface—to reveal and interpret for us dimensions of experience that are generally beyond our immediate comprehension. In gerontology, this is an awesome responsibility because the artifacts created serve to shape and define the way in which a society views its elders and the process of aging. At the same time, it is an opportunity for creativity, and a call for risk-taking in utilizing diverse literary and artistic forms to nurture the gerontological gaze that will frame our old age. The following two chapters open up vistas that may help us to see in new ways.

## REFERENCES

Achenbaum, W. A. (1989). Foreword: Literature's value in gerontological research. In P. Bagnell & P. S. Soper (Eds.), *Perceptions of aging in literature: A cross-cultural study.* Westport, CT: Greenwood Press.

Berman, H. J. (1994). *Interpreting the aging self: Personal journals of later life.* New York: Springer Publishing Company.

Browning, R. (1864). Rabbi Ben Ezra, in *Dramatis Personae.* London: Chapman & Hall.

Clark, E. (1995). *Aging is not for sissies II: Portraits of senior athletes.* San Francisco: Pomegranate Artbooks.

Denzin, N. K. (2000). The practices and politics of interpretation. In N. K. Denzin & Y. S. Lincoln (Eds.), *Handbook of qualitative research* (2nd ed., pp. 897–922). Thousand Oaks, CA: Sage Publications, Inc.

Grumbach, D. (1991). *Coming into the end zone: A memoir.* New York: W. W. Norton & Co.

Grumbach, D. (1993). *Extra innings: A memoir.* New York: W. W. Norton & Co.

Kastenbaum, R. (1994). *Defining acts: Aging as drama.* Amityville, NY: Baywood Publishing Company.

Kimble, M. (1993). A personal journey of aging: The spiritual dimension. *Generations, 17*(2), 27–28.

Leonard, J. (1993). Not losing her memory: Images of family in photography, words and collage. In D. Shenk & W. A. Achenbaum (Eds.), *Changing perceptions of aging and the aged* (pp. 3–9). New York: Springer Publishing Company.

Longfellow, H. W. (1890). Morituri Salutamus. *The poetical works of Henry Wadsworth Longfellow.* Boston: Houghton Mifflin.

Luke, H. M. (1987). *Old age.* New York: Parabola Books.

Maclay, E. (1977). *Green winter: Celebrations of old age.* New York: Reader's Digest Press.

Magilvy, J. K., Congdon, J. G., Nelson, J. P., & Craig, C. (1992). Visions of rural aging: Use of photographic method in gerontological research. *The Gerontologist, 32*(2), 253–257.

McLerran, J. (1993). Saved by the hand that is not stretched out: The aged poor in Hubert von Herkomer's *Eventide: A Scene in the Westminster Union. The Gerontologist, 33*(6), 762–771.

Pope, S. L. (1999). Meaning of life among persons with advanced cancer. Unpublished doctoral dissertation, College of Nursing, University of Kentucky.

Ravin, J. G., & Kenyon, C. A. (1998). Artistic vision in old age: Claude Monet and Edgar Degas. In C. E. Adams-Price (Ed.), *Creativity and successful aging: Theoretical and empirical approaches* (pp. 251–267). New York: Springer Publishing Company.

Scott-Maxwell, F. (1968). *The measure of my days.* New York: Penguin.

Schutz, S. P. (Ed.). (1974). *The best is yet to be.* Boulder, CO: Blue Mountain Arts.

Waxman, B. F. (1999). Nature, spirituality, and later life in literature: An essay on the romanticism of older writers. *The Gerontologist, 39*(5), 516–524.

Webb, E. J., Campbell, D. T., Schwartz, R. D., & Sechrest, L. (1966). *Unobtrusive measures: Nonreactive research in the social sciences.* Chicago: Rand McNally & Company.

Wyatt-Brown, A. M. (1993). Introduction: Aging, gender and creativity. In A. M. Wyatt-Brown & J. Rossen (Eds.), *Aging and gender in literature* (pp. 3–13). Charlottesville, VA: University Press of Virginia.

Yahnke, R. E. (1993). Representations of aging in contemporary literary works. *Generations, 17*(2), 83–86.

Yahnke, R. E. (1999). Aging, intergeneration, and community: *Waking Ned Divine* and *Tea with Mussolini. The Gerontologist, 39*(4), 504–508.

# CHAPTER TWELVE

# A Picture Is Worth . . . : The Use of Photography in Gerontological Research

## Dena Shenk and Ronald M. Schmid

P hotographs have been used in various ways as a research tool in the social and health sciences but sparingly in gerontology. Yet even the fields of visual anthropology and visual sociology remain relatively underdeveloped. The words of Howard Becker, published in 1979, still ring true more than 20 years later:

> Visual social science isn't something brand new, . . . but it might as well be. . . . One advantage of a field which has just reached that state is there has not been time for standard procedures and paradigms to get established. As a result, people come into the work with a great variety of backgrounds, training, and experience, and of necessity make a great variety of experiments (almost anything you do is an experiment at this stage), and the ration of novel ideas, procedures, and results to the total volume of work produced is very high (1979a, p. 7).

Despite the limited extent of use, visual methods have been employed effectively by a number of researchers in gerontology. Examples include Achenbaum and Kusnerz's (1982) collection that uses images to explore changing perceptions of old age in the United States (see also Achenbaum, 1993). Coles and Harris (1973) include photographs as an integral element of their portrayal of older adults in New Mexico. Joanne Leonard's (1993) photocollage and text on her autobiographical work using images of multiple generations from her family is an important example of the humanistic uses of visual images in gerontology. Magilvy, Congdon, Nelson, and Craig (1992) integrate photography in an ethnographic investigation of rural home care for older adults. One of the few efforts to "engage in a critical evaluation of the potentials and the limitations of the photographic modality" in gerontology was a symposium held at the San Francisco Gerontological Society of America meetings in 1991 on "Perceiving Beyond the Data: Photography as a Research Tool in Gerontology" (Howell, 1991).

Photography can be both a medium of inquiry and a mechanism for presenting research findings. As a medium of inquiry, photographs in tandem with other methodological approaches can provide a detailed record of a specific time and event. Photographs are also useful as an approach for effectively presenting research findings to a variety of audiences. They can generate a more comprehensive sense of an individual, context, or event than may be elicited through a verbal description.

> The photograph can give the viewer an emotional connection with—as well as an intellectual understanding of—the scene depicted. Photographs at their best do not simply make assertions; rather the viewer interacts with them in order to arrive at conclusions. . . . In our interacting sensitively to their detail and meaning, photographs can help us to see, feel, and understand in ways that words alone cannot (Aron, 1979, p. 67).

Photographic methods offer new "ways of knowing" and may correspond to different learning styles. While lecturing is effective for those who learn verbally, others learn more effectively through visual demonstrations. While interviews provide verbal data, photographs provide visual and spatial data. The different ways of knowing, verbal and spatial, are complementary. Both kinds can be used effectively to understand and elucidate aspects of the aging experience.

## Types of Photographic Research

Both the purposes of a study and the philosophical and theoretical framework will determine how photographs are utilized in a research project. Collier states that there are "three basic ways that photographs can be used scientifically, to measure, to count, and to compare" (1975, p. 213). Wagner suggests that in social science alone, there are at least five separate modes of photographic research: a) Photographs as interview stimuli, b) systematic recording, c) content analysis of naïve (not professional) photographs, d) native image-making, and e) narrative visual theory (1979, pp. 17–18). Each of these approaches could be used productively to help answer specific gerontological research questions, particularly in conjunction with other research methods.

A useful approach in effectively implementing photography as a research tool with a given population is to first consider how the people being studied use photographs (Shanklin, 1979). Photographs are a medium with which many older adults are familiar and comfortable, and thus could be used productively in a variety of ways in eliciting data, as well as illustrating research findings. Gerontological researchers often use family photographs informally as a way of developing rapport with older adults. Photographs can also be used in qualitative gerontological research to test and extend the findings from other research approaches and to generate useful discussion.

## The Nature of Photographic Data

Skepticism about the use of photographs in the social and behavioral sciences is related to numerous challenging methodological issues, although the difficulties are not unique to photographic work. "Visual materials simply make obvious the difficulties we have with every variety of data" (Becker, 1979a, p. 7). Careful consideration of the issues raised by the use of visual methodologies can help in critically assessing other research methods as well. For example, as interviews tell us nothing about topics not explored, photographs leave out everything outside the frame. The way in which photographs portray what *is* within the frame, however, is unique (Becker, 1979a). Similarly, the effect of the relationship between the photographer and subjects should be considered, as well as the effect of the relationship between investigator and the people involved in participant observation or interviews.

The unique relationship between the photographer and the subject raises interesting concerns. "It's often said that a photograph records, among other things, the relation of the photographer to the people in the picture. . . . Part of our concern is always to know how much time the photographer spent; we trust the sample more if we know it was a long time" (Becker, 1979b, p. 111). On the other hand, research subjects themselves can create self-portrait photographs, an approach that has been used successfully with a variety of populations (e.g., Ewald, 1985; Worth & Adair, 1997; Ziller, 1990). Photovoice is the current term for the strategy of using photography to have people document and discuss their life conditions as they see them (Wang & Burris, 1994, 1997; Wang, 1999). The process of creating the photograph and the roles of the individuals involved in that process must be carefully considered.

## Responsibilities of the Researcher

The proximity between the researcher and photographed subject gives rise to important ethical issues in the use of photography. Harper (1979) suggests that we gain the ethical right to tell a story or create an analysis when our knowledge has been formed by genuine involvement with the subjects we wish to portray. The relationship between the photographer and the subject of the image should be based, of course, on honesty and trust. While related issues are involved in any kind of interaction research, the extent of these concerns is affected by the visual nature of the data. These issues include securing adequate permission from research subjects, the process of creating the images, the legitimate uses of photographs, and issues of identification.

The process of obtaining permission to make photographs of people is a negotiation between the subjects involved and the photographer (Becker, 1979b, p. 111). While researchers always need to obtain permission from their subjects, a specific consent form should be developed for this type of data collection. Due to the fact that visual images can be recognized, and thus a certain portion of confidentiality cannot be protected, subjects must be fully informed about the consequences of providing such images.

The researcher usually has a strong influence on the composition, what gets included and what is left out, what background is chosen, and perhaps even the facial expression of the subject. These images are then frozen in time. Like the text itself, they do not age or change, and this has consequences for the future interpretation and reading of the research. Thus, it is essential to create such lasting images with a great deal of sensitivity, including making extensive use of the subject's input.

Another key issue is selection of the images to be used. Photographs can easily be selected to make a particular point and the researcher retains the ethical responsibility to be accurate in the way in which the images are used and likely to be construed. These issues are similar to those involved in using interview data (i.e., a photograph out of context may be as misleading as a decontextualized quotation), but are more sharply defined by the reflexivity of the use of photographs and the emotional responses photographs are likely to evoke. Decisions regarding the specifics of consent, creation of the images, how the photographs will be used, and how the subjects will be identified have to be considered carefully based on the parameters of the particular project.

## Uses of Photographic Data

The potential for visual methods to complement or enrich ethnographic work is great. The irony is that ethnographic reports are usually presented in the written mode, allowing language "to do the work of the eyes" (Ball & Smith, 1992, p. 6). Photographs are generally included in ethnographic reports more for evidential than analytical purposes. The photographs serve essentially presentational and illustrative purposes, rather than providing a focus for a more sustained analysis of the visual dimensions of the culture (Ball & Smith, 1992, p. 9). Bateson and Mead's (1942) classic *Balinese Character: A Photographic Analysis* is recognized as a major exception. Margaret Mead's on-site fieldnotes accompany the photographs, and the images and text together "present richer ("thicker") ethnographic descriptions than would be possible by words alone" (Ball & Smith, 1992, pp. 13–14).

An essential how-to guide to using photography in ethnographic research is available in *Visual Anthropology* (Collier & Collier, 1986), the first text on visual research. The authors outline various uses of photography in ethnographic research, including a) orientation and developing rapport, b) developing an overview of the community (mapping and surveying), c) developing a cultural inventory, and d) interviewing with photographs. Magilvy et al. (1992) used photographs in each of these ways in their study of rural home care for older adults. Photographs were used initially to develop rapport with the older adults and home-care workers in order to gain a familiarity with the two rural communities. Photographs were also used to develop a cultural inventory of approaches, techniques, and equipment used in rural home care and with the older adults and home-care workers to generate further data through reactions to the images.

In addition to providing an entrée into the community, photographs may serve as visual "field notes" (Shanklin, 1979, p. 145) and as memory aids (Fetterman, 1998). Photography provides a venue for capturing details that can later be studied and analyzed.

Approaches for analysis vary from open inquiry and macroanalysis to structured and microanalytic study (Wagner, 1979; Ball & Smith, 1992). As with all research endeavors, appropriate mode(s) of analysis will depend upon the mode of photographic research and the purpose(s) for which they are being used. Similarly, triangulation strategies that enhance analysis in other modes of inquiry may apply to visual data analysis. Using more than one analyst is a useful strategy to consider (Wagner, 1979, p. 152). Photographic data may accompany other data-collection methods, such as in-depth interviews. Wagner discussed this approach in terms of the Twin Rivers community study (1979):

> By moving back and forth between examination of the photographic contact sheets and a review of the verbal data, we were able to refine the meaning of each. The verbal data (were) no more valid than the visual, but taken together they gave us a useful triangulation for studying the community (p. 150).

The visual and verbal data can be used to support and strengthen each other and together can lead to a clearer understanding based on the combination of both approaches. This approach was employed by the authors—an anthropological gerontologist (Shenk) and a documentary photographer (Schmid)—in studying the lives of rural, older women.

## The Rural Older Women's Project

Schmid created documentary photographs of the 30 research subjects engaged in the Rural Older Women's Project, an ethnographic study of the daily lives and systems of support of rural, older women using a life-course perspective (Shenk, 1987, 1992, 1998; Shenk & Schmid, 1993). In addition to the creation of photographs of the participants, this multiphase project, undertaken in a rural four-county area in central Minnesota, collected life histories, information on social networks, and questionnaire data. A follow-up telephone survey was completed in 1990, 3 years after the other data were collected.

Photographic images were used to help capture, study, and present the essence of the rural aging experience as defined by the researchers and the older women themselves. Uses of the photographs include both realistic and expressive elements (Edwards, 1997). That is, the photographs were used for their realistic detail to garner additional data about the research subjects to support and supplement the other research findings. In addition, the photographs were used expressively to generate and share a deeper level of understanding of the research subjects and of the rural aging experience with the audience. The photographs provide depth, detail, and humanness to what might otherwise be abstract, and they provide a vehicle for transmitting what has been learned to a larger audience. Their unique power lies in evoking an emotional reaction that can enable the observer to reach a deeper understanding of the topic.

Photographs were an essential element in the creation and verification of each woman's story and assisted in interpretation of her definitions of meaning. Each of the 30 women agreed to have her photograph created as a final phase of the research project, and, as a companion method, the images were created based on the findings of the other approaches. The two researchers met in preparation for each photographic session. The ethnographer briefed the photographer about the woman he was going to meet. They discussed important aspects of the subject's life that had emerged in the interviews. The photographer used this information as the basis for developing a relationship with the subject.

Two elements were critical to developing the necessary level of rapport with each woman to make her a partner in the process. First, an unstructured conversation and exchange of personal information allowed each subject to become comfortable with the photographer. The photographer began each session talking with the participant in her home, exchanging information until she was comfortable with him and indicated she was ready for the photographic session. The sessions with the photographer lasted an average of 4 hours, depending on how long it took to develop a relationship of trust and sharing between the photographer and subject. Second, each woman maintained a sense of control over the photographic session. The participants gave him tours of their homes, yards, or farms, allowing the photographer as much access to their physical and personal space as the women considered appropriate. They discussed where to make the photographs, selecting a location that was special to the woman. Often this was a corner of her home that told of her existence, history, and identity. This level of comfort and sense of control were crucial to create meaningful visual representations of each woman.

The people involved in creating a picture create the reality portrayed. In this case, the photographer worked with each woman in a mutual, interactive process to translate and portray her reality. The images developed were based both on the woman's sense of self and the scholarly interpretation of her experience. The photographs also revealed elements that were unplanned or unintended, but became obvious within the visual frame.

The documentary photographer attempted to photograph each individual in an honest way, meaning a natural expression as opposed to an artificial scene contrived for the situation. They (photographer and subject) did not construct a picture by adding and subtracting elements or attempting to glorify or denigrate the subject. The focus was on using existing natural light to make an honest picture in a natural setting. The photographer's approach was to place an abstract two-dimensional frame around a three-dimensional reality, while attempting to illuminate and interpret an individual's life-experience. The viewer is encouraged, through details in the photographic frame, to derive his or her own interpretation about the subject. Communicating information about the subject is central, by photographing each woman in the midst of her chosen personal environment with her own objects or icons from her life.

As research data, photographs were used to complement the life-history, interview, and social-network data. The two researchers analyzed the visual images of each subject to discern previously unnoticed elements of her personal environment, as well as elements that confirmed or substantiated interview findings. We were looking both for themes and patterns of meanings for these rural, older women, as well as elucidation of each individual woman's life experience through settings and items that held special meaning for her.

The woman's choice of physical setting—artifacts included, activities portrayed, and pose—provided useful insights into what was important to her and how she saw herself. In terms of setting, one woman posed outside next to a favorite flower, another in her favorite reading chair in the living room, and one (whose hobby was woodworking) on her woodpile. One woman posed next to the bookcase that had been in her family for two generations and another in front of a painting of the family farm. The women portrayed themselves involved in favorite activities, including gardening, looking at family photographs, and cooking. One woman chose to dress in her gardening clothes and hat and posed on her knees in the garden. Finally, the women struck varying poses and stances that embodied their self-images. The photographs, therefore, provide visual documentation of artifacts and activities that held special importance for the rural, older women. They also provide an additional perspective on each woman's view of her own life and sense of self.

We viewed the analysis and use of photographic data as an interactive process or cycle involving the researchers, the older women, and audience. As a research tool, we initially used photographs to gain a deeper understanding of the life stories of the subjects and to support findings of other phases of the project. The triangulation of methods, as well as discussion and analysis of the photographs by the anthropologist, photographer, and research participants enhanced the credibility of the research findings. We then used the photographs to discuss and demonstrate our findings to both professional and public audiences. Through discussions with those who viewed the photographs, we gained a clearer understanding of what was displayed and the emotional reactions evoked by the images as the viewers recounted their own stories (Ewen, 1979, p. 56).

## Ethical Quandaries

We grappled with several issues related to the ethics of using photographs. Each subject provided written permission to allow the photograph to be created and used in the project. Furthermore, each subject agreed to allow us to use the photographs in future presentations and publications. The ethnographer and photographer grappled with how to identify the subjects in publications and debated the relative merits of using fictive or real names. We agreed that real names would not be used with the images and that the photographs would not be used with specific data that would allow them to be identified. We originally identified a photograph with a fictive first name, but later agreed to present the photographs without any name. We believed that this approach was more respectful than including a fictive name. Indeed, the subjects indicated that they preferred for us to use their real name.

Another major ethical concern was the selection of images to be used in presentations, publications, and exhibits. While the women chose the setting and pose for their photographs, we chose which photographs to include for educational purposes. Again, the two researchers engaged in extensive discussions and made these choices both on the basis of the visual and technical quality of individual photographs and on what the images portrayed. The most "effective" images were chosen for an exhibit or presentation on the basis of at least three criteria. We chose (a) technically strong images that were effective for (b) demonstrating a particular theme and (c) displaying characteristics of the individual's life experience.

In the remaining portion of this section, we present five photographs from the Rural Older Women's Project and discuss how these images were created and used.

## Catherine Becker

Catherine Becker reminisced about the summer kitchen that stood behind the farmhouse where she lived with her husband. Her husband had lived on the farm for all of his 86 years and she had joined him there when they had married 46 years ago. They no longer used the summer kitchen, but she shared her memories of cooking meals there.

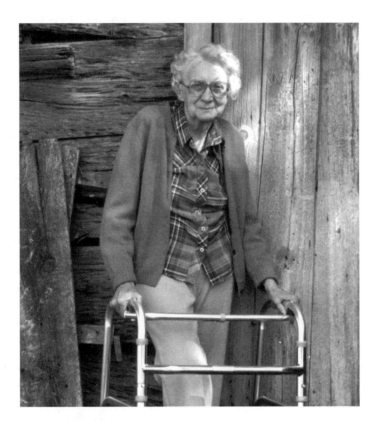

**FIGURE 1.   "Country kitchen."**

She talked about how, during the summer, they had used the summer kitchen to feed the farmhands and family alike to keep the heat of cooking out of the house. It was a rundown, yet sturdy, old structure, and was her chosen background for her documentary portrait. Aesthetically, we appreciated the way the grain of the wood paralleled the lines in her aging face. Her choice of an historical spot seemed particularly appropriate given her deep, personal interests in family history and genealogy.

This photograph of the summer kitchen represents the important theme of "women's work" on the farm. The visual image enhances words from the life story told by Dorothy Dreyfus:

> I fed thrashers and I'll never forget the first time I did that. Twenty-eight people. I asked Clifford's mother what I could do, because at that time she

was in charge of cooking, that was when I was first married and living on the farm. And she said, "You can peel the potatoes" . . . and she brought up a 12-quart pail of potatoes, heaping full. . . . And we fed the 28 men and then we did the dishes. And we barely got the dishes done when we took lunches out. And the first time I did that all alone, I had quite a few misgivings, but I managed it, after having helped her for several years I knew how to do it (Shenk, 1998, p. 15).

Photographs are not only visual representations of the deep, personal, life experiences of the individual subject, but also reflect themes and patterns that are descriptive of the rural aging experience.

## Ruth Rainer

Ruth Rainer posed with her handmade quilt spread across her lap in the living room of her home. Proudly, yet shyly, she looks out at the camera from beyond her creation. As the oldest girl in a farm family with 12 children, she helped raise 8 brothers and 3 sisters. She never married and she cared for both of her parents and her two aunts in the home where she now lived alone. Ruth remained at home to care for these family members, while her only other sister who did not marry chose a religious life. That sister can be seen in the first photograph on the left in the collection of family photographs on the table beside her. Although the family resemblance is striking, the divergence in the sisters' lifepaths is notable.

Ruth suffered from curvature of the spine early in life and explained that she was always self-conscious about her deformity. She talked about it in the following segment from her life-history narrative: "I had a very difficult time in school, because that's the time when the kids in school kind of made fun of me. I suppose the parents talked about it at home, how, that I was deformed." She talked about it extensively when asked about the biggest problem she faced on a daily basis.

Well, I suppose I should know how to handle this, but dealing with the deformity of my back. . . . It's well padded. When I was six years old I had curvature of the spine. It was probably caused from poor eating. My parents encouraged me to eat, but I just didn't. I spent one year going back and forth to Gillette Hospital, but they couldn't do much. It's always bothered me and affected me. I was very self-conscious of it when I was dating. I thought people were looking at me. When two of my older brothers got married, their brides didn't ask me to be in the wedding, but they asked a younger sister. I thought that it was because of my back. That always hurt me. Then,

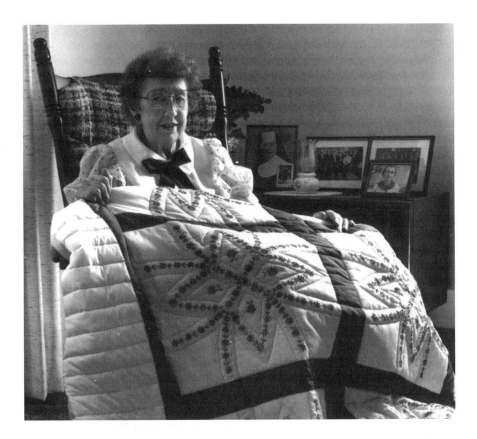

**FIGURE 2.   "Quilt."**

> when the younger brothers got married, their brides did include me in the wedding. That helped ease the pain. . . . I know I should know how to handle this. Being around new people is very difficult for me because of this. It has affected my whole life.

It does not seem accidental that Ruth chose to display one quilt that she is quite proud of, while sitting in a chair. As she looks out at the camera with a hesitant smile, the visual image is a clear reminder of her self-consciousness about her deformity.

### Irma Gardner

Irma Garner lounged comfortably in the swing on the front porch of her farm home at the western edge of Stearns County. She had lived

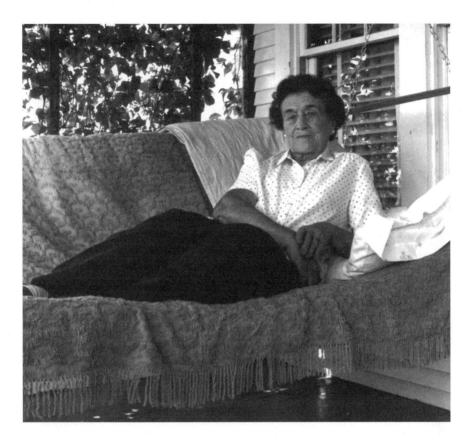

**FIGURE 3.** **". . . . in her special spot . . . ."**

on the farm for 60 years, alone since her husband died in 1974. Irma talked about her loneliness, her nervous breakdown, and bout of cancer, as well as raising six children, living through the Depression on a very low, fixed income, and her determination to remain in her home as long as she was "mentally and physically able." She proudly pointed out the gleaming porch floor, and talked about the mattress she was lying on in her portrait, in the following segment from her life history:

> The mattress that is on the swing is from the Depression when the government bought the cotton and gave the cotton to the people, but they would have to go, they would set up places. Like for Stearns County, it was at Richmond. We had to go there and make the mattresses ourselves. We had to beat the

cotton with boards. They furnished everything, the outer ticking, that striped ticking that was there. Nobody was applying, then Dr. O'Connor's wife from Eden Valley got up once and spoke and said, "The government is trying to help the poor people, the cotton farmers." Here the people were too proud to go and take it. She said, "There is not a family in the community that can't use a couple of new mattresses. You can deny it, but you might as well admit it. . . . " We two went and this neighbor here went along with us. We had to go to Richmond to get ours. We made two large and one for a cot. Then they told us when we had them made that we would get for as many mattresses that we had, we would get quilts. Then· this neighbor got mad, "I could use those." But then he couldn't get in on it. Then it was too late, they couldn't get it. Here we are, then we went to Litchfield, we had to help out. We packed the lunch. We beat it and sewed it with big needles. That one mattress is on the porch yet and the other one, I had some coil spring, I had box mattresses made out of it by a company. They took the cotton from those. You know what it would cost to get cotton like in those? So I always take care of the mattress. Last Sunday, I took it in to get it good and dry. If it isn't, then it lies on the floor, then I roll it up.

She struggled to make sense of her 60 years of living as she decided what to do next. She wanted to remain in her home, although her children urged her to move into town. Major themes of having lived a "simple" and difficult life are portrayed through a visual image that enhances these words from the beginning of her life-history narrative:

Then living here I have all of the memories of living here, the good and the bad. Then on everything went, we had six children, all of them at home, not one of them in a hospital. A lot illnesses at those times. The Depression hit us in '35, '36. The drought and several years close in there, we were hailed out. When I think of the Depression, I think of the farmers today. It was the same then. You just battled. It makes you grow stronger; all the problems you have in life are blessings. You don't look at them that way at the time. It gives you strength to go on.

This outlook gave her the strength that enabled her to live alone at the age of 80. Eventually, her arthritis became worse, and her deteriorating health necessitated a move to a nursing home, away from the comfort and security of her long-term farm home. She learned to accept the changes as she had met challenges throughout her life: "It isn't the greatest, but I make the best of it."

This photograph of Irma seated comfortably in her special spot captures her personal struggles and triumphs, and reflects aspects of the shared experiences of this generation of aging farmwomen.

## Ina Parker

Ina Parker and her cat, Baby, look out at us from a photograph taken in the room behind the kitchen in her home. Ina and Baby lived alone in one of the first houses built in Hanover, Minnesota, a deteriorating, midwestern town. Ina was proud that her grandparents on both sides were among the first to move to the town from Germany. In fact, her maternal grandfather had built the house Ina lived in. We located Ina through a listing of Hundred-Year Farms at the local county historical society.

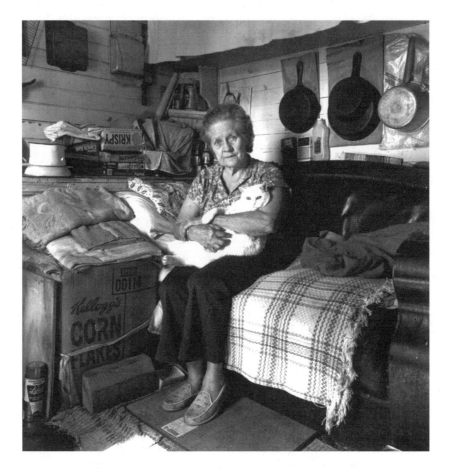

FIGURE 4. "Depth of living."

The depth of living that goes on in this room is evident in the photograph, as is her poverty. All of Ina's cookware hangs from nails on the wall. Additionally, she uses the large Corn Flakes box for storage. She naps every afternoon on the couch on which she and Baby are seated, covering herself with one of the carefully folded old blankets that are stacked atop the box. She has lived in this house since she was born, caring for each of her parents here until they died. She lives only on the first floor of the house now, unable to climb the stairs to the second story. She never married and has few family or friends. While she and Baby managed, Ina was quite lonely.

As a mechanism for presenting research findings, photographs from the Rural Older Women's Project have been incorporated into publications and have been used to develop a photographic exhibit. "Silver Essence: The Lives of Rural Older Women in Central Minnesota" stands alone as an artistic endeavor and educational tool for teaching about the rural aging experience. The exhibit includes several panels of explanatory text about the rural aging experience and elicited this remark from an observer:

> The photographs take advantage of picturing the women in their own settings. The photos were so sensitive that the person in the setting made the story come to life. The result is very powerful and you get a picture of the person's lifetime. It is more than the sum of the two parts. Something very exciting happens (H. Freshley, personal communication, May 19, 1989).

Viewers of the photographs commonly say that they remind them of people they know. In this sense, the photographs are not only images of specific individuals; they also generate emotional reactions and demonstrate themes and patterns within the rural aging experience in general. Thus, photographic images can be a useful tool as we wrestle with discerning both contextually grounded and universal features of human aging. Our efforts in the Rural Older Women's Project were focused primarily on assessing and displaying the contextually grounded experience of growing older in rural Minnesota during the 20th century. More recent work has sought to extend our research to other contexts.

### Cross-Cultural Comparison

We expanded the photographic aspects of our work to explore the visual representation of universal aspects of the human aging experience. Our first efforts in this regard involved photographing older individuals in

Dubrovnik and Zagreb, Croatia. What was then Yugoslavia was selected because it offered clear contrasts to the American Midwest and was a site where the first author had done some preliminary research.

There were obvious differences in the Croatian project. We had to work through translators and the language barrier limited interactions. We also had less time to spend with each subject. In Croatia, less was known about the research subjects at the time the photographs were created; the photography and basic interviews were done at the same time. We developed a second photographic exhibit. "Reflections on Aging: A Study from Yugoslavia and the U.S." was a comparative exhibit of aging in central Minnesota and Croatia. Ten visual images of older women in Croatia were paired with 10 photographs from central Minnesota, allowing the viewer to observe similarities and differences in the aging experience in these vastly different settings (Figures 5 and 6). Images were matched according to dominant visual themes in the two sets of photographs. The exhibit included a panel of explanatory text. Each photograph was marked simply "Yugoslavia" or "U.S.," and the images were allowed to stand on their own with no further description. The visual themes of the matched pairs of photographs included artifacts such as a piano, a television set, or tapestry wall hanging, and activities included subjects reading, doing handicrafts, living with disability, cooking, looking at old photographs, and showing their collections. The photographs ranged in tone from playful to serious, and represented similarities in the aging experiences in these vastly divergent cultural settings. These are the visual portrayal of universals in the human aging experience, including living with disability, and seeking continuity through ongoing activities and hobbies.

The set of photographs from the comparative exhibit, included as Figures 5 and 6, focus on the theme of reminiscence as an aspect of the aging experience. The American woman is viewing a family album while seated in the living room of the home where she and her husband raised their two children and now lives alone. The Croatian woman is looking at a photograph of her own mother as a young girl, while standing in the garden of her sister's home. These two very different images of two women growing old in vastly different environments highlight the shared element of remembering and connecting oneself to past and future generations. While each photograph evokes a distinct emotional response, the pairing is based on a key aspect of the aging experience.

## Conclusion

Using photography in conjunction with other methods can generate transcendent insights. Visual representations allow the researcher to

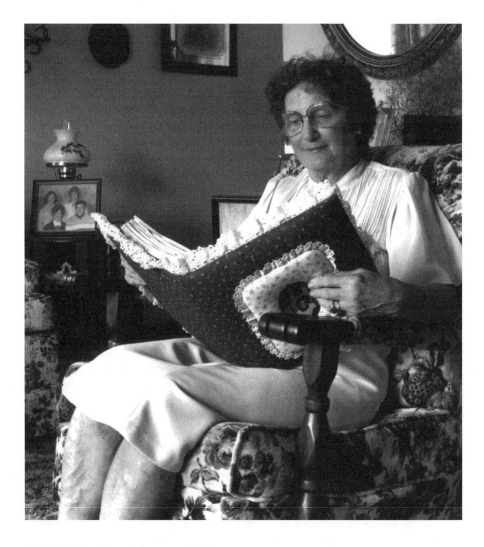

**FIGURE 5.   Reminiscence: USA.**

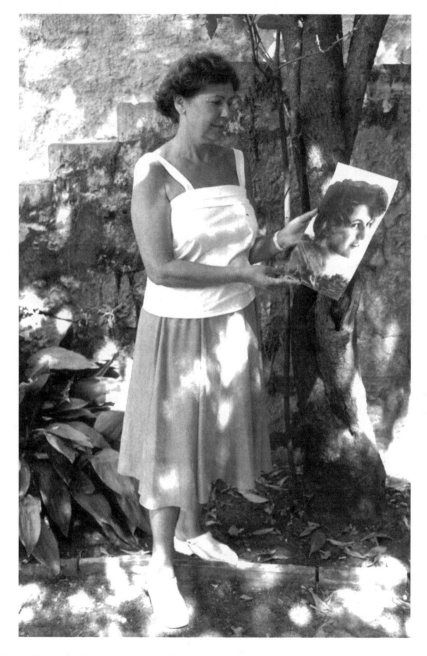

**FIGURE 6.** Reminiscence: Croatia

complement research findings and, at the same time, enable the observer to interact with the photographic data based on his or her own experience. The benefits of using photography as a research tool include providing evidence that is difficult to put into words (Ball & Smith, 1992). Photography can also be viewed as a way to portray the context within which other kinds of data can be analyzed and understood.

Some concerns regarding the use of photography as a research tool can be addressed by using photographs in conjunction with other qualitative methods. Visual data should be triangulated with findings from open-ended interviews, life histories, and/or participant observation, thereby strengthening the findings obtained from each of these approaches. By using photographs along with these other kinds of data, we can reveal the importance of particular findings that might otherwise be overlooked, and verify such findings. In addition, photographs can be used to demonstrate research findings effectively to professional and public audiences.

There are numerous issues to consider when deciding whether to use photography as a research tool. The decision should be made in light of the particular research question, with a clear understanding at the outset of how the visual images are to be used, and how they will be analyzed or interpreted. Anticipated uses of photographic data determine the way in which the photographs should be created. The quality of the images is a related issue and the intended purposes should determine who creates the photographs and influence how they are created.

Finally, and of tremendous importance, is the question of how subjects' privacy can be protected while respecting their true identity. Photography "is a tool which, like the tape recorder, can make a significant contribution in our search for knowledge" (Highley & Ferentz, 1988, p. 115). The challenges of effectively and responsibly using photographic data are great, but they are more than equaled by the possibilities.

## REFERENCES

Achenbaum, W. A., & Kusnerz, P. A. (1982). *Images of old age in America, 1790 to the present* (Rev. ed.). Ann Arbor, MI: Institute of Gerontology.

Achenbaum, W. A. (1993). Images of old age in America 1790–1970—After a second look. In D. Shenk & W. A. Achenbaum (Eds.), *Changing perceptions of aging and the aged* (pp. 35–39). New York: Springer Publishing Company.

Aron, B. (1979). A disappearing community. In J. Wagner (Ed.), *Images of information: Still photography in the social sciences* (pp. 59–67). Beverly Hills, CA, and London: Sage Publications, Inc.

Ball, M. S., & Smith, G. W. (1992). *Analyzing visual data.* Newbury Park, CA: Sage Publications, Inc.

Bateson, G., & Mead, M. (1942). *Balinese character: A photographic analysis.* Special publication of the New York Academy of Science, Vol. 2. New York: Academy of Science.

Becker, H. (1979a). Preface. In J. Wagner (Ed.), *Images of information: Still photography in the social sciences* (pp. 7–8). Beverly Hills, CA, and London: Sage Publications, Inc.

Becker, H. (1979b). Do photographs tell the truth? In T. D. Cook & C. S. Richards (Eds.), *Qualitative and quantitative methods in evaluation research* (pp. 99–117). Beverly Hills, CA: Sage Publications, Inc.

Coles, R., & Harris, A. (1973). *The old ones of New Mexico.* Albuquerque, NM: University of New Mexico Press.

Collier, J., Jr. (1975). Photography and visual anthropology. In P. Hockings (Ed.), *Principles of visual anthropology* (pp. 211–230). Hawthorne, NY: Mouton De Gruyter Publishers.

Collier, J. Jr., & Collier, M. (1986). *Visual anthropology: Photography as a research method* (Rev. ed.). Albuquerque, NM: University of New Mexico Press.

Edwards, E. (1997). Beyond the boundary: A consideration of the expressive in photography and anthropology. In M. Banks & H. Murphy (Eds.), *Rethinking visual anthropology* (pp. 53–80). New Haven, CT, and London: Yale University Press.

Ewald, W. (1985). Portraits and dreams—Photographs and stories by children of the Appalachians. New York: Writers and Readers Publishing, Inc.

Ewen, P. (1979). The beauty ritual. In J. Wagner (Ed.), *Images of information: Still photography in the social sciences* (pp. 43–58). Beverly Hills, CA, and London: Sage Publications, Inc.

Fetterman, D. M. (1998). *Ethnography: Step by step* (2nd ed.). Thousand Oaks, CA: Sage Publications, Inc.

Harper, D. (1979). Life on the road. In J. Wagner (Ed.), *Images of information: Still photography in the social sciences* (pp. 25–42). Beverly Hills, CA, and London: Sage Publications, Inc.

Highley, B., & Ferentz, T. (1988). Aesthetic inquiry. In B. Sarter (Ed.), *Paths to knowledge: Innovative research methods for nursing* (pp. 111–139). New York: National League for Nursing.

Howell, S. C. (1991). Perceiving beyond the data: Photography as a research tool in gerontology [Abstract]. *The Gerontologist, 31*(1), 16.

Leonard, J. (1993). Not losing her memory: Images of family in photography, words, and collage. In D. Shenk & W. A. Achenbaum (Eds.), *Changing perceptions of aging and the aged* (pp. 9–11). New York: Springer Publishing Company.

Magilvy, J. K., Congdon, J. G., Nelson, J. P., & Craig, C. (1992). Visions of rural aging: Use of photographic method in gerontological research. *The Gerontologist, 32*(2), 253–257.

Shanklin, E. (1979). When a good social role is worth a thousand pictures. In J. Wagner (Ed.), *Images of information: Still photography in the social sciences* (pp. 139–145). Beverly Hills, CA, and London: Sage Publications, Inc.

Shenk, D., & Schmid, R. M. (1993). Visual images of aging women. In D. Shenk & W. A. Achenbaum (Eds.), *Changing perceptions of aging and the aged* (pp. 71–74). New York: Springer Publishing Company.

Shenk, D. (1987). *Someone to lend a helping hand: The lives of rural older women in central Minnesota.* St. Cloud, MN: Central Minnesota Council on Aging.

Shenk, D. (1992). Someone to lend a helping hand: Older rural women as recipients and providers of care. *Journal of Aging Studies, 5*(4), 347–358.

Shenk, D. (1998). *Someone to lend a helping hand: Women growing old in rural America.* Amsterdam: Gordon and Breach Publishers.

Wagner, J. (Ed.). (1979). *Images of information: Still photography in the social sciences.* Beverly Hills, CA, and London: Sage Publications, Inc.

Wang, C. C., & Burris, M. A. (1994). Empowerment through photo novella: Portraits of participation. *Health Education Quarterly, 21*(2), 171–187.

Wang, C. C., & Burris, M. A. (1997). Photovoice: Concept, methodology, and use for participatory needs assessment. *Health Education and Behavior, 24*(3), 369–387.

Wang, C. C. (1999). Photovoice: A participatory action research strategy applied to women's health. *Journal of Women's Health, 8*(2), 185–192.

Worth, S., & Adair, J. (1997). *Through Navajo eyes: An exploration in film communication and anthropology.* Albuquerque, NM: University of New Mexico Press.

Ziller, R. C. (1990). *Photographing the self.* Newbury Park, CA: Sage Publications, Inc.

# CHAPTER THIRTEEN

# Seeing the Unseen: Literary Interpretation in Qualitative Gerontology

## Maria D. Vesperi

> I am knotted up to a single purpose now. What a relief! I am
> stripped down to nothing, needing no protection anymore.
> All needs have been fulfilled.
>
> May Sarton, *As We Are Now,* (1973)

Invisibility is a recurrent theme and concern in the study of aging.
Images of loss, fading, shrinking, disengagement, and stooping below the line of vision permeate the cultural construction of what it
means to be old in many societies. Kurt Vonnegut provides an extreme
example of loss and disengagement in *Fortitude,* a futuristic play in
which a 100-year-old woman is kept alive through the technological
machinations of a narcissistic, ethically compromised doctor. All that
remains of the person is a disembodied head, suspended a floor above
the room where her physical functions and emotions are controlled by
"pulsing, writhing, panting machines." A visitor, taken to this room
before he meets the patient, marvels at what she has endured to stay
alive. "What guts that woman must have!" he exclaims.

"You're looking at 'em," the doctor replies (Vonnegut, 1974, p. 1).

In the new millennium, Vonnegut's critique of bioethics seems less
like satire and more like prophesy; the quarter-century since *Fortitude*
appeared has been marked by medical discoveries and attendant quandaries that call into question what it means to be alive. Vonnegut's story
is fiction, but it is nonetheless fodder for gerontologists who seek to
appreciate aging in qualitative terms. In these pages, I hope to go

further, to explore how a culture builds all representations of aging—fictional or otherwise—from a storehouse of recognizable materials. "Students of culture, like poets, are engaged in constructing a worldview," writes Paul Friedrich in "The Culture in Poetry and the Poetry in Culture" (1996, p. 38). In anthropology as in poetry, he explains, "the objective is not only to get a worldview but to get inside a worldview, to construct texts of one's own that reveal maximum empathy and comprehension" (1996, p. 39).

No endeavor has been the source of more hope and more despair. Empathy and comprehension are hotly contested words, implying as they do that the Other can be known to such a degree, if at all. In Western literature, as in much ethnography, such assumptions have traditionally been linked to the colonial project of constructing the self by means of someone else. Toni Morrison offers strong examples of this link in her analysis of the Africanist presence in novels by White American authors (Morrison, 1992); Arnold Krupat identifies a similar dynamic in his discussion of Native American autobiography (Krupat, 1992). In *Fortitude*, which can be read as a cautionary tale about the violence inherent in constructing the Other, Vonnegut offers a cyborg less recognizable as an aged woman than as a fearsomely "material" witness to the arrogance of her creator and the society that spawned him. Lest anyone miss the reference to Mary Shelly's 19th-century meditation on the topic, Vonnegut named his renegade constructionist "Dr. Frankenstein."

Yet, as Daniel and Peck remind us in their discussion of the links between anthropology and literature, it is a mistake to regard the Other as "no more than a projection of one's fears, which then ought to be cured by one's 'understanding' of one's self" (Daniel & Peck, 1996, p. 12). Further, if one accepts Simone de Beauvoir's claim that old age is among Sartre's "unrealizables" (Sartre, 1966; Beauvoir, 1972), the phenomenon of aging presents a truly unique obstacle to the representation of "Otherness." Old age can be empirically identified as a social or demographic category; it is also possible to study how the label "old" is symbolically communicated to the person, who ultimately accepts or, less commonly, resists it. All the same, "old age" remains unrealized, beyond the internal time-consciousness of the individual (Vesperi, 1985, p. 151).

Patricia Mellencamp provides a clear example of this disjuncture in her contribution to Kathleen Woodward's *Figuring Age* (1999), a collection of essays by and about older women. On a cold winter morning in Milwaukee, Mellencamp took her little dog for a routine walk in a local park, where she fell and was knocked unconscious. "After ambulancing me to the hospital, the rescue squad had taken my dog to the humane society for safekeeping," she relates. "When my sister, Nancy, picked him up, she was given a manila envelope containing his sweater. She gave me the envelope six weeks later, when she decided I was sufficiently recovered. On it was written, 'elderly owner in hospital.' My nameless body had been given an identity."

Later, she muses: "One minute I was a middle-aged professor, taking a walk, the next I was elderly, unable to move" (Mellencamp, 1999, p. 311).

If individuals must struggle to apprehend for themselves what it means to be "elderly," how can an observer hope to represent their experience? Some would argue that the goal is naive, unattainable, or simply a conceit. Yet novelists, poets, and playwrights have provided nuanced portraits of older people, and qualitative researchers have offered thickly textured descriptions of their lived experience. Many authors would agree with Elliot Liebow, who opens his study of homeless older women, *Tell Them Who I Am*, with this candid assertion: "I do not mean that a man with a home and a family can see and feel the world as homeless women see and feel it. I do mean, however, that it is reasonable and useful to try to do so. Trying to put oneself in the place of the other lies at the heart of the social contract and of social life itself" (1993, p. xv).

To complicate matters further, the line between ethnographic and literary genres has become increasingly fuzzy, blurred, and vague. Some greet this news with apprehension and renewed attention to policing disciplinary boundaries; others see opportunities for territorial remapping, borderland mischief, even outright trespass. Daniel and Peck find it necessary to engage this dilemma in the very first sentence of their introduction to *Culture/Contexture*: "The presence of the literary in anthropology is best described as 'uncanny'—a nonscientific drive lodged in the heart of a putative science, a presence both desired and dreaded, a Freudian *unheimlich*" (1996, p. 1). *Culture/Contexture* is a collection of essays that survey the trampled fences between these fields and, in the process, delineate new areas for interdisciplinary scholarship.

Qualitative gerontologists have long recognized that the study of aging cannot be limited to expression through a single medium; the topic is much too complex and much too pervasive, if often hidden. The task of interpretation is a daunting one, but I take heart from Arnold Krupat's reminder that, "If we cannot be objective, we can still be scientific" (Krupat, 1992, p. 77).

## Visible in the Margins

"The distasteful metaphor of 'over the hill' implies being out of sight, invisible and hence out of mind," writes Kathleen Woodward in her introduction to *Figuring Age* (1999, p. xii–xiii). Woodward's project in editing this book is to create an "arena of visibility" (1999, p. ix) for older women, a phrase she attributes to Barbara Myerhoff. The reference comes from " 'Life Not Death in Venice': Its Second Life," where Myerhoff analyzes the response to a tragedy that occurred on the boardwalk outside the California senior center she described so vividly in *Number Our Days* (1978). Here a young bicyclist, claiming later that he "didn't see her," collided with an 86-year-old woman who subsequently died. Myerhoff dubs the incident a case of "death by invisibility." In many cases, she says, the extremely marginal are not consciously ignored or abused; they are simply not seen (Myerhoff, 1992, p. 259, pp. 264–265).

Marginality is indeed an undeniable symptom of the well-identified, culturally constructed constraints that have such pervasive social and economic consequences for older people. How qualitative researchers situate their subjects within this cultural construction of age and interpret its meaning is another matter. (For example, the aged nomads in recreational vehicles who appear in Dorothy and David Counts' *Over the Next Hill* (1996) might well disagree with Woodward. For them, "over the hill" means up and gone—release from conventional expectations and responsibilities.)

Death by invisibility could certainly be viewed as one end of a continuum comprised largely of less literal but cumulatively devastating social deaths. Woodward, for one, seizes upon Myerhoff's tale as an apocryphal rallying cry. She states that " . . . this small story with its appalling consequence is a parable of generational ignorance and the invisibility of older women in everyday life" (Woodward, 1999, p. ix).

Yet parables can be dangerous when used to craft cultural representations. In his discussion of ethnography as "a performance emplotted by powerful stories," James Clifford points out that all qualitative descriptions "simultaneously describe real cultural events and make additional, moral, ideological, and even cosmological statements" (Clifford, 1986, p. 98). No matter how unvarnished their presentation, such accounts are always at least doubly mediated—first when they are chosen as narrative vehicles from a repertoire of fieldwork experiences, then again when the reader apprehends them as both locally representative and imbued with transcendent meaning. Clearly, Myerhoff's (1992) story represents the invisibility of one older woman at a particular place and time. To explicitly stretch this to "older women"—and even more alarming, to identify broad "generational ignorance"—is not only to essentialize these categories but the relationship between them as well.

Parables of marginalization are particularly volatile because, despite the best of motives, focusing too tightly on loss and exclusion robs individuals of agency and decontextualizes their experiences. Much of the recent discussion in this area has focused on revisiting how racialized categories are constructed in the social sciences, and rightly so, given the traditional focus on "race" and the concomitant lack of attention to how whiteness is constructed (Baker, 1998; Frankenberg, 1993; Gibson, 1996; Harrison, 1998, 1994; Hartigan, 1997; Morrison, 1992; Mukhopadhyay & Moses, 1997; Page & Thomas, 1994; Smedley, 1998). The call for a more reflexive approach is not new. In their 1972 book, *Racism and Psychiatry*, Thomas and Stillen cautioned:

> "Studies of the black person usually focus on what is abnormal in his life. He is viewed as a package of problems. . . .
>
> "This lopsided emphasis on pathology, even when motivated by sympathy, results in dehumanization. Seen narrowly as a 'victim,' the black man appears in the learned journals as a patient, a parolee, a petitioner for aid, rarely as a rounded human being. Small wonder that the black community is fed up with being 'researched' by investigators who can see only the deforming marks of oppression" (1972, pp. 45–46).

It is easy to see how such an investigative framework could be even further distorted in studies of aged African Americans, and in studies of old age itself as a broad construction. At the close of the century, Sue Taylor still finds it necessary to critique the representation of African American elders in social scientific literature as "vulnerable, at risk of impoverishment and suffering from multiple chronic ailments" (Taylor, 1998). In contrast, her own recent work on older African Americans in small midwestern towns is attentive to the positive view of self that is so notable among this group (see also Deppen-Wood, Luborsky, & Scheer, 1997; Groger, 1995; Peterson, 1997; Shenk, Croom, & Ruiz, 1998; Vesperi, 1998). As Thomas and Stillen (1972) pointed out, and as many have noted since, research paradigms often encode implicit, unexamined comparisons that do violence to the experience of research subjects.

Myerhoff avoids this trap masterfully in her discussion of the bicycle accident outside the Israel Levin Senior Adult Center. She notes that the tragedy's symbolism was not lost on the deceased's peers, who organized a protest parade complete with a mock coffin. After prayers at a nearby synagogue, the group returned to the center to dance in celebration of another member's 100th birthday. Myerhoff stresses the death-to-life continuity of these events: " 'It's a good way to finish such a day,' people agreed, clearly aware of the symbolic propriety of juxtaposing a funeral and a birthday to assert their continuing vitality and power despite injury and loss. The ceremony had been an enactment of their historical vision and their rejection of the assigned position of helpless victim" (1992, pp. 265–266).

Myerhoff describes the occasion as "profoundly reflexive," an example of what she labels cultural mirroring. The process involves a definition of self that begins when people exert agency on the symbols that generate stereotyped identities and reflect them back in an altered form. She explains: "They displayed and performed their interpretations of themselves and in some critical respects became what they claimed to be. By denying their invisibility, isolation, and impotence, they made themselves seen, and in being seen they came into being in their own terms, as authors of themselves" (1992, p. 259). Drawing on Turner's concept of social drama, Myerhoff stresses the role of the anthropologist and the journalists who covered the day as witnesses to this transformation. Hence a "small story" about invisibility becomes a story about the individual and collective agency of so-called marginal people.

Myerhoff writes that the people in her study became visible through "the canny deployment of their symbols, consciously manipulated" (1992, p. 258). Her casual description of her subjects as canny is the only such reference I have found, and an apt one. Representation was no Freudian mystery to the elders of the Israel Levin Senior Adult Center. There was nothing uncanny about their life circumstances; the social meaning of old age was obvious to them. Blunt acknowledgment guided them to craft symbols that left little to the public imagination.

It is important that Myerhoff describes herself and the journalists as "witnesses." Journalists, in particular, are often cast as machiavellian characters who shape public opinion to meet their own needs. In stressing the role of the journalist as witness and mirror, Myerhoff restores the newspaper or television to its place as a medium of communication.

In *The Education of Harriet Hatfield* (Sarton, 1989), a sympathetic newspaper story serves as the catalyst for cultural mirroring. The novel's title character has been a background figure until the age of 60, shielded from public life by material comforts and the high social standing of her life's partner. It is only as an older woman that she is transformed into someone visible, when she moves to a working-class neighborhood and opens a women's bookstore. "I have changed a lot, I guess," she observes to friends who marvel at her courage in revealing her private life to the *Boston Globe*. "Some people would say not for the better" (1989, p. 114).

Like the real people in Myerhoff's story, Harriet invites a reporter, Hetty Rinehart, to "witness" her bookshop after the store is threatened by homophobics. And like Myerhoff's informants, she challenges the public with its own labels:

" 'I don't get it,' says Hetty flatly, 'except,' and she looks me in the eye, 'you are a lesbian yourself, aren't you?"

"It was bound to be asked, that question, and there are a hundred ways I could fail to answer it. Joan's shadow crosses my mind—none of their damn business, she would say. 'It's odd that no one has asked me that question before. When I was young it was not asked. Now it is and I must say yes' " (1989, pp. 100–101).

It is interesting that Sarton uses the same name, Harriet Hatfield, both for this heroic figure and for the deeply unsympathetic, middle-aged owner of the retirement home in her well-known earlier novel, *As We Are Now* (1973). The characters and their circumstances could not be more different, but transformation is a key to understanding each. In *As We Are Now*, the main character, Caro Spencer, speculates that Harriet might have been a better person before she was corrupted by the privilege of absolute power over her frail charges: "I try to separate what Harriet has become from what she may have been ten years ago. Her face is now that of a greedy and sullen pig—small eyes, a mean little mouth" (1973, pp. 10–11). Harriet is introduced from the start as a looming, intimidating presence: "Then an enormous woman filled the doorway, wiping her hands on her apron" (1973, p. 6).

Using a dominant figure to display the agency of a seemingly power-less one is a delicate challenge, but Sarton achieves it to stunning effect in *As We Are Now*. She first establishes that 76-year-old Caro loses her freedom and much of what identified her as a person when she is confined to an old folks' home. " . . . suffice it to say that it has taken two weeks for me to obtain this notebook and a pen," Caro remarks in the book's opening passage (1973, p. 3). Yet she gathers strength throughout the story, until finally, "stripped down to nothing," she wields power over her surroundings in a devastating way.

"Sybil," a short story by A. Manette Ansay, plays subtly on the line between visibility and invisibility. The tale opens as its title character, who is aphasic and partially paralyzed due to a stroke, sits helplessly while her twin granddaughters spike her hair with pink mousse. Fleeting concerns for her well-being are quickly dismissed by the young girls. For the most part, they treat her like a favorite doll, fantasizing about her feelings and speaking *for* her, rather than *to* her. As Krupat reminds us in his introduction to *Ethnocriticism* (1992), even well-meaning efforts to speak *for* the underrepresented encode a risk of reproducing the conditions of their domination.

> " 'She's crying," says the first twin.
> The second twin peers into Sybil's face, small pink mouth agape. . . .
> 'No she's not,' says the second twin. 'She's just thinking, that's all.' "

And later:

> " 'She looks bea-u-tee-ful,' says the first twin serenely.
> 'I don't think she likes it.'
> 'She looks just like a movie star' " (Ansay, 1995, pp. 116–117).

If nothing else, Sybil is spectacularly visible at this point in the story. Her daughter-in-law, the twins' mother, is startled by the vision she presents:

> "Margie gets home from work at five, and the first thing she sees is Sybil at the table with spiked, rosy hair. The twins are nowhere in sight. Ants cluster on the table where drops of mousse have fallen.
> 'Oh, God,' says Margie. 'Where are they? Where'd they go? Oh, Sybil, I'm so sorry! It washes out though, I've used it on my bangs. It'll rinse away in a jiffy, I swear' " (1995, p. 117).

Margie has a date, however, and despite her conciliatory words, her first priority is changing into a red sundress. Then she feeds Sybil her dinner—cottage cheese straight from the container. Soon enough:

> "It's too late: Johnny thumps up the porch steps and swings his head through the doorway.
> 'Hey,' he says to Margie. Then he sees Sybil. His gaze sticks to her, caught in a rosy web of mousse" (1995, p. 119).

One irony of this brief tale, which begins in late afternoon and ends the following day at breakfast, is that Sybil's striking appearance soon becomes normalized; she never does get her hair washed. Another irony is that the twins, Sybil's powerful if unwitting tormentors, are structurally equivalent from their mother's perspective. Like Sybil, they exist somewhere below Margie's line of sight, despite her distracted efforts to keep track of them. Ansay's description credits them with transparency at best: "They are solemn little girls with pale yellow cheeks and yellow pony tails and their voices are pinched and whispery" (1995, p. 116). In contrast, Margie and Johnny are fleshy and substantial.

Like Myerhoff's, Ansay's "small story" could be interpreted as a parable of "generational ignorance." Yet just as Myerhoff's story is *about* the aged protesters—not the bicyclist or even the dead woman—Ansay's story is *about* Sybil. The other characters and their actions serve simply as devices to reveal her to the reader. The presence of Johnny, for instance, stirs sexual memories for Sybil; she is free to stare at him as he eats breakfast in his underwear precisely because he regards her as insignificant. Sybil is reminiscent of Jean Genet's beleaguered prostitute in *Our Lady of the Flowers,* or Genet himself as interpreted by Jean Paul Sartre in *Saint Genet, Actor and Martyr.* Genet's paradoxical assertion that he is free to be what others have made him is applicable to Sybil, and to many real and imagined characters who must operate within essentializing cultural constructions.

## *Objects in the Mirror May Be Closer Than They Appear*

Daniel and Peck explain that, "The German word used by Freud for "the uncanny," *unheimlich,* signifies a breach of *heimlich,* which in turn has the double meaning of homeyness and secrecy" (1996). They are not alone in finding this term suggestive; the uncanny pops up with cautionary frequency in the qualitative literature. In her discussion of Japanese nativist ethnology, for example, Madeline Ivy explains that, "The uncanny effect does not arise from a simple lack of knowledge . . . it instead erupts from an *excess* of what was supposed to be kept hidden and repressed (what Lacan would call the 'real') . . . it is the horror of being confronted with this excessive and terrible certainty . . . that accounts for the anxiety of the uncanny" (1996, p. 309, emphasis in original; see also Geertz, 1973).

The uncanny is hidden, repressed, and yet disconcertingly familiar—for our purposes, not unlike the cultural construction of old age. Kathleen Woodward offers a thorough treatment of this subject in *Aging and Its Discontents* (1991). Her book frames a useful model for qualitative researchers who want to analyze how older people are represented in western fiction. Woodward points out that dehumanizing caricatures and stereotypes of aging can be linked to anxiety and denial, emotions that are keyed to culturally based notions about aging and death. She posits, for example, that Marcel Proust's famously grotesque description of the elderly party guests in *The Past Recaptured* is an effort to avoid the foreshadowing of a disconcertingly familiar future. Woodward points out that Proust is only partly successful; he writes that "the experience greatly perturbed me . . . their old age made me desperately sad as an announcement of the approach of my own" (Proust, 1959, p. 260, cited in Woodward, 1991, p. 59). Woodward explains that "to see, like Marcel, one's own aged body with a shock of recognition is to experience the *uncanny*" (1991, p. 63).

Both Ivy and Woodward relate the "excessive and terrible certainty" of the uncanny to Lacan's mirror stage of development: the point where infants, watching themselves in a mirror, perceive the mirror image as whole and coordinated, while experiencing the self as unperfected and clumsy. Woodward then suggests that the reverse is true for older people: "If the psychic plot of the mirror stage of infancy is the anticipated trajectory from insufficiency to bodily wholeness, the bodily plot of the mirror stage of old age is the feared trajectory from wholeness to physical disintegration" (1991, p. 67). As Woodward and many others have observed, cultural stereotypes about aging prompt the individual to reject this image, to experience the self as alienated from the body.

The uncanny and the mirror stage of old age are both well exemplified in Stephen King's masterfully crafted short story, "My Pretty Pony" (1993). Perhaps King is more at ease in the realm of the uncanny than most writers, but whatever the reason, "My Pretty Pony" provides one of fiction's rare, appreciative portraits of the aged person as an integrated whole. The omnisciently narrated story begins when George Banning, an aged farmer with serious heart trouble, observes a boy cheating at hide-and-seek by counting too fast. The scene prompts Banning to invite his young grandson, Clive—the loser in the game—for a walk in the apple orchard to "take instruction" on the subjective nature of time.

As the story takes shape, King offers a description of Banning from the young boy's perspective: "There were apple blossoms caught in Grandpa's long hair, still only half white, and the boy thought the old man was beautiful in the trees" (1993, p. 39). Throughout the story, apple blossoms link the old man's beauty and the present moment: "One caught in the dent below his Adam's apple, caught there like a jewel that was pretty simply because some things *were* and couldn't help it, but was *gorgeous* because it lacked duration; in a few seconds it would be brushed impatiently away and left on the ground where it would become perfectly anonymous among its fellows" (1993, p. 440, emphases in original).

Later, the reader sees Clive as he is reflected in the gaze of his grandfather: "He wasn't a good-looking boy and never became the sort of man women exactly consider handsome, but as he smiled in complete understanding of the old man's rhetorical sleight-of-hand, he *was* beautiful, at least for a moment, and Grandpa ruffled his hair" (1993, p. 446, emphasis in original).

Banning begins his lesson by transferring a legacy; he gives Clive his pocket watch. In another twist on psychoanalytic theory, Woodward fruitfully applies the concept of the transitional object to a discussion of Beckett's *Malone Dies* (Woodward, 1991, pp. 131–145); the idea of the "transitional last possession" could certainly be applied to Banning's watch. King plays with the comparison between the "lively" ticking of the watch "beneath its metal skin" and the triphammer of Banning's diseased heart, which he refers to as his "ticka." Banning's grandson plays a reluctant role in this transition; he fears dropping the watch and he knows "that people and watches both stopped someday" (1993, p. 442). An apple blossom, once again, marks the transition in owner-ship, and a change in Clive's acceptance of mortality as well: "But it was still Grandpa's watch: of this he was quite sure. Then, as he had this thought, an apple blossom went skating across the crystal and was gone. This happened in less than a second, but it changed everything. After the blossom, it was true. It was his watch, forever . . . or at least until one of them stopped running and couldn't be fixed and had to be thrown away" (1993, p. 443).

With regard to time, Banning speaks first to the boy's own experience of summer vacation, when time seems endless. "Clive thought of that highway of days and nodded so hard his neck actually popped" (1993, p. 449). Clive is skeptical but accepting when Banning explains that from adolescence into middle age he will experience "real" time: "It ain't long like it was or short like it gets to be" (1993, p. 451). Soon, however, Banning offers glimpses of the uncanny. He speaks of times that "go on forever" when a person is injured, and of his own first, momentary confusion about whether it was summer or fall. This oc-curred when he was in his 40s and he remembers it as a moment of "dismay," elaborating further with a telling metaphor: "It was like step-pin up to the bathroom mirror meanin to do no more'n shave and seein that first gray hair in your head" (1993, p. 458).

King keeps the locked gaze of Banning and his grandson from becom-ing maudlin by allowing Clive to catch glimpses of the uncanny on his own, to experience "the horror of being confronted with excessive and terrible certainty" identified by Ivy. Clive's worst moment comes when his grandfather briefly loses his grip on the present: "He sighed, looking around, as if to remember where exactly it was that they were. His face had a momentary look of utter helplessness that disgusted the boy as much as it frightened him. He didn't want to feel that way, but couldn't help it. It was as if Grandpa had pulled open a bandage to show the boy a sore which was a symptom of something awful. Something like leprosy" (1993, pp. 461–462).

Repelled or intrigued, Clive is continually awed by Banning's power. He can light a cigarette with a single match on a windy day; he can question God's wisdom without being struck by lightening. Most significantly, the old man's vitality remains grounded in his physical presence. "Grandpa fixed him with his eyes, a dark autumnal blue utterly unlike Clive's Mediterranean brown ones. He put one of his gnarled hands on Clive's shoulder. It was knotted with arthritis, but the boy felt the live strength that still slumbered in there like wires in a machine that's turned off" (1993, p. 444). Clive, in contrast, is barely visible to his distracted parents and physically dominated by his older sister. Only with his grandfather does he become a whole person.

A radically different relationship between grandparents and grandchildren is explored in "Who's Irish?", a short story by Gish Jen (1998). The narrator is a 68-year-old Chinese immigrant, "Chinese age almost seventy," who clashes repeatedly with her fully Americanized daughter and Irish American son-in-law over childrearing, gender roles, and the meaning of family. This time, the mirror is a broken one; the gulf between generations and cultures is refracted in each interaction between the narrator and her granddaughter, Sophie. The child refers to her grandmother as "Meanie"; the grandmother wonders what happened to Sophie's "nice Chinese side." Sophie "looks like mostly Chinese," she observes. "Nothing wrong with Sophie's outside, that's the truth. It is inside that she is not like any Chinese girl I ever see" (1998, p. 81).

"Who's Irish?" is told from a single perspective; no omniscient voice weighs the grandmother's pronouncements about her family, her surroundings, or herself: "I am work[?] hard my whole life, and fierce besides" (1998, p. 80). It is clear from what she relates of Sophie's behavior, however, that the child sees no reason to respect her in the role of grandparent or even as a babysitter. "As if good example mean anything to Sophie. I am so fierce, the gang members who used to come to the restaurant all afraid of me, but Sophie is not afraid" (1998, p. 82). The continuity of experience that unites Clive and his grandfather in "My Pretty Pony" is broken here; there is no uncanny opportunity to move beyond a surface assessment of youth and age.

## Conclusion

In the nonfiction memoir, *Brothers and Keepers*, John Edgar Wideman constructs a mirror that reflects two images: his own and his younger brother's. Wideman is a professor of literature; his brother, Robby, is serving a lengthy prison term for murder. What Wideman sees in the mirror frightens him, in part because the things that distinguish him from Robby make him uneasy about himself. Ultimately, he is frustrated in his effort to understand and represent Robby for who he is: "Despite my attempts to identify with my brother, to reach him and share his troubles, the fact was I remained on the outside" (1985, pp. 199–200). Wideman also learned that writing a book about his brother did not make Robby more visible; in fact, it accentuated his lack of agency, his status as a prisoner: "Robby's story would be 'out there,' but he'd still be locked up. . . . Though I never intended to steal his story, to appropriate it or exploit it, in a sense that's what would happen once the book was published.

"His story would be out there in a world that ignored his existence" (1985, pp. 199–200).

Social scientists who study aging often find that the invisibility of their subjects extends to their own research findings and theoretical contributions. The studies are "out there," but the walls remain. It has been more than 50 years since sociologist Leo Simmons used the Human Relations Area Files to identify aspects of aging across 71 cultures (Simmons, 1945), and the subsequent development of a comprehensive literature has been truly impressive. Yet as recently as 1995, a guest columnist lamented the state of the frail elderly and exhorted readers of the *Anthropology Newsletter* to take responsibility for "the shape of aging in the US." She concluded, "For anthropologists, this is a pressing issue: it is in the domain of our interests and it will be part of all our lives" (Simonelli, 1995, p. 46). There was no mention of the extensive qualitative and quantitative literature on the subject; one can only conclude from a statement, such as "It is time that we took a long look at what life will be like the 21st century," that existing studies in her own field were invisible to her.

Indeed, while the many excellent ethnographic studies of aging are read with enthusiasm by students who pursue "special topics" courses, they are rarely adopted as general fare for introductory classes in anthropology or sociology. Colleagues may know these books and admire them, but ironically, they do not seem to regard the universal experience of aging to be among the basics of social life along with kinship, gender relations, subsistence, ritual, or even death. Yet associations among age, health, and social connectedness are vital and quite straightforward;

explanations of biological and social phenomena are mutually reinforcing.

For example, among residents of the independent Polynesian nation of Niue, elders who exhibit signs of extreme physical debility or dementia are left increasingly to fend for themselves (Barker, 1997, pp. 407–424). In her discussion of this distinction between socially active, healthy elders, and the decrepit Niue elderly—who are mostly men—Judith Barker notes: "Facial tics, involuntary vocalizations, and limb palsies in old age are regarded as belated punishments for evil-doing. Elders with these problems were held up as examples for children: 'Old Togia makes noises like a chicken all the time now. That's because when he was young he must have stolen chickens and never confessed to doing so' " (1997, pp. 412–413). And further, the demented elderly are firmly situated within the Niuen understanding of the life cycle and the transition from life to death. "Decrepit elders . . . especially those who no longer look or behave like competent adults, who rave incoherently, who speak of long-past events or converse with long-dead kin, are being actively courted by *aitu* [spirits of the dead], are *mati*, in transition. They are 'the nearly dead' " (1997, pp. 422–423).

Within the small group of elders identified by Barker as neglected, many were never married or had spent decades working as out-migrants. While their limited social ties to the community and their inability to contribute to the family economy by performing household chores were functions of their present frailty, this social profile was also characteristic of their status at earlier life stages. "People who took no time to raise a family, to help siblings and other family members through life, to establish a bond of love between themselves and younger kin have no one to call on in old age, have no one who is obligated to assist" (1997, p. 415).

Barker's description is powerful because it traces the relationship between social behavior and worldview. The defining aspect of qualitative research is, after all, its concern with qualities—the textures, shapes, and values of human interaction and material life. Phenomenological attention to qualities is central to the task of an anthropologist. A lifelong aspect of the fieldworker's project is the attempt to apprehend the truly arbitrary nature of the symbolic frames through which the world is perceived and ordered. In appreciating how powerfully and pervasively culture shapes our vision through—to quote Myherhoff once again—the stories we tell about ourselves to ourselves, we will become more attentive to the qualities that are isolated and defined in others' views.

# REFERENCES

Ansay, A. M. (1995). Sybil. *Read this and tell me what it says.* New York: Avon.

Baker, L. D. (1998). *From savage to negro: Anthropology and the construction of race.* Berkeley, CA: University of California Press.

Barker, J. C. (1997). Between humans and ghosts: The decrepit elderly in a Polynesian society. In J. Sokolovsky (Ed.), *The cultural context of aging: Worldwide perspectives.* Westport, CT: Bergin & Garvey.

Beauvoir, S. de. (1972). *The coming of age.* (P. O'Brian, Trans.). New York: G. P. Putnam & Sons.

Clifford, J. (1986). On ethnographic allegory. In J. Clifford & G. E. Marcus (Eds.), *Writing culture.* Berkeley, CA: University of California Press.

Counts, D. A., & Counts, D. R. (1996). *Over the next hill.* Peterborough, Canada: Broadview.

Daniel, E. V., & Peck, J. M. (Eds.). (1996). *Culture/Contexture: Explorations in anthropology and literary studies.* Berkeley, CA: University of California Press.

Deppen-Wood, M., Luborsky, M. R., & Scheer, J. (1997). Aging, disability and ethnicity: An African-American woman's story. In J. Sokolovsky (Ed.), *The cultural context of aging: Worldwide perspectives.* Westport, CT: Bergin & Garvey.

Frankenberg, R. (1993). *White women, race matters: The social construction of whiteness.* Minneapolis, MN: University of Minnesota Press.

Friedrich, P. (1996). The culture in poetry and the poetry in culture. In E. V. Daniel & J. M. Peck, (Eds.), *Culture/Contexture: Explorations in anthropology and literary studies.* Berkeley, CA: University of California Press.

Geertz, C. (1973). Religion as a cultural system. *The interpretation of cultures.* New York: Basic Books.

Gibson, J. W. (1996). The social construction of whiteness in Shellcracker Haven, Florida. *Human Organization, 55*(4), 379–388.

Groger, L. (1995). Health trajectories and long term care choices: What stories told by informants can tell us. In J. N. Henderson & M. D. Vesperi (Eds.), *The culture of long term care: Nursing home ethnography.* Westport, CT: Bergin & Garvey.

Harrison, F. (1998). Introduction: Expanding the discourse on "race." *American Anthropologist, 100*(3), 609–631.

Harrison, F. (1994). Racial and gender inequalities in health and health care. *Medical Anthropology Quarterly, 8*(1), 90–95.

Hartigan, J., Jr. (1997). Establishing the fact of whiteness. *American Anthropologist, 33*(3), 495–505.

Jen, G. (1998, September 14). Who's Irish? *The New Yorker.*

King, S. (1993). My pretty pony. *Nightmares & dreamscapes.* New York: Viking.

Krupat, A. (1992). *Ethnocriticism.* Berkeley, CA: University of California Press.

Liebow, E. (1993). *Tell them who I am: The lives of homeless women.* New York: The Free Press.

Mellencamp, P. (1999). From anxiety to equanimity: Crisis and generational continuity on TV, at the movies, in life, in death. In K. Woodward (Ed.), *Figuring age: Women, bodies, generations.* Bloomington, IN: Indiana University Press.

Morrison, T. (1992). *Playing in the dark: Whiteness and the literary imagination.* Cambridge, MA: Harvard University Press.

Mukhopadhyay, C. C., & Moses, Y. T. (1997). Reestablishing "race" in anthropological discourse. *American Anthropologist, 99*(3), 517–533.

Myerhoff, B. (1992). *Remembered lives.* (M. Kaminsky, Ed.). Ann Arbor, MI: University of Michigan Press.

Myerhoff, B. (1978). *Number our days.* New York: E. P. Dutton.

Page, H., & Thomas, R. B. (1994). White public space and the construction of white privilege in U. S. health care: Fresh concepts and a new model of analysis. *Medical Anthropology Quarterly, 8*(1), 109–116.

Peterson, J. W. (1997). Age of wisdom: Elderly black women in family and church. In J. Sokolovsky (Ed.), *The cultural context of aging: Worldwide perspectives.* Westport, CT: Bergin & Garvey.

Sarton, M. (1989). *The education of Harriet Hatfield.* New York: W. W. Norton.

Sarton, M. (1973). *As we are now.* New York: W. W. Norton.

Sartre, J.-P. (1966). *Being and nothingness.* New York: Washington Square Press.

Shenk, D., Croom, B., & Ruiz, D. (1998). Discussion of African American women aging after Jim Crow. In R. J. F. Elsner (Ed.), *Voices of experience: Listening to our elders* [Tech. Rep. No. UGAGC-98-001]. University of Georgia Gerontology Center.

Simonelli, J. (1995, March). Out on the floe. *Anthropology Newsletter, 46,* 48.

Simons, L. W. (1945). *The role of the aged in primitive society.* New Haven: Yale University Press.

Smedley, A. (1998). "Race" and the construction of human identity. *American Anthropologist, 100*(3), 690–702.

Stine, R., Cafferata, G. L., & Sargl, J. (1987) Caregivers of the frail elderly: A national profile. *The Gerentologist, 27,* 616–626.

Taylor, S. A. (1998, July). *Place identification and positive realities of aging.* Paper presented at the 14th International Congress of Anthropological and Ethnological Sciences, Williamsburg, VA.

Thomas, A., & Stillen, S. (1972). *Racism and psychiatry.* New York: Bruner/Mazel.

Vesperi, M. D. (1985, 1998). *City of green benches: Growing old in a new downtown.* Ithaca, NY: Cornell University Press.

Vonnegut, K. (1974). Fortitude. *Wampeters, foma and granfaloons.* New York: Delacorte.

Wideman, J. E. (1985). *Brothers and keepers.* New York: Penguin.

Woodward, K. (Ed.). (1999). Introduction. *Figuring age: Women, bodies, generations.* Bloomington, IN: Indiana University Press.

Woodward, K. (1991). *Aging and its discontents: Freud and other fictions.* Bloomington, IN: Indiana University Press.

# PART VII

# Perspective

# CHAPTER FOURTEEN

# Forward to the Past

## Nancy E. Schoenberg and Graham D. Rowles

> "No man can have in his mind a conception of his future, for the future is not yet. But of our conceptions of the past, we make the future."
>
> Thomas Hobbes

"In 1907, when the first ball began its descent into Times Square, approximately 3.7 million persons 65 years of age or older in the United States potentially could have enjoyed the event (Schick, 1986). Ninety-three years later, about 35 million older Americans might have tuned into their television sets and vicariously participated in the revelry as, completing its descent, the ball flashed its greeting to the new millennium . . . "

And so we end where we began. While in the year 2000, few observers could fail to be impressed by these exponential increases in the aging population, when the ball drops again during the next decade, this wonderment is likely to recede. We are more accustomed to the "graying" of Western society. If we ourselves have not entered "old age," then most certainly we will know many older adults and, quite possibly, several centenarians. Aging, with all of its varied representations, will be no stranger to any of us given the unprecedented projection that one fifth of the population will have reached age 65 by 2030. In outlets ranging from the popular media to consumer industries to the biomedical world, few alive in Western society are unaware of the increased current and future presence of an aging population.

We anticipate that over the next decade, society will have sufficient exposure to these demographic trends to shift attention from current preoccupation with the skyrocketing population of elders in favor of a second stage, a deeper-level focus on the quality of aged lives. This focus will dwell on the potential to enhance the lives of elders by improving our understanding of the experiences and meanings of aging. Thus, when the ball first fell around the turn of the century, scientific inquiry was guided by the formidable task of extending life expectancy, a challenge that continues to this day as we battle the scourges of heart disease, cancer, and Alzheimer's disease. More and more, however, attention has begun to focus on the qualities of aging lives.

To examine the qualities of aging lives necessarily involves developing multiple ways of exploring and mining the riches associated with old age, particularly among an aging population that is vast and increasingly diverse. The chapters presented in this volume have been inspired by scholarly traditions in many disciplines, by need to fill the void of tools useful to capture varying facets of aging, and by a great deal of creativity. The chapters embrace some of the most fundamental premises in qualitative inquiry—the celebration of "outliers," the embrace of ambiguity and seeming inconsistency, the acknowledgement that science is a mirror of an ever-changing society, and the obligation to engage in scholarly work with a commitment to the highest ethical standards.

Part and parcel of upholding ethical responsibilities in research is to uncover insights that are capable of improving the lives of the individuals who comprise the focus and substance of our research. While the precise objective of such improvement may be specific to the population group, there is an increasing recognition that qualitative approaches have the potential to inform policy, to increase awareness of structural inequities among the aging population, and to contest inaccurate and demeaning images of aging. Inspired by postmodernism, critical gerontology, and feminist perspectives that offer alternative ways of thinking, and by accompanying methods that offer new ways of knowing, we issue a call to readers to activate their research by unpacking long-maintained but possibly erroneous assumptions about aging. We challenge readers to replace such assumptions with unconstrained creativity that gives a voice to those unheard, sheds light on phenomena yet unseen, and provides useful insights that touch the hearts and minds of those who, from their positions of power, influence the lives of so many elders.

This is no easy responsibility; however, undertaking creative and inspired research that makes a difference is not without its heritage and precedents. Acknowledging and integrating the scholarly work of those who have come before us in creating radically new vistas to explore is our best hope of being able to truthfully represent the complex ways in which perceptions of the past, a position in the present, and the promise of the future are integrally intertwined in the lives of our elders. It offers the best hope of probing beyond the superficial and perhaps revealing what it means to grow old.

While we must acknowledge the past, the making of the future is in the present, and it is in our hands. We are at a point in history where, to an unprecedented degree, we have the freedom and opportunity to shape our old age. On a far more modest level, we also have the opportunity to guide the future of the way in which we think about aging and of qualitative gerontology. The two are not unrelated. Certainly, we need to harness the ever-growing array of methodological resources at our disposal, many of which have been considered in this volume. But perhaps even more important, we must not shy away from committing the full range of our intellectual and emotional (empathic) resources and investing our spirit in the quest for deeper insight into the aging experience as, through the conduct of our lives, we help to forge what aging will become in the upcoming decades. A passionate commitment to affecting positive change and a willingness to be liberated from limiting conventions offers an exciting vista. It is our belief that we sit poised to enter an era of openness and receptivity to new ways of seeing and understanding, and to engaging in partnerships with those whose lives we are attempting to understand and to enhance. As we probe evermore deeply and creatively into the lives of elders it is our hope that:

> We shall not cease from exploration
> And the end of all our exploring
> Will be to arrive where we started
> And know the place for the first time.
> T. S. Eliot (1943)

## REFERENCES

Eliot, T. S. (1943). Little Gidding V. *Four quartets.* London: Faber & Faber.
Hobbes, T. (1888). *The Elements of Law: Natural and Politic.* Oxford: James Thornton.
Schick, F. L. (1986). *Statistical Handbook on Aging Americans.* Phoenix, AZ: Oryx Press.

# Index

Conflict, family *(continued)*
  recognition of dementia symptoms,
    224–225
Constructed meaning, collaboration to
  make meaning, distinguished,
  146–149
Constructs of aging, evolution of, 4
Context, actively using age in construc-
  tion of, 165–168
Control of interview, locus of, 105
Count, Dorothy and David, 266
*Culture/Contexture,* 265

Data
  storytelling as, 32–33
  triangulation of, 183
Death, experience of, in U.S., 73–92
Debriefing sessions, 204
Dementia, 9, 109–128, 213–232
Dialysis, use of, 81–85
Dichotomous view, of quantitative,
  qualitative methods, 182
Dimensions of aging experience,
  expansion of, 6
Disengagement theory, 166
Disputes, about recognition of symp-
  toms, 227
Do not resuscitate orders, 76
  policy of hospital regarding, 86
Documentary photography, 241–262

*Education of Harriet Hatfield,* 268
Elderly population in U.S., 3
Environment, online, sense of self
  and, 112
Epistemological perspective, nature of
  knowing, 7–14
Essayists, representation of aging expe-
  rience, 233–280
Ethical issues
  with guided autobiography, 47–49
  with interviewing, 133–134
  with photography, 244, 249
*Ethnocriticism,* 270
Evaluators, as key informants, 202–203

Experience, meaning, relationship between, 143–145

Facility, spatial order, effect of, 97
Facticity, in guided autobiography,
  38–39
Family conflict
  over response to symptoms, 227
  recognition of dementia symptoms,
    224–225
Fiction, representation of aging experi-
  ence in, 233–278
Field journals, 204
*Figuring Age,* 264, 266
Focus group, 213–232
Folk-disengagement theory, 166
Footpath metaphor, use of, 53
*Fortitude,* 263

Genet, Jean, 271
Gerontological Society of America, San
  Francisco, 242
Gerontology, maturation of, 4
Gould, Stephen Jay, contribution of,
  10
Grounded theory, 161–163
Group debriefing sessions, 204
Group dynamics, online
  dementia caregivers, 109–128
  virtual community, dementia caregiv-
    ers, 109–128
Group setting, use of, 58
Guided autobiography, 37–50, 58–60
  adaption of, 41
  arbitrariness, of recall, 63
  distortion, of recall, 63
  dynamics of, 43
  facticity in, 38–39
  insights of, 41
  longitudinal data over lifespan, 62
  memory-priming questions, 59
  method, 58–59
  personal interpretation of events, 63
  reasons for preparing, 59
  sequence of sessions, 59
  topic sequence, themes, 59